Sovereign Bodies, Sovereign Spaces

Critical Indigeneities

J. Kēhaulani Kauanui (Kanaka Maoli) and
Jean M. O'Brien (White Earth Ojibwe), *editors*

Critical Indigeneities publishes pathbreaking scholarly books that center Indigeneity as a category of critical analysis, understand Indigenous sovereignty as ongoing and historically grounded, and attend to diverse forms of Indigenous cultural and political agency and expression. The series builds on the conceptual rigor, methodological innovation, and deep relevance that characterize the best work in the growing field of critical Indigenous studies.

A complete list of books published in Critical Indigeneities is available at https://uncpress.org/series/critical-indigeneities.

Sovereign Bodies, Sovereign Spaces

Urban Indigenous Health Activism in the United States and Australia

. . . .

MARIA JOHN

The University of North Carolina Press Chapel Hill

This book was published with the assistance of the Lilian R. Furst Fund of the University of North Carolina Press.

Set in Charis by Westchester Publishing Services
Manufactured in the United States of America

Library of Congress Cataloging-in-Publication Data
Names: John, Maria (Maria Katherine), author.
Title: Sovereign bodies, sovereign spaces : urban Indigenous health activism
     in the United States and Australia / Maria John.
Other titles: Critical indigeneities.
Description: Chapel Hill : The University of North Carolina Press, [2025] |
     Series: Critical indigeneities | Includes bibliographical references
     and index.
Identifiers: LCCN 2024044813 | ISBN 9781469680408 (cloth) |
     ISBN 9781469680415 (paperback) | ISBN 9781469680422 (epub) |
     ISBN 9781469680439 (pdf)
Subjects: LCSH: Health activism—United States—History. | Health activism—
     Australia—History. | Indians of North America—Health and hygiene—
     United States. | Aboriginal Australians—Health and hygiene. | Indian
     activists—United States—History. | Activists, Aboriginal Australian—
     History. | BISAC: SOCIAL SCIENCE / Indigenous Studies | SOCIAL
     SCIENCE / Sociology / Urban
Classification: LCC RA424 .J57 2025 | DDC 362.1/042—dc23/eng/20241128
LC record available at https://lccn.loc.gov/2024044813

Cover art designed by Ashley Muehlbauer.

This book is dedicated to all those fighting
for the health of their loved ones.

Contents

Illustrations

Acknowledgments

This book exists because of the generosity, insistence, support, and patience of so many people. My deepest and most important thanks go to the many health activists and their families—past and present—whose stories, memories, histories, and teachings provide this book with a purpose. Whether it was in interviews I conducted myself, or in archival materials and interviews I was granted access to, learning about the enduring impact left by health activists on their families, communities, and nations, has been the single most important historical lesson to give this book its shape. At a certain fundamental level, this book is about the great lengths to which people will go to protect the health of their loved ones—which is also to say, at a certain fundamental level, this book is simply about love. While it is surely an impossible task, I can only hope I've done some, even partial, justice, to those who have shared, carried, and lived these histories.

Long before I could say I was writing a book, the ideas and questions that set this project in motion were expertly engaged and encouraged by beloved mentors whose handprints are still all over this work. At Columbia University, where I first began to explore the historical connections between Indigenous health and settler colonialism, I had the honor of calling myself a student of people I affectionately dubbed "the dream team." Audra Simpson has taught me so much about many of the biggest questions that drive my work, and over the years, her mentorship has continued to influence so many of the ways I think and teach, and how I understand what it means to be a good mentor, colleague, to be accountable, and to be rigorous. Her sense of humor is completely unmatched, and I will always be grateful that it saw me through some of the bumpiest moments in graduate school. Mae Ngai, an impossibly attentive mentor, was the very best historian for me to work with as I struggled to figure out my academic home. Her gravitation toward students thinking across and outside of national frameworks, and her embrace of historical approaches that engage the questions, tools, and methods of other disciplines gave me the confidence to pursue the research that has laid the foundation for this book. As a scholar and as a mentor, she has inspired me to love history in new and critical ways. I could not have done any of this without her. Karl Jacoby, in his completely modest way, has been a steadfast champion, source of support, and constant inspiration. He is the very best person to talk to about writing, and he shows such continuing care toward his students as they navigate the profession. His thoughtful and honest guidance on these matters have left me so much better prepared for this work than I think he will ever know. Back home in Australia, at Monash University, Bain Attwood was entirely responsible for opening my eyes to the problems and politics of historical study—a preoccupation that drives me still. Of all mentors, it is hardest to express adequate thanks to Bain, whose scholarship, teaching, and encouragement are responsible in so many ways, for having set me on this path over twenty years ago. Even as he continues to be a trusted advisor, Bain's friendship now enlarges the many gifts I have received from him. The depth of my appreciation for all he has done will always be impossible to convey.

Elsewhere at Columbia University, and more broadly in New York City, I was surrounded by people—faculty and my peers—whose interests in critical questions about health, race, place, colonization, power, and resistance centrally shaped my thinking. I learnt so much from being a student of Elizabeth Blackmar, James Colgrove, Mary Marshall Clark, Barbara Fields, Eric Foner, Alice Kessler-Harris, Nara Milanich, Samuel K. Roberts, David Rosner, and Kavita Sivaramakrishnan. The mentorship of Sue Mendelsohn, Jason Ueda, and Nicole Wallack completely changed the way I write. And Bill McAllister remains one of the best readers and sounding boards I've ever had. So much of the excitement and joy of these years was due to the friendships and intellectual companionship of a tremendous graduate community. About Native studies and settler colonialism, I learned so much from fellow travelers and treasured friends: Tamar Blickstein, Chris Clements, Margaux Kristjansson, Mikinaak Crystal Migwans, Teresa Montoya, Hayley Negrin, Trevor Reed, Aurélie Roy, Les Sabiston, Kristen Simmons, Anne Spice, and Adam Spry. About health and colonial medicine, my horizons were forever expanded by Elisa González, Charlotte Legg, and Jessica Pearson. About writerly things, my spirits were carried by Sarah Goldberg, Tejan Green Waszak, and Kat Savino. And without the camaraderie of Kyoungjin Bae, Emma Baumhofer, Samuel Fury Childs Daly, Andre Deckrow, Debra Glasberg Gail, Romeo Guzmán, Masako Hattori, Nick Juravich, Suzanne Kahn, Mookie Kideckel, Jessica Lee, Weiwei Luo, Liz Marcus, Daniel Morales, Cara Rock-Singer, Ollie Murphy, Ian Shin, and Jeffrey Wayno, there is no way I would have survived the demands of those years. Entirely responsible for making me feel at home in this time are dearest friends, Claire Edington, Hi'ilei Hobart, Katherine Johnston, J. T. Roane, Sarah Runcie, and Natasha Wheatley.

A project like this required that I spend significant time travelling—to archives, to libraries, to meet people, and to visit places. Several institutions funded and made this research possible over the years: the American Philosophical Society Philips Fund for Native American Research; the Anti-Discrimination Center in New York City; the Mellon Interdisciplinary Fellows Program; the National Library of Australia's Seymour Scholarship (gifted by John and Heather Seymour); the Columbia University Center for Oral History's Summer Institute; the Columbia Teaching Scholars Fellowship and travel grants from Columbia's Graduate School of Arts and Sciences; as well as the Dean's Research Fund at the University of Massachusetts Boston. Of all the archives, my most memorable time was at the National Library of Australia, where I spent several productive months buried in manuscript collections and was hosted by the exceptionally generous Margy Burn, Robyn Holmes, Beth Mansfield, and their extended team. Staff at the National Archives and Records Association in Seattle were also instrumental in my research efforts, particularly Patty McNamee. At the National Archives and Records Association II in Maryland, I owe many thanks to Joseph Schwarz for making my time there so productive. At the University of Washington Archives in Seattle, I would have been completely overwhelmed without the guidance of Carla Rickerson and her team. In Australia, special thanks are owed to Naomi Crago of the Sydney City Archives, and at the State Library NSW, to Lynne Hewitt and to Melissa Jackson and Ron Briggs of the Indigenous Services team.

More personally, my travels were made possible by the generosity of so many individuals. I am grateful to David Northover, Minty Longearth, and Katie Schultz, without whom my time in Seattle could not have been the same. Teresa Brownwolf-Powers, who shared both knowledge and excitement with me as we spent many an afternoon and evening discussing the AIWSL, was the most gracious guide. For all her help in finding sources, and for all her own research shared, I am eternally grateful. For helping me find my bearings in the contemporary work being done for Native health in Seattle, I am also thankful for the early guidance of Shelly Means, Aren Sparck, and Janeen Comenote. Both Ian Crowfeather and Jania Garcia have my deepest thanks for their time and extended correspondence, and for sharing their important memories of their parents. In Sydney, Ross and Selvi Macleod welcomed me into their lives at a difficult time, making their generosity even more profound. Cavan and Mira Hogue gave so openly of their home, making my research in Sydney entirely possible. In Melbourne, Gary Foley kindly spent an afternoon in conversation with me and later shared documents and items from his personal archive, all of which enlarged my understanding of Aboriginal politics in the 1970s. In Canberra, having the honor of spending time with Jilpia Nappaljari Jones and Julie Tongs, and learning from their life's work in service of Aboriginal health was a privilege I can still hardly describe. While all those who shared an interview with me are too numerous to list individually here, their names are in this book, and their voices are at its core.

Upon leaving New York City, it was my great good fortune to spend a year as an Andrew W. Mellon Postdoctoral Fellow in Indigenous Studies at Wesleyan University, in the American Studies Department. There, I began the work of reshaping this research into a book. Incredible colleagues, mentors, and students at Wesleyan helped me see my research in important new ways and pushed my thinking on essential questions with their encouragement, curiosity, and feedback. At the center of it all, in this time I had the incomparable honor of being mentored by J. Kēhaulani Kauanui—this was just the kind of path-shaping and explosive intellectual experience that anyone who knows Kēhaulani and her scholarship might imagine. Kēhaulani's mentorship and investment in my work has been truly transformative and continues still—it is responsible in so many ways for the shape that this book has finally taken. Building the beginnings of the Indigenous Studies Research Network at Wesleyan was also a joy and a privilege to work on with Kēhaulani. Within this network and beyond, important readers and interlocutors on campus included Abbie Boggs, Laura Grappo, Anthony Hatch, Patricia Hill, Indira Karamcheti, Marguerite Nguyen, Paula Park, Joel Pfister, Stephanie Prieto, and Margot Weiss. I was also tremendously lucky to find myself in a cohort of other earlier career folks at Wesleyan, all of whom formed an essential community—intellectual and otherwise—at such an important time: Long Bui, Jacob Doherty, Corinna Zeltsman, Marla Zubel, and most of all, Diana Schwartz Francisco, Luis Francisco, and Khalil Johnson.

The final stretches of the marathon this book became were completed during my time as an assistant professor at the University of Massachusetts Boston. On campus, I have met such inspiring, dedicated, and supportive colleagues—people who are truly heroic in the amount they take on and in their dedication to our students. I feel inspired by and honored to work alongside people with so much integrity, each and every day. And while I cannot thank each of my colleagues by name, I will say how fortunate I feel to have joined UMass Boston's history department, where everyone is a friend. Among my history colleagues, I owe special thanks to Tim Hacsi and Heidi Gengenbach, who have both served tirelessly as department chair in my time at UMass Boston, and who have been unwavering champions in their support and encouragement. In my work as director of the Native American and Indigenous Studies program at UMass Boston, I have also spent the last six years in deep, meaningful collaboration and partnership with beloved Native American and Indigenous Studies program colleagues on campus: Ping-Ann Addo, Daniela Balanzátegui, Christopher Fung, Jamie Morrison, Blaire Morseau (when we had her!), Stephen Silliman, Rachel Winters, and Cedric Woods. They have been my sounding board and my sense of home on campus. Elsewhere in Boston, both on and off campus, my appreciation runs deep for new friends and colleagues this city has connected me to and allowed me to spend time with, if only for a season: Cassandra Alexopolous, Martin Blatt, Nicholas Brown, Kevin Bruyneel, Leanne Day, Christine DeLucia, Nick Estes, Isabel Gómez, Andrés Fabián Henao Castro, Renee Hudson, Nedra Lee, Jami Powell, and Heike Schotten. A junior faculty colloquium organized by wonderful UMass Boston colleagues Sari Edelstein and Aaron Lecklider allowed me to workshop a chapter in its final stages and, most crucially, meant that I was read by the magnanimous Brianna Theobald, whose insights and questions helped me position and understand my own work in new and transformative ways. Finally, my students at UMass Boston must be thanked. Without the assistance of Emma Lovejoy, I would not have been able to complete the permissions process for images used in this book. More broadly, our students inspire and give me purpose every day. I am tremendously lucky to be in their classrooms.

There are also so many intellectual heroes who have popped in and out of the frame consistently, and who have been essential at many different stages of the journey this book has taken. Dian Million first saw this project in its infancy. I owe so much to the early enthusiasm she expressed for what I was doing. Ever since, her sense of urgency that this work must be published, and the supportive ways in which she has expressed this both in person and in writing over the years, has been the most powerful form of encouragement I could imagine. Ned Blackhawk, who at various junctures has gone out of his way to engage my work and open up opportunities, has left me completely humbled and forever grateful. For their engagement and encouragement at turning points both small and large, I have been deeply moved by the friendliness and wisdom of Warwick Anderson, Kevin

Bruyneel, Phil Deloria, Sandy Grande, Jean M. O'Brien, Jeffrey Ostler, Josh Reid, Coll Thrush, and Traci Brynne Voyles. Their scholarship has accompanied me at every stage of this book, and their generosity as intellectual giants in our field has taught me so much. For their expertise, encouragement, advice, invitations to present my work, or in some cases, comments on papers and drafts, I also owe special thanks to a remarkable list of brilliant scholars in both the United States and Australia: Seth Archer, George Aumoithe, Merlin Chowkwanyun, Miranda Johnson, Doug Kiel, Emma Kowal, Juliet Larkin-Gilmore, Nhu Le, Sana Nakata, Andrew Needham, Laura Rademaker, Joanna Radin, Samuel Kelton Roberts, Naomi Rogers, Tim Rowse, Kim Tallbear, Brianna Theobald, Kelly Wisecup, and Amy Zanoni. In a category of her own is Hi'ilei Hobart, my long-suffering, ever faithful "conference wife" and confidante. We've traveled almost every road this profession has offered us together—sometimes in ways we've dared only dream about! I have been inspired by her greatness from the moment we met and have learned more from her than she will probably ever know. I am always laughing, inspired, and well fed when I am with her. There isn't much more you can ask for in a friendship.

Finishing a book in the middle of a pandemic meant many things. For one, it is no exaggeration of the truth to say that this book was revived back into existence by Jean O'Brien and J. Kēhaulani Kauanui. When I was at a total loss, they provided the steady assurances, guidance, and patience that were responsible for setting me back on track. Their belief in this project from the moment they invited it into the Critical Indigeneities Series at The University of North Carolina Press has been the best kind of encouragement and honor for a first-time author. It is humbling to find yourself supported by your intellectual heroes, and even more grounding when you learn the extent of their greatness on a human level. I truly don't have the words to express the depths of my gratitude for their care—over my words, ideas, and well-being. They met me exactly as I was in multiple moments of personal crisis and never let me lose sight of the path ahead. I owe them so much. The very same depths of human and professional kindness were extended my way elsewhere at The University of North Carolina Press. Mark Simpson-Vos has the patience and compassion of a saint. More than this, he is the very best kind of editorial voice of reason a writer needs. No question was ever too small or big for Mark, and no email or request was ever met with anything but the most positive, supportive, thoughtful, and generous response. It has been a dream to work with him and his extensive team. I am especially grateful to Mark for lining up such careful readers for the manuscript in the review process. The critiques and encouragements of these readers helped sharpen and deepen this work so much. My thanks as well, to Michelle Witkowski and her team, for their expertise in combing through the entire manuscript, and to Mary Ann Lieser, who thoughtfully created a superb index for the book.

In closing these thanks, I feel it is important to reflect on the fact that this book was also completed at a time of collective grief. I have no doubt it has been shaped by this, in ways I may not yet fully understand. Also important to say is that for me, this book was finished at a time of immense personal grief. Just as I was to begin revising the manuscript that became this book, my beautiful, wise, quirky, and courageous mother, the most exceptional and resilient human being I know, got diagnosed with frontotemporal dementia (FTD)—an aggressive and degenerative brain disease that can strike much earlier than other forms of dementia. Being Maisy's daughter has been my greatest gift and privilege in life. The pain of slowly losing her in a thousand small and big ways over such an extended journey of loss has, at times, been far more than I have felt able to bear. All the complexity of care that has accompanied her diagnosis and transformed my life ever since has meant that I have had to ask a lot of certain people in my life. My family in Hong Kong are my bedrock and my anchor to all that matters most. Without them I wouldn't know who I am, nor would I have been able to complete this book. Aunties, uncles, sisters, and cousins—in all the ways those relations are made—have picked me up and reminded me who I am when I've needed it most: Lucy, Fanny, Kitty, Eva, Eddie, P. Y., Kar Yan, Kar Chun, Pia, Secilia, Graham, Tess, Viv, Div, Joyce, Lydia and Eddy, and Pam. In the United Kingdom and Australia, where all my other family resides, I am grateful for the loving support, always on hand, from my aunty, uncle, cousins, and in-laws: Ingrid, Stewart, Anna, Magnus, Simon, Chris, Emma, Mano, Mio, Lucinda, and Lloyd. Sugiati, who we affectionately call "AhD," has made absolutely everything possible in these last four years.

No less essential in my life are the friends who have made the United States a home in the most meaningful ways: Charmaine DeMello and Michael Clark, Justin Fauci, Diana Schwartz Francisco and Luis Francisco, Katie Johnston, Chris Muir, Sarah Runcie and Dale Runcie, and Varun Prasad and Claire Krebs. Friends who reside far in terms of distance remain closest to my heart: David Hollingsworth, Tom Kenny, Laetitia Smoll, Megan Whitty, and Pat Wilson. And friends who inspire me daily with their wisdom and capacity for care, are Stephanie Gaydon and Simon Sleight—they will always deserve my deepest thanks for knowing me best and simply knowing best. Three incredible women in Boston who helped me find my feet as a new mother, and who filled the role of surrogate mothers and sisters to me in ways they could probably never understand, are Heather Robinson, Anna Hourihan, and Gabriellys Rivera-Romero. Maria Kent Beers and Rachel Martinez, fellow travelers on the FTD road and leaders in the advocacy space for frontotemporal dementia have taught me so much about health activism and have my utmost respect and gratitude for all they continue to do for our community.

To my parents, Maisy Cheung and Karl John, I simply owe everything. The older I get, the more I understand and admire them, and the more I treasure the adventurous, open-minded, unimposing, and supportive environment they created for me to find my own way in this world. To my little brother Kai, I feel tremendous love—he is a wish fulfilled. To my chosen sisters, Charmaine, Pia, and Steph, you women are everything my heart always needs. And to my brother and sister-in-law, Andres and Shannon, who have filled our lives with so much love in the last few years, I am eternally grateful for the family we are together.

At the end of all this, and at the end of every single day in our beautiful, complicated life, the person who I want and need to thank the most is Emilio Mora, with whom I now share the unbridled joy of parenting our radiant son, Rafael. Only two years on this earth as I write these words, Rafael has already moved mountains in our world. Of all the things I need to thank Emilio for, I need to thank him most for making it possible for me to be both the mother and the daughter that I've needed and wanted to be in these past few unparalleled years. His love and his generosity know no limits and are the only reason I had any time to write and to rest. He is home to me, and so to him, I owe the kind of thanks one properly needs a lifetime to express. It is a lucky thing that time is already on our side.

Sovereign Bodies, Sovereign Spaces

Introduction

Structural Violence in Indigenous Health Care

· ·

It was an unfathomable story to most who caught the headline, but within Native American communities, the macabre incident struck a chord: "Native American health center asked for COVID-19 supplies. It got body bags instead."[1] This was March 2020, during the earliest days of the COVID-19 pandemic, but for the Native health workers who opened that unexpected package at the Seattle-based clinic, this moment transcended time, connected as it was to a much deeper history. The body bags weren't just a reminder of chronic government mismanagement of Native health care, of persistent funding shortfalls, broken treaties, and inadequate support over a period spanning hundreds of years. Nor were they simply a poignant symbol of just how little the United States continues to value Native lives. Perhaps more than anything, the body bags demonstrated the ongoing affronts to their survival that Native peoples continue to face in the United States today.

In health data, these realities present themselves in other ways too. American Indians and Alaska Natives die from diabetes at more than twice the rate of non-Indigenous populations. A recent report from the Centers for Disease Control and Prevention shows Native Americans have significantly higher rates of obesity, high blood pressure, cancers, and general poorer health status than other Americans. The suicide rate in Indigenous communities is also about 43 percent higher than that of non-Indigenous communities.[2] The staggering and disproportionate impact that COVID-19 wrought on Native communities in the United States is yet another marker of this history. Underlying all forms of injustice and inequality that Indigenous people have faced, we might view the unbroken history of their peoples' inability to maintain a level of health equal to those of their compatriots to be the most basic impediment and form of disparity they face, and which necessarily, precedes any other efforts to participate, on equal terms, politically, economically, or otherwise, in society.

Over the course of centuries, Native peoples' health in the United States has been under attack. Within US historiography, the recounting of this history often begins with the so-called virgin-soil epidemics.[3] This phrase was first made famous in an academic essay published in the 1970s by Alfred Crosby, but the idea has since been popularized thanks to pop histories such as Jared Diamond's runaway bestseller, *Guns, Germs, and Steel*.[4] In brief, the theory argues that when Europeans arrived in the Americas, they carried diseases (such as smallpox) that Indigenous peoples had never experienced, and to which they therefore lacked any immunity. The idea that disease effectively served as a handmaiden of European colonization has since become a familiar trope. Yet what is seldom considered is how this way of framing the history completely disregards how colonization itself made Indigenous populations vulnerable to disease in the first place. The virgin-soils theory and the all-too-simplistic refrain that early colonial epidemics all but "wiped out" Native populations displace the violence of colonial settlement from the actions of colonizers and conveniently attribute the wide-scale catastrophic deaths of Indigenous populations to blameless pathogens.

Contesting its simplicity, scholars have more recently pushed back against the virgin-soils framework.[5] Paul Kelton, David S. Jones, and Andrés Reséndez, among others, underscore that Native peoples were more often crippled by contextual factors surrounding the introduction of disease, such as the damaging (sickness-producing) impacts of war and Indigenous enslavement.[6] Roxanne Dunbar-Ortiz has highlighted the inadequacy of crude "immunity" explanations for Indigenous depopulation, noting, "If disease could have done the job, it is not clear why the European colonizers in America found it necessary to carry out unrelenting wars against Indigenous communities in order to gain every inch of land they took from them."[7] And as Jeffrey Ostler highlighted in an article reflecting on COVID-19 in the context of Native histories of epidemics, "Native vulnerability had—and has—nothing to do with racial inferiority or, since those initial incidents, lack of immunity; rather, it has everything to do with concrete policies pursued by the United States government, its states, and its citizens."[8]

As the COVID-19 pandemic unfolded, much of mainstream media used the vernacular of a "crisis" to report on the disproportionate impact being experienced by Indigenous communities. By contrast, Indigenous reportage and historical analysis of the pandemic framed its devastating impact on their communities as a matter of Indigenous sovereignty, and as evidence of an unbroken history of underfunded and underresourced health systems, limited access to health services, poor infrastructure, and underlying health disparities.[9] This was no crisis or moment of aberration, in other words. It was, as Ostler wrote, a result of the fact that "Native communities' vulnerability to epidemics is not a historical accident, but a direct result of oppressive policies and ongoing colonialism."[10] It matters tremendously that we understand COVID-19 as an issue of Indigenous sovereignty and historical continuity because this helps us fit this latest historical moment—unexpected body bags and the larger pandemic alike—into a much longer (indeed, systemic) pattern of medical neglect and abrogation of federal government responsibility. Over the course of centuries, the persistent neglect of Indigenous health has become a form of structural violence in the United States.[11]

This book, much like the work of the health activists it chronicles, is focused on bringing the history of this structural violence to light. In equal measure, this book also aims to show that this kind of structural violence toward Indigenous peoples in health care is not unique to the United States but rather has been a long-standing and core feature of settler-colonial societies. Nations such as Canada, the United States, and Australia are settler-colonial societies. They are built on a foundation of what Patrick Wolfe calls a "structure" of invasion.[12] As Wolfe explains, settlers never leave the lands they seek to colonize; their goal is to build a new society for themselves by displacing the prior occupants on whose lands they have set their sights. Wolfe identifies that precisely because the lands on which they seek to build their new society are already inhabited (by Indigenous people), the success of the settler-colonial project ultimately depends upon the eradication and replacement (elimination) of Indigenous peoples by settlers. Therefore, Wolfe famously asserted, when Indigenous people survive (as they invariably have), there is a need to recognize that settler-colonial invasion is "a structure[,] not an event." What he meant by this is that "logics" and "structures" of Indigenous elimination pervade within settler society and must continually do the work of invasion (Indigenous elimination) over and over, across time, to confront the "problem" of Indigenous survival. What was once violent confrontation and open warfare on the frontier thus becomes more "genteel" forms of elimination in policies and practices such as child removal, residential schooling, blood quantum requirements for federal recognition of Indigeneity, or simply the broader project of Indigenous assimilation writ large.[13] Together, and over the course of history, these invariably violent policies and practices have shifted ground and reinvented their techniques of erasure and elimination but never ceased. This book analyzes specific, chronic structures of neglect, violence, and invisibility within health care that have been born of and maintained by settler colonialism as part of a structure of invasion, and which can best be understood by situating present-day Indigenous health disparities in their historical context.

This kind of analytical approach resembles what Indigenous health scholars do when they consider "historical determinants of health." For example, in the Canadian context, Charlotte Reading explains that "to fully appreciate the current health disparities facing Aboriginal peoples, we must first explore the historical roots upon which current structures have evolved."[14] Current structures—or what might otherwise be labeled the "social" or "proximal" determinants of health—might, for example, include things like the quality of infrastructure in communities, or access to educational, employment, or other social goods like food or housing. Historical determinants can be likened, Reading explains, to the roots of a tree: "Like the roots of a tree, these deeply embedded determinants represent the historical, political, ideological, economical, and social foundations . . . from which all other determinants evolve."[15]

Though the details of distinct national histories differ in important ways, Indigenous health scholars recognize that across the settler-colonial contexts of the United States, Canada, and Australia, the health impacts of settler colonization, conquest, and attempted assimilation of Indigenous communities into the dominant society has produced nearly universal health outcomes for Indigenous people across these nations. It is here in this history, scholars like Reading would argue, that we discover the "roots" of contemporary or proximal determinants of Indigenous health are deeply embedded in a settler-colonial structure. Canada, the United States, and Australia are societies fashioned from what reads like a checklist of settler-colonial policy: the centralization of Indigenous peoples into remote communities and reservations; the oppressive nature of federal recognition policies involving blood quantum or other divisive requirements; the damaging legacy of assimilation policies and institutionalization (whether in residential or boarding schools, or in adoption programs); and racial discrimination in social environments and the labor market, as well as a chronic lack of public or private investment in economic development for Indigenous communities, whether reservation, rural, or urban. All these historical experiences, health and medical scholars tell us, have had a long-lasting impact on the health and well-being of Indigenous populations in these nations today.[16]

Health and medicine have also been wielded as blunt instruments of settler colonialism. As Mary Jane McCallum and Adele Perry have shown in the context of Canada, hospitals and health care fall within "a range of institutional systems shaped by Indigenous dispossession and marginalization," settler "nation-building," and "the maintenance of white settler prosperity and priority." To be sure, they note that hospitals differ in important ways from jails, foster homes, and residential schools, yet they do still have a particular place within the network of institutions that "continue to regulate, and not infrequently imperil, Indigenous lives" in settler-colonial nations.[17] The practice and discourse of medicine has also been key in shaping ideas about Indigenous peoples and their communities, and in perpetuating a medical discourse that has empowered institutions and people to treat Indigenous populations as inherently pathological. Mary Ellen Kelm argues that the prevailing ideology across settler-colonial nations that health could only be guaranteed to Indigenous people through assimilation meant, in turn, that Indigenous bodies became sites of colonization.[18]

Many of these analytical frameworks have been applied, with great rigor, to the Canadian context. In addition to McCallum, Perry, and Kelm, scholars such as Sherene Razack, Sarah de Leeuw, Lisa Stevenson, Gary Geddes, Maureen K. Lux, and Margo Greenwood are leading voices in this research space.[19] While Canada is not included in the present study, I do bring the Australian and United States contexts together under the same sort of scrutiny that has already been applied to Indigenous health and health care in Canada. I do not engage in a meaningful comparison with Canada in this book, but the parallels between what has occurred there and what I discuss of Australian and US history are worth mentioning here. Taken together, these overlapping histories reflect the pervasiveness of systemic neglect, erasure, invisibility, abandonment, and abuse faced by Indigenous people in settler-colonial medical contexts—features we can group together as forms of structural violence within Indigenous health care.

By identifying logics and structures of elimination and violence that are pervasive throughout the history of Indigenous health care, I argue that a more critical and urgent understanding of present-day Indigenous health disparities becomes not simply possible but required. As Reading has put it, "If we neglect to consider the most profoundly influential determinants of Aboriginal health (historical determinants), we are not only ignoring what is now a critical mass of (epidemiological) evidence, but we are complicit in the perpetuation of structural inequities that will impact the health and well-being of future generations of Aboriginal peoples."[20] To this I would add, if we are attuned to the specific ways in which present structures of inequality are actually *continuous of* past attempts at colonial control or domination, the moral significance of combatting structural inequalities in the present thereby takes on a more urgent character since the injustice is not isolated to the present but rather is actually continuous with, and constitutive of, the past colonial project in the present; that is, the lack of regard and response to the "root" (historical) determinants of Indigenous health are not simply conspicuous and suspect, they are complicit in the persistence of settler-colonial structures of neglect and violence (elimination) in the present.

These analytical frameworks add to the important conclusions of scholars such as Jaskiran Dhillon, Caroline Fidan Tyler Doenmez, Glen Coulthard, Hi'ilei Hobart, Tamara Kneese, Emma Kowal, Margaux Kristjansson, Tess Lea, Dian Million, Irene Watson, and Aileen Moreton-Robinson, among others, whose research has revealed the persistence, in multiple contexts, of settler colonialism's destructive impacts on contemporary Indigenous peoples via regimes of "recognition" and "care" and within the legal, child welfare, and education systems.[21] I think about my own work in relation to this scholarship and the way it has drawn our attention to continuing forms of settler-colonial power and violence operating in these contemporary settings. However, my work shifts our gaze more directly toward histories of neglect and abandonment in the context of health and medicine, where so often discourses of "care" have masked the bare imposition of colonial power.

The concepts of neglect and abandonment so central to the history in this book are influenced by the work of Elizabeth Povinelli, who helps us understand the banal nature of suffering and survival under late liberalism's unique modes of governmentality. My analysis of Indigenous health struggles can be read as a historical engagement with Povinelli's provocation that state violence in late liberalism is often exerted not through overt killing by the state but rather through death by exhaustion and abandonment.[22] To this day, the overrepresentation of Indigenous people in hospital emergency care remains a significant problem within settler-colonial nations and signals the abandonment of these communities on numerous fronts. The low rates of primary and preventative care accessed by Indigenous people that these high emergency care rates reflect are a direct historical legacy of the kinds of discrimination and neglect that this book addresses. A history of mistrust, abuse, and abandonment at the hands of the medical system has understandably produced high levels of medical avoidance and consequent poor health in many Indigenous communities today. Recounting these histories and making their widespread (and ongoing) nature clear as part of a structural analysis of settler colonialism makes this book, in many foundational respects, a history of medical racism.

Yet importantly, this is also a book about Indigenous resiliency, ingenuity, and activism in the face of this medical neglect. By bringing a structural analysis of settler-colonial violence to bear on the history of Indigenous health struggles, we not only see how pervasive and persistent these violent structures of elimination and erasure are in the present and the different forms they now take, but likewise, how tenacious Indigenous survival and radical care in the face of such persistent neglect has been. Equally then, this book is a history of Indigenous health activism. In this vein, it bears underscoring that Indigenous wellness has long been an affront to the settler-colonial structures of elimination in health care that I critique. As J. Kēhaulani Kauanui has written, any analyses of settler colonialism must account for enduring Indigeneity; first, that "Indigenous people exist, resist, and persist; and second, that settler colonialism is a structure that endures indigeneity, as it holds out against it."[23] A related point, as Audra Simpson has noted, is that settler colonialism "fails at what it is supposed to do: eliminate Indigenous people, take all their land, absorb them into a white, property-owning body politic."[24] The health activism of the communities and individuals in this book provide a striking example of how Indigenous people have and continue to not just defy but, in Simpson's language, "refuse" the logics and structures of elimination and violence that have been couched in the language of "care" and embedded in policies and discourses of health and medicine. Fighting for the health of their people and creating alternative structures of radical care in the teeth of chronic settler-colonial neglect and abandonment has been one way that Indigenous people have made sure of their own survival. In their health politics, Indigenous communities in settler-colonial nations have therefore embodied the political axiom that "existence is resistance."

Indigenous Health Struggles, Activism, and Sovereignty in the United States and Australia

At the Seattle Indian Health Board (SIHB), where the body bags arrived, the Native community was not unaccustomed to the kind of neglect and abandonment that such a delivery—mistaken or not—signaled. Reflecting on his time as an activist, SIHB cofounder Bernie Whitebear (Colville) remembered how rare preventative health care was for Native people in Seattle during much of the twentieth century. Whitebear frequently raised concern over the fact that Native people in Seattle would only seek out care "in emergency or life-threatening circumstances" due to rampant levels of discrimination within mainstream medical care and a pernicious issue of structural invisibility he described as "ping-ponging":[25]

This situation was the result of our people being ping-ponged from one hospital to the next under the mistaken assumption that the Federal government was responsible for the welfare of all Indians. Hospitals mistakenly thought the government took care of our health care even after we leave the reservation and because of that denied to treat us. In reality . . . the Bureau of Indian Affairs (BIA) and the Indian Health Services (IHS), had developed a policy that [by denying all government services to nonreservation Indians] in effect meant that "once you left the reservation, you were no longer Indian.[26]

What Whitebear described, whether we call it ping-ponging or medical neglect, was, by the middle of the twentieth century, such a common experience for Indigenous people in US cities that a well-known joke circulated in the 1960s about an urban Indian seeking a room at a hospital: "Did you hear the one about the Indian who couldn't get a room? He didn't have a reservation."[27]

Even in cases where medical treatment was accessible, the oftentimes openly racist treatment that Indigenous people endured to receive medical care in cities frequently meant that most preferred to go without. Across the United States, this history of medical neglect, discrimination, exclusion, and invisibility has characterized the experiences of so many Indigenous people within mainstream health care settings that it is referred to across time not simply in jokes but in the very way that Indigenous health services today represent themselves. Until recently, the image and message (shown in figure 0.1) greeted visitors to the Seattle Indian Health Board's Facebook page. The "Rez or no rez, we've got you covered" tagline (see figure 0.1) references the very history of "ping-ponging" and neglect to which Whitebear referred.

Yet, while these histories are seldom taught about as a part of broader narratives about health (in)justice and activism, the Indigenous communities that have long endured and survived this kind of medical neglect and discrimination have always spoken up about their experiences. In the twenty-first century we are seeing the impact that technology and social media are now having on exposing these cases of medical abuse and abandonment—in some cases, in real time. The names Joyce Echaquan, Brian Sinclair, Georges-Hervé Awashish, and Marylynn Matchewan are sadly known to us because their medical abandonment or abuse was caught on camera.[28] While the technology exists today to bring widespread attention to these cases of medical neglect, in the time that preoccupies

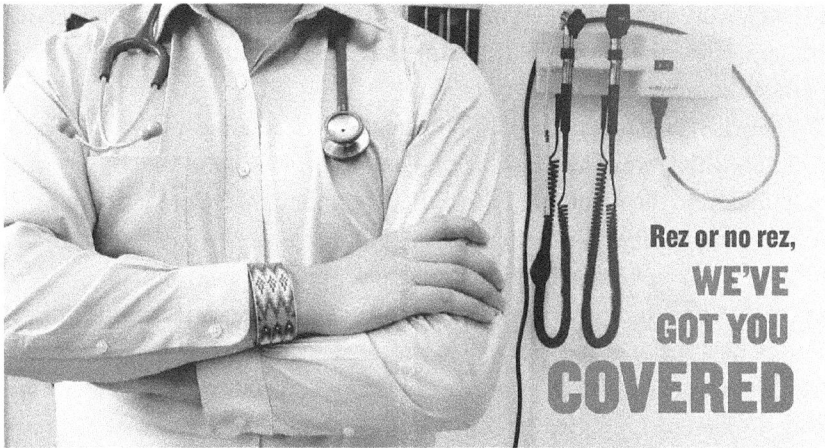

FIGURE 0.1 Seattle Indian Health Board banner ad. Seattle Indian Health Board, Facebook, May 11, 2017.

much of this book these histories were largely invisible to the mainstream. Starting in the post–World War II decades, however, it is striking that Indigenous people across Australia and the United States were avoiding mainstream medical care in urban settings for very similar reasons.

In Sydney, there was no "ping-ponging," but structural racism of a different form worked just as effectively to exclude Aboriginal patients from medical care. There, hospital workers and administrators often insisted on upfront cash payments from Aboriginal people—a condition of treatment not imposed on non-Aboriginal patients. Health care providers also discouraged and turned away Aboriginal patients, not on the erroneous assumption that the provision of their care legally fell upon another institutional entity or branch of government, but simply as a matter of bold-faced indifference and racism. Naomi Mayers (Yorta Yorta), who helped establish the Aboriginal Medical Service (AMS) Redfern in Sydney, wrote of how for a long time, due to intolerable levels of "racism" and "ignorance of Aboriginal people and where they came from," Aboriginal people in Sydney "only went to hospital at the last gasp."[29] Central to the story of Indigenous health activism that this book tells is how this dire standard of treatment (or rather nontreatment) led to a full-blown health care crisis by the 1970s. In most American and Australian cities by this time, Indigenous people found themselves without access to any health care at all. And in the cases where people were being "ping-ponged" from one institution to the next, as the activists themselves underscored at the time, this health crisis was in fact government created. These stories are well-known within Indigenous communities, but too few of these injustices have captured the attention of broader audiences.

Likewise, the quiet triumphs of the health activism this book examines—most of which was the work of Indigenous women, and much of which culminated in the creation of the Indigenous community-controlled health services I have already mentioned—are vitally important stories within the broader history of Indigenous politics and activism in the twentieth century. But these health stories are often missing from these activist histories. This book aims to be a corrective to that absence as well. At the same time, the history of this activism provides a unique opportunity to underscore how Indigenous politics at this time bore the hallmarks of broader currents—most especially, antiracist advocacy in the context of medical care, and the democratization of health care itself being expressed in contemporaneous political movements like the Black Panther Party's People's Free Medical Clinics, the women's health movement, the barefoot doctors, and the community health movement. Rarely do we see Indigenous actors represented in wider histories of health politics and activism; the history in this book therefore connects Indigenous people to broader health histories, activism, and the medical struggles of other communities at the time.

This book reflects on remarkable parallels between not simply the struggles but also the political solutions of Indigenous health activists in the United States and Australia. In particular, it accounts for the remarkable appearances, mere months apart, of a new kind of Indigenous social and political organization across the urban landscapes of the United States and Australia in the early 1970s. At this time, urban Indigenous communities in places like Seattle, Washington; Minneapolis, Minnesota; and Sydney and Melbourne in Australia began establishing their own grassroots, community-controlled health services. Under an ethos of self-determination, these clinics aimed to provide medical care by Indigenous people, for Indigenous people. Two of the first such clinics to be formed—and which are the focus of this book—were the clinics in Seattle and Sydney: the Seattle Indian Health Board in 1970 and the Aboriginal Medical Service Redfern just six months later, in 1971. To this day, these two clinics are still operational and are indeed leaders in their field, not simply for the health care they provide but as sites of and for Indigenous political organizing and health research.

The proliferation of community-controlled health services well into the twenty-first century as *the* health care model for Indigenous primary care in both the United States and Australia attests to the profound influence these clinics have had in transforming the delivery of medical care to Indigenous communities in these countries. In both the United States and Australia today, Indigenous community-controlled health clinics serve both rural and urban populations, and it is widely recognized that these services have been essential not only in terms of improving Indigenous access to health care but also as significant providers of Indigenous employment, and as centers of urban Indigenous social and political life.[30] Recognizing their political significance, this book brings the histories of the Seattle and Sydney clinics together for the first time in order to ask new questions, not simply about Indigenous health struggles starting in the mid-twentieth century but also about Indigenous political activism in this period, as well as the ramifications of postwar urbanization on Indigenous peoples' political projects—particularly that of Indigenous sovereignty.

Sovereignty—the issue at the heart of Indigenous history in the United States and Australia alike—is typically framed in terms of the maintenance of land holdings and independent tribal governments. What the history of urban Indigenous health activism underscores, however, is that a host of new and pressing questions about Indigenous sovereignty arose from the shifting demography of Indigenous communities after World War II. In both the United States and Australia today, over 70 percent of all people self-identifying as Indigenous are now urban-dwelling.[31] The need for health care to serve these growing diasporic and pan-Indigenous urban communities in the mid-twentieth century posed enormous political questions: What does Indigenous sovereignty mean in cities where members of different tribal nations are coming together in a setting where there is no tribal government to represent them? Perhaps more pointedly, What does Indigenous sovereignty mean for diasporic and pan-Indigenous communities that are located on another people's territory? How under such conditions can an urban center be transformed into a pan-Indigenous space without the people of the land falling out of the frame? What new forms of sovereignty arise in such settings? The realities of medical exclusion and neglect experienced by so many Indigenous people in American and Australian cities at this time sharpened these questions in a very particular way: What should happen to Indigenous people's rights off the reserve, and off the reservation? As Whitebear explained, Indigenous people who left their reservations for cities in the postwar era suddenly found themselves cut off from rights they had previously enjoyed (health care) because the government effectively ceased to recognize them as Indigenous outside of the reserve/reservation space. But as numerous activists expressed at the time, What had changed apart from their address? Weren't urban, pan-Indigenous, and diasporic communities owed the same rights and recognitions as reserve or reservation communities? On what basis could they suddenly be denied these obligations? The history shared in this book reflects how in the late twentieth century, Indigenous health activists were forced to confront these questions. For them, sovereignty came to be seen and reimagined as portable and redefined around the idea of self-control over one's own body—an idea I suggest we can think about as the "reterritorialization" of Indigenous sovereignty.

Deterritorializing and Reterritorializing Sovereignty

A comparison of shared health struggles across two different settler national contexts reveals a much larger political challenge faced by pan-Indigenous urban communities in the mid-to-late twentieth century: they were unable to gain federal government support and recognition *as* Indigenous peoples. As a result of moving into cities (and thereby "assimilating"), it was argued by the national governments of the United States and Australia that Indigenous people who relocated from reserves/reservations into cities had forfeited any rights *as* Indigenous peoples. Put simply, when urban pan-Indigenous communities in US and Australian cities tried to make their health struggles known in the late 1960s, they were told by municipal and federal authorities alike that they could and should access mainstream health services like all other citizens, or else they should access resources set aside for other "minorities." Not satisfied with being told they had essentially "lost" their Indigenous rights and identities simply by virtue of relocating into cities, and not content to let the health issues of their communities worsen, activists in Seattle and Sydney were compelled by the early 1970s to take measures into their own hands, creating their own free grassroots medical clinics run by, and exclusively for, their own people. The stories of how these clinics got off the ground and eventually won government support are at the center of this book. But so, too, is the question of how we might understand these clinics to be evidence of, and the embodiment of, a political vision that has enlarged the political project of Indigenous sovereignty to encompass matters beyond land and government.

In both the United States and Australia, sovereignty has long been the central concept around which Indigenous social movements have formed and political agendas for decolonization and social justice have been articulated. It is notable, however, that after World War II, the meaning of sovereignty within Indigenous discourses expanded and came to encompass a multiplicity of legal and social rights thought conducive to political, economic, and cultural self-determination. Whereas the language of sovereignty was invoked within Indigenous political discourse almost exclusively in relation to legal and territorial claims until around the 1990s, even a cursory glance at recent protest placards from Indigenous political rallies across the globe, or at new monograph titles containing the word "sovereignty" within the field of Indigenous studies, reveals a vastly broadened discourse around this term. Diverse concepts of sovereignty, including cultural, intellectual, visual, and sexual, to name a few, have now become prevalent within Indigenous politics. This book asks what the role of health struggles has been in this broader process of reimagining Indigenous sovereignty.

To the extent that health struggles have contributed to a process of reconceptualizing what Indigenous sovereignty means, this book argues that urban Indigenous health activists in the United States and Australia blazed a distinctive trail in Indigenous political culture. It was in the context of health struggles that activists came to recognize that if the goals of Indigenous sovereignty were to successfully meet the needs of pan-Indigenous urban communities (who were distinct from those urban communities whose traditional homelands *were* the cities), then as a political, intellectual, cultural, and social project, Indigenous sovereignty could—indeed had to—be *deterritorialized*. This is not to suggest that territory ceased to matter, nor that all Indigenous peoples within these different national contexts and who formed diverse communities in cities shared the same understanding of sovereignty. Rather, I begin with the observation that in both nations the proliferation of sovereignty's meanings and deployment by more diverse configurations of Indigenous people and communities since World War II has reflected an increasing turn away from a singular idea of Indigenous sovereignty as a legal construct, denoting mainly jurisdiction over territory. Instead, what we see in the settler-colonial contexts of the United States and Australia is that the struggle for sovereignty is increasingly about creating multiple possibilities for self-governance and self-determination, for multiple configurations of Indigenous communities and in many areas of life. Moreover, these visions for achieving sovereignty have increasingly taken forms that need not resemble formal government. Hence in the twenty-first century, it is common to refer to efforts to revive Indigenous languages, to revitalize traditional forms of food consumption and production ("food sovereignty"), to reinstate forms of traditional education, to assert control over the use of Indigenous artwork ("artistic sovereignty"), or to protect Indigenous cultures from pernicious forms of cultural appropriation or misrepresentation ("visual sovereignty" or "cultural sovereignty") as being different ways of engaging with the struggle for sovereignty.[32] As Joanne Barker has pointed out, "What is important to keep in mind when encountering these myriad discursive practices is that sovereignty is historically contingent. There is no fixed meaning for what sovereignty is."[33] The benefits of approaching sovereignty in this way are, I believe, twofold. First, we gain a richer understanding of the political project of Indigenous sovereignty itself—how it has changed over time, been adapted by various communities for their shifting goals and circumstances, and what, if anything, has remained constant across the various engagements with it. Second, if we make a point of thinking about the goal of Indigenous sovereignty in this way—as a shifting and responsive target—then it also becomes possible for us to use the discourse and practice of Indigenous sovereignty as a means of measuring or registering other important historical changes. For example, in the case of this study, the more expansive conceptions of sovereignty pressed for by urban pan-Indigenous communities reflect the impact of urbanization on political conceptions of community and belonging in this context.

Within Indigenous studies, some scholars push for a different language to describe the many political projects that now fall within an understanding of Indigenous sovereignty, citing a concern that the concept of sovereignty can never be wholly freed from its Western roots to sufficiently express or include Indigenous forms of sovereignty that both predate and prevail settler-colonial domination. Another approach, perhaps, is to think of how understandings of sovereignty might be indigenized. Aileen Moreton-Robinson, for example, describes what is different about the way in which sovereignty is understood in an Indigenous Australian context: "Our sovereignty is embodied, it is ontological (our being) and epistemological (our way of knowing), and it is grounded within complex relations derived from the intersubstantiation of ancestral beings, humans, and land. In this sense, our sovereignty is carried by the body and differs from Western constructions of sovereignty, which are predicated on the social contract model, the idea of a unified supreme authority, territorial integrity, and individual rights."[34] This concept of "embodied" sovereignty is evident in the health activism this book describes.

The title of this book, *Sovereign Bodies, Sovereign Spaces*, thus holds double meaning: It gestures toward a significant political and discursive shift around ideas of Indigenous sovereignty pursued by health activists as they sought to drive home the importance of embodied and mobile forms of sovereignty. As urban diasporic communities found their Indigenous identities under attack, a concern for embodied sovereignty also reflected health activists' attunement to the fact that Indigenous peoples' physical bodies, and not just Indigenous lands, were the target of colonization. Yet the concept of sovereign bodies and spaces is also a reference to the fact that in cities following World War II, instead of focusing solely on securing rights to land and waterways, increasing activist efforts were directed toward the creation of Indigenous-run institutions (bodies) that could enact self-governance regardless of their location on or off recognized Indigenous territories. Through the creation of their community-controlled health clinics and in the ideal of a reconceptualized Indigenous sovereignty that these organizations modeled, this book contends that urban Indigenous health activists were at the forefront of a process of not simply deterritorializing but more pointedly, of *reterritorializing* Indigenous sovereignty. Instead of grounding their claims to sovereignty in nationhood or land, they mapped their sovereign status and claims onto their literal, physical, flesh and bone bodies, and onto the self-governing institutions they created to protect the health and well-being of their people.

It is important to understand too, that this process of reterritorialization (onto their own bodies and institutions) did not seek to supplant or replace the territorial claims of the Indigenous nations for whom the cityscapes were sovereign homelands. On the contrary, health activists often fought in solidarity alongside these communities for their territorial claims.

The Spatial Logics of Settler-Colonial Governance

The central problems of structural invisibility, neglect, and elimination at the heart of this book cannot be understood without taking into consideration the longer history of settlement and the colonial production of city spaces in relation to Indigenous people. In both the United States and Australia, the settler-colonial construction of towns and cities was not just a physical process. It also involved the imposition of a moral order and a symbolic system on land and people. For much of Australian and American history, the presence of Indigenous people in towns and cities was seen to be incompatible with this order and system; Indigenous people and communities who built camps in and around colonial settlements compromised European pretensions to cultural superiority and signified the intrusion of the "untamed wild." Indigenous people who lived in these liminal spaces between the settled and the unsettled zones were thus widely perceived in threatening terms as "fringe dwellers" in Australia,[35] and less euphemistically in the United States as "wandering Indians," "problem Indians," or "vagabonds."[36] Regarded as completely demoralized communities, with neither the nobility of savagery nor the willingness to assimilate, the spectacle these people represented in nineteenth-century cities so disturbed settlers that their presence became a theme within popular discourse and culture at the time.

The artwork of Anglo-American painter Augustus Earle typifies this settler unease over the presence of Aboriginal people in Sydney. Earle lived in Sydney for two years during the 1820s, and his paintings and sketches of Aboriginal people, such as his famous 1830 painting *Natives of New South Wales as Seen in the Streets of Sydney* is a reference point for the nineteenth-century settler perception of Aboriginal fringe-dwellers.[37] In this famous image of George Street, Earle depicts a group of Aboriginal people sitting in the street with no apparent purpose, some dressed in the discarded clothing of whites and with bottles and clubs. They are represented doing things in public—sitting, chatting, drinking—that, according to colonial morality, should have been performed in private.[38]

"Fringe-dwellers" and "wandering Indians" inhabited an ambiguous cultural space between Indigenous and European life. The central goal of Indigenous Affairs in both the United States and Australia across much of the nineteenth and twentieth centuries was therefore to remove them from this state of cultural limbo and thus clearly demarcate the colonial from the "Native" in either one of two ways. In the "protection" era of the nineteenth and early twentieth centuries, this involved isolating Indigenous people to allow them to recover a semblance of traditional life on government-apportioned reserves and reservations. In later twentieth-century "assimilation" policies, the goal became reversed, as cultural absorption and integration into the mainstream was pursued to transition Indigenous people to modern ways. These protectionist and assimilationist approaches, followed (in turn) by both US and Australian governments, enacted a common process of symbolic geographic ordering, whereby "authentic" indigeneity was associated only with nature/remote areas. Once Indigenous people entered towns, villages, or cities, they were seen as problematic remnants of their former traditional selves, or as being in an awkward process of transition.[39]

The discursive, legal, and cultural reinforcement of this trope—that Indigenous people and their cultures are incongruous with modern life—has long been the subject of scrutiny by scholars.[40] In one of the most influential studies on the matter, Jean M. O'Brien argues, "Historical narration implicitly argued that Indians can never be modern because they cannot be the subjects of change, only its victims."[41] In public ceremonies and symbols, in artistic representations, in scholarly and professional writing, and in fictionalized accounts (both written and visual) of Indigenous peoples in urban (or otherwise "modern") spaces, we have seen this idea repeated again and again.[42] The association of "authentic" Indigenous identities with nonurban, nonmodern locations, positions urban Indigenous cultures and lifeways as inauthentic and less legitimate. This has led to what Laura M. Furlan calls a "dominant narrative" about Indigenous people in the city: that they do not and cannot belong (*as* Indigenous peoples) in these urban spaces.[43] As Douglas K. Miller also notes, the assumption built into this dominant narrative is that whenever Indigenous people do end up in urban spaces, they are "always moving deeper into assimilation."[44]

In *Indian Cities: Histories of Indigenous Urbanization* (2022), coeditors Kent Blansett, Cathleen D. Cahill, and Andrew Needham have termed this long-standing and ongoing history of disassociating the urban from "authentic" Indigeneity as the "deurbanization" of Indigenous peoples. In their words, "A deurbanization of Indigenous people has been central to both the discourse and reality of colonization. In other words, settler societies have denied the existence of Indigenous urban pasts—and presents and futures—insisting that urbanity and Indigeneity are antithetical."[45] The deurbanization of Indigenous people to which these scholars refer obviously ignores a vast history in which Indigenous peoples built and lived in cities long before the arrival of European colonizers. Much work has been done, for example, about the ancient metropolises of Cahokia, Pueblo Bonito, and Tenochtitlan, to name a few. But as the editors of *Indian Cities* note, the "links between the inhabitants of those cities and subsequent Indigenous populations were all but erased from most historical narratives."[46] As scholars of Indigenous urban histories like Coll Thrush, Grace Karskens, and others also show, so many of today's cityscapes are built on the traditional homelands or early urban blueprints of Indigenous nations.[47] For those communities, the settler's urban landscape came to them, or else it was built on a foundation they had already laid.

When looking at the postwar twentieth-century histories of Indigenous urbanization in the United States and Australia, it is therefore important to underscore that while I am taking the post–World War II urbanization boom as a departure point, my intention is not to reproduce an understanding of Indigenous urbanization that erases a much longer history of Indigenous urban life that preceded the twentieth century, and indeed, that predates colonial times. Nor do I wish to sideline the important and continuing histories of the Indigenous communities whose homelands were the destinations of pan-Indigenous urban migrants—communities such as the Tongva in Los Angeles, the Duwamish in Seattle, or the Gadigal people in Sydney. As most histories of twentieth-century Indigenous mobility and urbanization will note, though, after World War II unprecedented numbers of Indigenous people from across the United States and Australia began migrating into major urban centers. Cities like Chicago, Los Angeles, and Seattle in the United States, and Adelaide, Melbourne, and Sydney in Australia were popular destinations because of government-sponsored relocation programs or due to preexisting networks of family and migration. Although the urban journeys of these twentieth-century Indigenous migrants were made under quite different circumstances to the "fringe dwellers" and "wandering Indians" of the nineteenth century (who were in many cases refugees from frontier wars), it is important to understand the long shadow cast by the colonial construction of urban space and the cultural categories that were used to make sense of the presence of Native American and Aboriginal people in cities. As this book shows, the health struggles of pan-Indigenous urban communities in the United States and Australia expose the continuance, well into the twentieth century, of these longer histories of spatial and cultural categorization—that deemed the rural as the locus of Indigenous tradition and authenticity, and the urban as the site of cultural transformation and permanent "loss" of Indigenous authenticity.

With respect to how this dynamic played out in the context of health care, it is hard to ignore how the geographic barriers to accessing health care that urban Indigenous people routinely faced in the mid-twentieth century effectively enshrined a spatial logic of colonial governance in health policy, since this worked to confine Indigeneity to specific locales (the reserve/reservation). The problem of historical continuity that this brings into focus might be understood in the following terms: until the 1970s, the structural (spatial) impediments preventing urban Indigenous people from accessing government-provided health care were not simply *productive* of structural racism within health systems and health outcomes; they were also based on, and thus continuous of, past governmental policies stretching as far back as the earliest settlement of colonial towns, and that were explicitly expressive of a racializing and assimilative agenda.

Expanding Current Frameworks

At a more basic level, my work seeks to expand the ways in which we think about the terms "political" and "activism" in the context of Indigenous history. In trying to think expansively about how these terms describe the actions taken by urban Indigenous people who sought to protect and improve the status of people's health within their communities, I take my cues from several sources. The first is the work of scholars who have thought about how we can look for the political voices and actions of people in various contexts of disempowerment. Historians, political theorists, and anthropologists like Steven Hahn, Robin D. Kelley, James C. Scott, John Gerring, Mark J. Leff, Sherry B. Ortner, Loretta Fowler, and Mabel Berezin have all, in one way or another, shown that our understandings of politics and the political must be relational and historical.[48] As Steven Hahn writes artfully, "the appropriate conceptual universe" of any study seeking to understand how people constitute themselves as political actors in societies that refuse them that part, must be determined by the specifics of social and historical context: "What could sensibly be regarded as political activity at one time and place might not be regarded as political activity at another, while different forms of activity in any one time and place assume political character in relation to other forms of activity."[49] In Hahn's by now classic example, he explains how a defiant slave in the antebellum US South does something markedly different from a free worker who defies the authority of an employer: "For slavery is a relation of direct personal domination in which there are few institutionalized avenues of negotiation."[50] As Hahn explains, the enslaved person's position within this historical context makes their defiance, by its very nature, a challenge "to the fictions of domination and submission around which slavery was constructed." It is thereby imbued with "a political resonance" that would not necessarily be true for the worker's defiance, which is mediated chiefly by the market.[51] By seeing such acts—individual and uncoordinated as they may be—as what might be termed a "collective struggle for socially meaningful power," Hahn provides a framework that can be applied to many historical contexts in order to bring politically meaningful forms of behavior into view where they might otherwise be overlooked—including, in this case, the health struggles of urban Indigenous communities after World War II.

In postwar cities across the United States and Australia, where government policies intentionally denied any recognition to urban pan-Indigenous people as a distinct social and political group but rather, actively treated them as assimilated minorities within the mainstream, Hahn's framework allows us to recognize the amplified political significance of many acts and exchanges that took place in everyday life. I argue that by simply drawing attention to the deficiencies of mainstream health services to cater to their needs in the postwar era, urban Indians and Alaska Natives in Seattle and Aboriginal people in Sydney engaged in acts that were, by their very nature, political. Calling attention to the medical neglect they faced in cities allowed urban Indigenous people in Seattle and Sydney to challenge the national romance of Indigenous people enjoying the full benefits of citizenship through assimilation, integration, and equality in the cities. To use Hahn's language, their actions and their words calling attention to medical discrimination, or in support of more adequate health care for their people—uttered to each other, to journalists, or in letters they wrote to the mayor—challenged the "fictions" around which assimilation, termination, and relocation policies were constructed. The political resonance of their health grievances and refusals to accept inadequate health care during the 1950s, '60s, '70s, and beyond are therefore the focus of the following chapters.

My use of a second key concept, activism, has been shaped by another body of scholarly writing that looks at what this means, both in the context of health struggles and in relation to Indigenous political goals. Sociologists Stephen Cornell and Alondra Nelson, and communications theorist Heather M. Zoller, all contribute valuable understandings to the ways in which we can make sense of people's efforts to address inequalities, either as stand-alone acts, or as part of broader activist frameworks and networks. Their categorizations of different forms of political engagement have influenced my understanding of the examples of urban Indigenous health activism discussed in this book. For Zoller, health activism, whether promoted as part of community development projects or through social movement activity, is "an alternative means groups use to assure their needs and grievances are heard."[52] Zoller also differentiates between health advocacy and health activism: Advocacy involves groups that work within the existing system and biomedical model, uses tactics other than direct disruptive action, and tends not to push for lay knowledge to be included into expert knowledge systems. Activism, on the other hand, involves activist-oriented groups that engage in direct, sometimes disruptive, action, challenge current scientific and medical paradigms, and pursue increased democratic participation in scientific or policy knowledge production by working largely outside the system.[53]

We can fruitfully compare Zoller's model to the way in which Alondra Nelson has written about the health politics of the Black Panther Party during the 1960s and 1970s.[54] Nelson distinguishes between advocacy and activism in ways that echo Zoller's framework, but she also purposefully uses these terms in fairly interchangeable ways to describe the initiatives of the Black Panthers—in particular, the development of their People's Free Medical Clinics.[55] In part, she writes, this is because "in investigating Party health initiatives, I perceived that its activism both reflected and amplified the distinctiveness of a tradition of black health advocacy in which pragmatic matters of disease and healing (e.g., the founding of health institutions) were coextensive with broader political matters (e.g., challenges to racism)."[56] Unlike Zoller, in other words, Nelson makes the crucial observation that health politics often marry the goals of advocacy and activism in inseparable ways—that is, against a backdrop of exclusion and neglect, advocacy in Zoller's sense can constitute a form of activism (again in Zoller's sense). Like Nelson, I perceive a union of advocacy and activism in the efforts of the people who strived to improve urban Indigenous health in the United States and Australia. In their case, assuring access to health care for urban Indigenous people was coextensive with the broader political project of asserting Indigenous territorial sovereignty in the city and beyond. In addition, I am also concerned with expanding the ways in which we can recognize urban Indigenous communities engaging in politically meaningful action—particularly to incorporate less visible forms of behavior that might fall under Zoller's definition of "advocacy." Like Nelson, I therefore use these terms throughout my work as if they were often two sides of the same coin.

I set these models for approaching health activism and advocacy against a helpful schema offered by Stephen Cornell in his work on different forms of political action that have served Native American social justice goals in the twentieth century. Cornell distinguishes, on the one hand, between "reformative" and "transformative" goals, and on the other, between "integrative" and "segregative" goals.[57] He writes, "Reformative goals seek to improve Indian-White relations; transformative goals seek to transform the structure itself."[58] Cornell describes the difference between integrative and segregative goals in the following way: "Goals are integrative in that they endorse, in effect, the integration of Indians into the dominant institutional patterns and culture, either as individuals or as groups." Segregative goals, on the other hand, in effect advocate "a separation of Indian communities from the institutions of larger society and the values they represent and the preservation or adoption of distinct institutional patterns specifically tailored to distinctive Indian needs, concerns, and historical experience."[59] As I show at different times and in different quarters of the loosely bound health movements I examine, the advocacy and activism of urban Indigenous health reformers in the United States and Australia truly reflected all elements of these various goals. In Seattle, I demonstrate that differences of opinion and outlook seemed to fall along gendered and generational lines, with an older cohort of female community leaders being more resistant to the idea of acquiring federal funds, whereas in Sydney, differences of opinion fell along more idiosyncratic lines.[60]

Finally, in thinking about the many things that might come under the umbrella of "health," or that were understood to be inextricably tied to the improvement of Indigenous health in these two national contexts, I am perhaps most influenced by, and attentive to the words and voices of people both past and present who were involved in this advocacy work at one time or another. These people—Pearl Warren, Adeline Garcia, Naomi Mayers, Ruby Hammond, Gordon Briscoe, and countless others—rarely described the significance of good health outcomes within their communities as goals that were disconnected from wider political, social, and economic aspirations. Hence securing reliable access to health care, fighting disproportionately high rates of disease and infant mortality, and advancing the cause of Indigenous patient empowerment within mainstream medical institutions were all significant "health" goals. But according to the activists who worked to attain them, these health outcomes were also unreachable without complementary efforts to improve social attitudes, political representation, or to reform housing or education policy. Nor were these health outcomes only desirable for health reasons. Simply put, urban Indigenous health activists understood from the outset that a health "problem" in their community was rarely an isolated issue. Therefore, quite often, activists approached their health goals as stepping-stones toward other important social, economic, or political outcomes, or else they treated these other goals as a means toward advancing health outcomes: "How are our children meant to do well in school if they can't see a doctor when they get sick?" was how one Indigenous woman expressed this point in 1969.[61] As I discuss in the following chapters, solutions and approaches to the health issues afflicting their community thus often reflected or incorporated other connected political concerns.

Reflecting this "intersected" approach to health issues, it is noteworthy that Indigenous health activists rarely explained the inequalities their people faced as matters of individual or community failing but instead sought to approach the existence of health problems in a way that addressed social and historical context first. A classic articulation of this approach was reflected in *The People Speak: Will You Listen?*—the 1978 report of the Indian Affairs Task Force of Washington State. In this report, the task force summarized its expansive views on health when accounting for why health continued to be "a problem of considerable gravity to Indian people." They reported, "Discriminatory treatment, sometimes to the point of negligence, has been experienced by Indians at existing health delivery systems by professionals who seem not to have any understanding of Indian health needs. Indian directors and citizens believe, generally, that this discrimination is much larger than simply a White-Indian issue. It is based on lack of contact, followed by a tendency to stereotype rather than an attempt at understanding. It is, therefore, one of the important functions of nearly every Indian agency to make it easier for the non-Indian professional to deliver sensitive health care to Indian patients."[62]

As this remark suggests, Indigenous health activism could just as easily (and importantly) focus on the work of breaking down stereotypes and increasing contact between Indigenous and non-Indigenous people, as it might focus on more anticipated projects, for example lobbying local politicians for funding to support their own clinic. In writing about the history of Indigenous health activism, I have let this expansive view of health guide my approach.

Methodology/Sources

Understanding the history of urban Indigenous health activism in both the United States and Australia has involved many moving parts and so demanded that I examine sources that reflect multiple perspectives, including those of Indigenous and non-Indigenous activists; national, state, and local government officials; medical and nonmedical experts on Indigenous health; attendees and conveners of national public forums and their local subdivisions; representatives of Indigenous and non-Indigenous political and/or social organizations; rural and urban Indigenous community leaders; and urban Indigenous patients and migrants themselves.

Most of my written sources were housed in national, state, municipal, and institutional archives. I was also fortunate to be given access to a few private collections, including papers from the American Indian Women's Service League and the Seattle Indian Health Board. In addition, by necessity, the research for this project also relied on oral history interviews. Oral history interviews were necessary to uncover the experiences of urban Indigenous health activists, patients, and migrants for several reasons. First, such interviews gave access to histories that defy archives. Many postwar urban Indigenous migrants were reluctant to "bite the hand that fed them"—that is, many wanted to be seen as trying to assimilate, or some were genuinely keen to "pass." Many urban Indigenous relocatees were at first hesitant to speak up about the bad conditions they faced in cities, lest they be accused by state officials of not assimilating and thus have what limited benefits they were given withdrawn. The written traces left by urban Indigenous migrants about the poor health conditions they faced are thus scarce. In even a small sampling of oral history interviews with former urban Indigenous migrants and their descendants, however, health conditions were notably cited when accounting for the reasons their families struggled prior to and during the process of relocating to cities. Also, because I am interested in less obvious forms of politically meaningful action, many of the indicators of poor health conditions do not register as part of a paper trail, even though they are ever-present in community memory; that is, in many instances the forms of "protest" or resistance that I am interested in consisted of forms of nonbehavior (e.g., *not* going to hospital). Events that are often private and hidden from public view can nonetheless be momentous and significant in shaping a community's behavior, whether it is a rumor about discrimination at a certain hospital, or the experience of going through an illness so devastating that it compels a person to move to where the health conditions might be better.

Oral history also has particular value for scholars working with and on the histories of Indigenous communities. This is because it is a particularly powerful tool for documenting the experiences of people who remain on the margins of the historical record. Moreover, it becomes especially important when considering communities whose cultural traditions privilege oral rather than written expression. Oral tradition and history remain central to Indigenous knowledge and social systems and to Indigenous people's understanding of their own histories. Using an oral history methodology was therefore important as I attempted to engage this history in ways that reflect Indigenous historical experiences and perspectives. In this sense, oral history has also been especially valuable for me as a historian committed to the intellectual project of decolonizing historical scholarship, by which I mean I have approached the history of urban Indigenous health activism by placing Indigenous peoples' experiences and perspectives at its center.

Several collections of relevant oral histories and memoirs have been published or deposited in libraries across the United States and Australia. In addition to these collections, I was also fortunate in being given access to a private collection of unpublished video interviews conducted and recorded by Teresa Brownwolf-Powers (Standing Rock Sioux), a Seattle filmmaker who worked on a project about the American Indian Women's Service League. This private collection, which I have referred to in citations as the Teresa Brownwolf-Powers Collection, contains rare interview material with many of the service league women, including some who were active in the Seattle Indian Health Board and many who have since passed on.

In both Seattle and Sydney, I conducted original interviews with urban Indigenous health activists and advocates (both current and former) and/or their descendants. This included medical/health workers of various kinds who have spent some portion of their lives dedicated to the cause of improving Indigenous health in these cities and elsewhere. I conducted the interviews in person, and in some cases where face-to-face meetings were not possible, I held interviews over the phone. For the most part, when interviewing, my method was to allow the interviewee to set the conditions for our interview, including both length and topics for discussion. In many instances this involved my traveling to their home, office, or some other place of convenience. I relied on a good deal of luck when reaching out to potential interviewees after I identified them through current or former activist networks. Once I secured an initial set of interviews, I let one contact lead to another. Many vital leads were established through invitations I received from community members and friends of friends in 2012–14. In addition, I also had the benefit of receiving guidance and contacts in Seattle through the University of Washington's American Indian Studies Department and the Indigenous Wellness Research Institute, and in Australia from staff at the National Library of Australia, the State Library of New South Wales, and the University of New South Wales Muru Marri School of Public Health and Community Medicine.

Like everyone working with Indigenous communities and histories, but especially as a non-Indigenous scholar, I have a responsibility to work in line with the ethics and expectations of Indigenous research methodologies, which are discussed rigorously by Linda Tuhiwai Smith in her foundational text *Decolonizing Methodologies*.[63] This has meant, for example, deferring to the preferences and requests of my interviewees regarding anonymity and also regarding access conditions on their interviews for the future. In Australia, my project was also reviewed and approved for ethics clearance and exemption by the Aboriginal Health and Medical Research Council's Ethics Committee. Since some of my informants wished to protect the privacy of their personal and family stories, and others simply preferred not to have their names in print, some of my informants' names have been changed. When I have done this, I indicate in the footnotes. As Mary Jane McCallum and Adele Perry also remind us in their careful work on Aboriginal health in Canada, in recounting traumatic histories, especially of communities that are not our own, it is incumbent upon researchers to "hold in balance" our sense of urgency in elevating difficult, oftentimes buried histories, and the "politics and ethics of rehashing, and the inherent risk of re-inflicting, Indigenous trauma."[64] McCallum has also noted that "we need to frame our recognition of trauma in an understanding that Indigenous history was and is much more than a story of loss; multiple forms of experience can and do coexist."[65] An attention to this final point is precisely why this book is both a history of structural violence within health care and a history of Indigenous activism and triumphs within it.

Aside from working within a decolonizing approach in these ways, my practices as an interviewer were also shaped by the Oral History Association's guidelines for best practices. Every interview had two parts: for example, a preinterview meeting or conversation during which I explained my research project and answered any questions, followed by a recorded session. I gave all interview participants the opportunity to review the interviews afterward and place any restrictions that they felt were needed. I took as much care as possible to select interviewees who represent diverse perspectives from within the various communities of stakeholders, participants, and actors involved in this history. In other words, I interviewed non-Indigenous and Indigenous health care providers, Indigenous and non-Indigenous activists, men and women within each of those groups, and overall, as much of an intergenerational cohort as I was able to gather. I did this in the hope of ending up with an interview group that would be as representative as possible. Nevertheless, given that a great deal of my contacts were made through other contacts, there was a limit to how much I could control for a breadth of experiences. Reflecting my interest in the ways that oral history can help the historian to fill in important gaps in knowledge that archives are ill-equipped to speak to, I have relied on the material gathered through my interviews for both the unique insight into experiential knowledge that they provide, and also for the more basic information about events that have escaped the notice of written records.

Chapter Outline

The ensuing chapters are structured chronologically. They also unfold with an oscillating focus on the United States and Australia respectively; thus chapters 1, 2, and 5 discuss the United States and Australia concurrently, while chapter 3 deals with Seattle exclusively, and chapter 4 with Sydney exclusively.

Chapter 1 starts in the 1950s and introduces the burgeoning migration of Indigenous peoples from rural areas and reservation/reserve communities into major urban centers in the United States and Australia. Utilizing sources ranging from government publications to oral histories, I show that multiple factors compelled Indigenous people to relocate in the postwar period. Access to employment and education were of course crucial, as were government incentives and programs that actively encouraged movement into the cities. But I also introduce the idea of "medical migration" by showing that desires for access to better health services and to escape the abysmal health conditions in rural areas were also crucial. This chapter sets up a key tension between what was promised by the policies of the US Bureau of Indian Affairs Direct Employment ("Relocation") Program and the work of the Australian Aborigines Welfare Board, and the grim reality of overcrowded and scarce housing, lack of jobs, and inadequate access to health services in the cities.

Chapter 2 picks up the story of bureaucratic mismanagement. I explain how the federal and state governments of both the United States and Australia approached Indigenous health services between 1950 and 1970, and how they intended for health care to be a key site for assimilating urban migrants. Drawing especially on government reports and personal papers of key government spokespeople, I show how in both nations the goal of assimilating these new urban populations came at the expense of access to health services they could actually use. This chapter also sets up the problem of structural invisibility as it was articulated at the time by urban Indigenous patients who found themselves to be effectively locked out of health care in cities.

Chapters 3 and 4 deal most heavily with the history of medical racism and structural violence pervading US and Australian health care in the twentieth century. These chapters also trace the emergence and evolution of grassroots Indigenous health activism in Seattle and Sydney that arose as a response to this medical discrimination. Each chapter leads up to the early 1970s, at which point the Seattle Indian Health Board and the Aboriginal Medical Service (Redfern) were founded. In contrast to chapters 1 and 2, which integrate a discussion of both national contexts, each of these chapters takes the story of one city as a representative case in a larger national story. Among other sources, these chapters draw on oral history interviews I conducted with Indigenous health activists in Seattle and Sydney, including central players in the founding of the SIHB and AMS. I demonstrate that the political strategies and solutions pursued in Seattle and Sydney were remarkably similar but also differed in certain respects. In these chapters we clearly see how the health struggles of urban Indigenous people in the United States and Australia forced them to justify their claims to an Indigenous identity, and to any rights and obligations owed to them because of those identities. I argue that to legitimize their claims, activists turned to a concept of sovereignty rooted in identity rather than territory.

Chapter 5 brings the discussion of the two locales back together. I compare the SIHB and the AMS in order to show how these clinics embodied the concept of a distinctly urban, nonterritorial form of Indigenous sovereignty. The new geography they represented was not inconsistent with forms of sovereignty expressed by Indigenous communities tied to traditional homelands, but it was premised on an understanding of community imagined at a different spatial scale; one that was diasporic, pan-Indigenous, and that traversed both urban and rural homelands. This chapter expounds on the concept of a "reterritorialized" sovereignty and makes the case that urban Indigenous health activists have been far more important to the development of Indigenous politics more broadly than has thus far been acknowledged. Reflecting on the long history of structural violence within Indigenous health care, and an equally long history of Indigenous adaptation and survival in and against these medical contexts, this chapter concludes by considering how in their health activism, urban pan-Indigenous communities in the United States and Australia have long been pressing for a more expansive and inclusive model of Indigenous sovereignty since at least the mid-twentieth century.

Concluding the book, an epilogue brings us, briefly, to the very recent past and reflects on how the strength of Indigenous community responses to COVID-19 in the United States and Australia can be traced to the traditions of health activism and sovereignty at the heart of this story.

1 For the Sake of Our Health

Post–World War II Indigenous Medical Migration
in the United States and Australia

• •

When Bill's family left the Yakama Reservation for Seattle in the 1950s he was only a young boy, but he remembers how his mother seemed "so pleased with herself" for "getting us boys away from all the health traps we could fall into on the rez."[1] What Bill meant here, he explained, was impossible to understand without knowing that his father and mother had been alcoholics: "It's a hereditary disease," Bill often said to me. "I was born with alcohol in my blood."[2] Therefore, from his mother's perspective at the time they moved, Bill explained that "she was sure her sons would fall into all the same traps as she did, if we stayed, and so she took us to the city in part for her, in part for us. She needed to get straight too."[3] Bill even recalled his mother telling him one time, many years after they had settled in Seattle, and at a time when he seemed to be "mixing with the wrong crowd," that "she said she brought us here so that we could have a healthy future, and not to be getting ourselves sick and in trouble like we were doing. . . . She reminded me that we had moved here for the sake of our health. . . . That really stuck with me," Bill recalled.

Bill's story stood out among my other informants who also recalled their families moving to Seattle for health reasons, because unlike most, his life's story seemed to center so distinctly around this idea that the city was meant to be a place of refuge, escape, and where one came to "get" or "be" healthy. Indeed, much of Bill's adult life, which has been spent moving back and forth between Seattle and Yakama, has been tempered by a constant struggle between getting healthy and falling off the wagon. Despite his mother's best intentions, Bill indeed suffered from alcoholism for much of his adult life. Celebrating his "tenth sober birthday" in the year that I met him, Bill was keen to narrate his life's story as one that was structured around a struggle to get healthy. And for him, the city continued to function as a place where he constantly returned in an effort to get well. For Bill, this meant distancing himself from unhealthy habits, conditions, and influences on his reservation. But it also meant being able to access vital support services like the Seattle Indian Health Board, the Thunderbird Treatment Center, and Alcoholics Anonymous, which he viewed as fixtures of the city.[4] Since becoming sober Bill has spent much of his time volunteering for various organizations in Seattle that seek to help Indians get "clean and sober and healthy."[5] And for him the city really seems to hold a key to unlocking this promise. Even outside of addiction issues, in the context of his own family (who visited him in the time I was in Seattle), Bill explained that he was trying to convince one of his daughters, who has diabetes, to come and live in the city "because she can get the best treatment here."[6]

Bill's story, like many descendants of migrants whom I spoke with in Seattle, touched upon a set of themes that we see repeated in the Australian context too; that is, in recalling the health struggles of his mother, himself, and his daughter, Bill spoke of his reservation as a place where it was difficult to stay healthy, not simply because of economic or social barriers, but because it was harder to get the specialized or accessible medical treatment that was available in the city. As reflected in many Australian stories as well, Bill's family had also moved to Seattle because his mother had wanted a brighter and healthier future for her sons. It is notable that Bill now wants the same thing for his daughter.

Bill's story reminded me of an Aboriginal woman's account I was told in Canberra. In sharing her life's story one Saturday afternoon in her suburban home in Belconnen, Dot wasted no time in explaining that she had initially regretted her family's decision to move to Sydney when she was only nine years old. As a result of that decision, Dot said, "I think mum was never happy, and always a little embarrassed to go home even though things were tough for us growing up in the city. And plus I think she always blamed herself too."[7] When describing the reasons that had initially compelled her mother to relocate their family into the city, Dot expressed a mixture of sadness and some shame over the fact that her mother had genuinely believed things would be better in the cities: "I guess their generation were more hopeful in a way," she said. "But they were also definitely naïve—I remember mum had said that we would be treated better if we left the country, but we weren't."[8] Dot's younger brother, whom she recalled had been "sick all the time," was one of their main reasons for moving, she said. As it turned out, her brother had a heart condition that took his life at a very young age. But Dot recalled that before he passed, and before they had moved to Sydney to try and improve his chances at getting specialized medical treatment, her mother had been adamant that "there will be good doctors in Sydney."[9] Dot said she was unsure about how her mother had formed these beliefs, but she suspected she had naively trusted the "stories you would hear at that time" about the cities offering "better jobs, and a better life."[10] While Dot didn't specify whether these "stories" her mother chose to believe had originated from the government or from other family or community members, it was clear that she felt both a little embarrassment and anger at the thought of her mother's ill-informed or trusting outlook: "I always wish I could have told her that things would be no different in the city," she lamented, "but I was only a kid then."[11] In her descriptions of their life settling into the Aboriginal community in Sydney during the 1960s, Dot spoke a lot about how "let down" and embarrassed her mother had seemed for much of her early childhood, "but she was too proud to take us home as well," she recalled. "This only got worse once [her brother] passed away."[12]

As an adult, Dot has dealt with her fair share of health issues too—she recently recovered from a cancer scare and is managing some mental health issues too. While she no longer lives in Sydney, she told me she often reflects on how different her life might have been if her mother had never moved them. "It's funny," she told me, "but especially after the cancer I feel lucky now to be living in a city, and I know my health is better taken care of here, so maybe mum was right in the end, even though it was too late for her, and too late for [my brother]."[13] Like many of my other Australian informants, Dot's story showed a side of Aboriginal urban migration that can often be hard to come by in written records. Many who moved (especially if they had done so with any genuine belief that conditions would improve) were often deeply embarrassed or concerned that their subsequent difficulties in attaining the "better life" that had been promised in cities must have been their fault in some way.

Bill and Dot, though they couldn't have possibly known it at the time, underwent a kind of migration experience as Indigenous children that was not unique to their family nor even their particular national contexts at the time. I refer to their experiences (and those of other Indigenous people with similar stories) as examples of Indigenous medical migration. Historians in both the United States and Australia have typically framed Indigenous peoples' migration experiences into cities during the twentieth century in terms of a choice to pursue upward social mobility and economic opportunities. However, the experiences of individuals like Bill and Dot, as well as their families, who migrated because health reasons had compelled them to seek out cities in the postwar period, adds an important new dimension to the standard economic accounts of Indigenous urbanization. While they have yet to receive much attention from historians in either the

United States or Australia, such experiences challenge us to rethink the motivations for postwar urban Indigenous migration, as well as to reframe our understanding of Indigenous struggles in the city. In later chapters I discuss how urban Indigenous health struggles in the 1960s and '70s might be read, not as evidence of maladjustment, but as deliberate strategies for negotiating the city on their own terms. Importantly, departing from the vast majority of histories focused on the experiences of young men looking for employment in cities, cases of medical migration also draw our attention to the experiences of women and children in particular, who made up the majority of medical migrants.[14] These observations became clear to me over the course of oral history interviews I conducted with descendants of families who had migrated to Seattle and Sydney in the postwar period. In addition to recalling their various struggles with health care and medical issues in these cities and the coping strategies they came up with in order to deal with medical neglect, many people also spoke about the health reasons that had compelled their families to move from the reserve/reservation in the first place.

Cases of medical migration are a particularly important subset of the economic story that accounts for people leaving rural areas. Perhaps an even better way to put this is to say that the economic and policy stories that have long dominated our understandings of postwar Indigenous urbanization are actually health stories.[15] The attention to health adds a degree of color to our understanding of this rural-urban movement, highlighting just how bad conditions were in rural areas. Medical stories also highlight that urban migration often entailed continuing connection to home communities, as well as significant movement back and forth as people sought out the most accessible care. This perhaps makes the urban medical migrant a more transitory figure than historians have thus far acknowledged in the case of postwar urban Indigenous migrants more generally. This kind of migration also indicates what mattered to people about their quality of life and shows that health was indeed an important part of people's evaluative framework in deciding where to live. Finally, these stories also bring into focus how for many women (mothers) in particular, health conditions were a paramount factor that drove their relocation, which challenges both the American and Australian stereotypes of the postwar Indigenous migrant as a young male looking for a job. By considering the significant health factors that both drove and drew Indigenous people into American and Australian cities during the postwar years, we might more readily be able to understand why health became such a politicized issue, and especially so for women, among both sets of urban Indigenous communities in later years, which is a story I tell in subsequent chapters.

· · · · · ·

For some time now, scholars interested in twentieth-century Indigenous histories in both the United States and Australia have been attentive to a significant shift in the geographic locus of these communities following World War II. At the midpoint of the twentieth century, an unprecedented number of Indigenous people in both the United States and Australia started migrating into major urban centers like Chicago, Los Angeles, Adelaide, Melbourne, Seattle, and Sydney. Of course, Indigenous urbanization both predated and outlasted this particular historical moment, but what is notable about this wave of migration is that federal government policies in both nations played a significant role in encouraging these unprecedented numbers of migrants and were seemingly motivated by very similar goals. In the United States, the federal government's Bureau of Indian Affairs (BIA) encouraged and facilitated a significant amount of this postwar migration by developing and implementing a relocation policy for American Indians in the 1940s, which later crystallized in the 1956 Indian Relocation Act. Initially, the policy was developed in response to conditions on the Navajo and Hopi reservations. The winter of 1947–48 produced a blizzard that gripped the Southwest, leaving Hopi and Navajo communities in grave danger due to freezing temperatures. This situation compelled the federal government to airlift food and other supplies, as well as hay for livestock, in order to provide temporary relief to these communities. Ultimately, the federal government made the decision to temporarily relocate Navajo families to Salt Lake City, Denver, and Los Angeles, providing them with housing and jobs. This became an early precursor to the formal relocation policy of the 1950s. The adverse conditions on those reservations also led the BIA to conclude that the reservation land bases were too small to support the Native population.[16] The BIA subsequently advanced a theory of overpopulation until it became a generalization for all reservations. In conjunction with the introduction of formalized "termination" policies in the 1950s, this concept of overpopulation on reservations led in turn to the policy of relocation, directed toward Native people from all parts of the country.[17] Federal rhetoric cast termination as an emancipatory project of giving Indians full civil rights by removing them from supposedly backward reservation communities. In reality, termination-era policies (including relocation) had been based on the economic needs of the United States; as policymakers looked at Indian reservations, they did not see sovereign nations or communities deserving of federal support on the basis of historic obligations so much as isolated communities of unassimilated Americans, some of whom occupied resource-rich or strategically useful lands.

In Australia, while there was no formalized government relocation program, the federal government did actively encourage Aboriginal movement into the cities as part of its turn toward a broad policy of "assimilation" in Aboriginal Affairs in the 1950s. Indeed, much like the philosophy behind termination-era policies in the United States, it was also the Australian government's intention at this time to curtail specialized services for Aboriginal people once they moved to cities, as part of a push to assimilate them into the Australian mainstream. While Aboriginal sovereignty was never quite at stake in the same way as Native American sovereignty was under termination, assimilation policies in Australia sought to produce the same material outcomes as termination, insofar as this was intended as a means to destroy Aboriginal "dependency" on government support. While no formalized relocation program therefore existed in Australia, interestingly the Aborigines Welfare Board (AWB) did initially relocate "worthy" Aboriginal families as a response to Indigenous population pressures in rural areas. Unlike in the United States, Aboriginal people were sometimes relocated to suburban homes, some in country towns, but many in cities like Sydney. While not a formalized relocation program like that enacted by the BIA, in Australia the AWB's senior officers did actively select families for such assistance in the hope they would serve as a model for others to follow. Apart from those initial families that were "officially" selected by the AWB, the vast majority of Aboriginal people were strongly encouraged by the government to move into cities as a means of "freeing themselves" from the shackles of their "wardship status," which they "remained in as long as they lived on reserves, missions and stations."[18] The parallels in these two national governments' actions and their reliance on a very similar language of liberation is certainly striking, and the first of numerous parallels worth highlighting between the United States and Australian contexts.

In addition to broadening our existing understandings of why Indigenous people moved to cities in the postwar era, this chapter highlights how very similar the strategies of the United States and Australian governments were in encouraging this inward urban Indigenous migration. With respect to individuals and families who relocated into cities for health reasons, I focus in this chapter on showing how the roles played by federal policy and propaganda in creating false expectations of what urban life would be like for

Indigenous migrants were especially consequential. This becomes relevant in later chapters because many of the health struggles endured by urban Indigenous communities in the 1960s and '70s were understood by those communities at the time to have been the product of irresponsible and damaging government policy. Hence activists eventually insisted that the United States and Australian governments accept responsibility for the health care needs and demands of their people. Toward the end of this chapter, I also suggest that health reasons forged bonds of connection and continued contact between rural and urban Indigenous communities in the postwar era. In these three registers—(1) highlighting the experiences of medical migrants; (2) emphasizing how an attentiveness to health matters lays bare the transnational continuities in settler-colonial government approaches to Indigenous urbanization; and (3) showing how health issues served as connective tissue between rural and urban Indigenous communities—this discussion not only enlarges our approach toward histories of Indigenous mobility and urbanization in the twentieth century, but it also shows that a greater attentiveness to health issues is merited in our attempts to understand Indigenous politics and community formation in the twentieth century.

Postwar Indigenous Urbanization Arrives in Seattle and Sydney

In August 1956, the US Congress passed PL 959, the Indian Vocational Training Assistance Act. This legislation authorized the appropriation of $3.5 million "in order to help adult Indians who reside on or near Indian reservations to obtain reasonable and satisfactory employment." In Senate Report No. 2665, it was stated that the act "should be of great value in preparing and orienting participants in the Indian relocation program." The service provided through the act not only assisted Native peoples in the provision of employment assistance and vocational training but also would "supply skilled workers now needed by our industry and thereby utilize one of our most dormant manpower resources."[19] It was also hoped that industries would establish plants and factories close to reservations in order to take advantage of the labor that would become available through the training programs. To implement PL 959, the BIA therefore established employment assistance offices in the late 1950s. In 1963, the act was amended; it was broadened to include placement on or near reservations as well as in seven urban centers (Chicago, Cleveland, Los Angeles, Oakland, San Jose, Denver, and Dallas). Though Seattle was not named as one of the first urban centers, the BIA established the Seattle Orientation Center in July 1963 in response to the high numbers of Alaska Natives and Native Americans moving to the city from nearby areas. The Portland, Oregon, and Billings, Montana, areas were also served through the Seattle office. In 1965, the BIA also established the first prevocational training program for Native people in Seattle, which focused on the provision of basic education services to trainees prior to placement in training programs funded by PL 959. Initially the prevocational training program was open to Washington State Indians only; however, this restriction was lifted in the latter part of the 1960s when the site was converted to an employment training center for Native people from all parts of the country.

By 1960, after an initial wave of postwar migrants had made its way to Seattle, it was estimated among members of the community that there were approximately 12,000 American Indian/Alaska Native people living in the Seattle-King County area.[20] Official estimates in the census put this at approximately half this figure, but as community leaders later explained, this was likely a gross underestimate given that the Seattle urban Indian community was so dispersed, transient, and hard to locate given the tenuous nature of many people's housing.[21] On the issue of housing, longtime Seattle resident Abe Johnny (Cowichan) recalled that in the postwar years many Native people in Seattle, including his father, "usually worked a couple of jobs," in part because "it was kind of hard getting a place to live back then." As Johnny recounted, Seattle's Native community often faced discrimination in finding housing, in part due to the large size of their families: "The only people that would really rent to us were the Italians," he remembered, "because they had big families too, so they kind of understood that it was hard for us to get a place. So, a lot of the places that we moved into were owned by Italians." If they failed to find rental housing, then according to Johnny, many of Seattle's Native community would move between temporary housing and staying with "relatives in the community," or else they would stay in hotels in the downtown area. For a lot of people—especially men—in the community, Johnny recalled how these difficulties often meant that "a lot of the Indians used to hang around Pioneer Square [downtown] because there was a lot of drinking back then, because . . . there was no jobs for a lot of people, and nowhere for them to go." In turn, he described how this fed a cycle of discrimination: "There was always a lot of signs on the doors that always said, 'No Indians' or 'No dogs' in this restaurant, this building, whatever. So—primarily because they used to see a lot of Indians sleeping and drinking on the benches back then. . . . They kind of looked at us all the same way."[22] These living conditions also meant that enumerating the Native population in Seattle was not at all easy at this time. Nonetheless, even accounting for unreliable figures, the jump to even 6,000 by 1960 signaled an extraordinary increase from the figure of only 1,700 in 1950.[23] In spite of these significant numbers, because they no longer lived on reservations and were thereby deemed part of the "mainstream," urban Indians at this time were largely ignored by governmental organizations such as the BIA after their initial period of training or placement was over. Urban Indian migrants were also marginalized by the city of Seattle due to their smaller population and wider dispersal in comparison to other minority groups. In time, this neglect would have disastrous consequences for the health of urban Indians since it meant that their medical struggles also went largely undetected.

In Australia, the precise pattern and rate of Aboriginal people moving to Sydney during the mid-twentieth century is harder to ascertain. This is mainly because until 1971, Aboriginal people were not included in the census data that was collected every five years, although some limited statistics were gathered in 1961 and 1966. Until its repeal in Australia's momentous 1967 referendum, Section 127 of the Commonwealth Constitution stated that "in recording the number of people of the Commonwealth, or of a State or other part of the Commonwealth, Aboriginal natives shall not be counted."[24] The Aborigines Welfare Board periodically collected demographic data about those living on government-run reserves (also called "stations" or "missions") but not about those living in unofficial camps or in cities and towns.[25] All of this makes accounting for Aboriginal demography before the 1970s extremely challenging. Quite apart from the issue of the census, it is difficult to pinpoint the size of the Sydney Aboriginal population at any one point in the 1950s and 1960s because of the high level of transmigration between the cities and rural areas in this time. This meant there was always a high turnover of residents, of people moving to and fro as seasonal employment and community and cultural obligations led many city dwellers to return to their homelands regularly and often for extended periods.[26] Prominent Australian ethnographer Charles Rowley wrote in the 1960s that the move to the city "remains experimental for many, who may come and go until assets in the metropolis, social and economic, will so far outweigh those in the areas of origin that the city becomes the home."[27]

Nonetheless, various estimates of the size of the Sydney population were made by academics at the time. In 1950, E. Wait reported that an AWB informal census in 1945 revealed there were 2,500 Aboriginal residents in the metropolitan area. The author believed that this had grown to 3,000 by 1950.[28] The influx from that point was quite rapid. Other estimates had put 12,000 Aboriginal people living in just the Redfern area in 1965, but F. Wells assessed the entire metropolitan population in the mid-1960s at "between 10,000 and 11,000."[29] Anthropologist Pamela Beasley's extensive study of Aboriginal households in Sydney in the late 1960s found that there were "at least 6,000 (possibly as many as 10,000) people of Aboriginal descent living in Sydney."[30] In 1971, Frances Lovejoy cited an unpublished University of Sydney study, which found approximately 12,000 residents in the state's capital.[31] Records from unofficial surveys carried out in the late 1960s also show that half of the Aboriginal population in Sydney at this time were under the age of fifteen as compared with 30 percent for the Australian population as a whole. Seventy-one percent were under thirty years of age.[32] Early anthropological research found these family groupings tended to be matrifocal, which was also reflected in the fact that many of my interviewees recounted stories of their mothers being the driving force behind family relocation into the city.[33] Whatever the precise makeup and total of the Aboriginal population in Sydney by the late 1960s, it is clear that much like in Seattle, the numbers had grown rapidly in the twenty-five years after the end of World War II.

By moving into the cities, Aboriginal people had supposedly opted to "exempt" themselves from their legal wardship status and opted into "citizenship." It is important to underscore that before 1967 "citizenship" for Aboriginal Australians was still an ambiguous and highly contested status since control of Aboriginal Affairs was still in the hands of the individual state governments. By virtue of the Nationality and Citizenship Act of 1948, Aboriginal people were technically already citizens by birth, and to that extent, citizenship was their birthright. Yet of course, the more salient point is that the enjoyment of rights depended not on the formal status of citizen but on the specific provisions of state and federal legislation.[34] When the AWB encouraged urban Aboriginal migrants to opt into "citizenship," it was therefore more in reference to their social than legal status.

For much of this period, the Aborigines Welfare Board thus had very little effective oversight or even knowledge about Aboriginal people who lived in metropolitan enclaves.[35] While in the country, town district welfare officers played an important surveillance role over those Indigenous people who lived off reserves, their influence over the ballooning population in inner Sydney was limited. This neglect was such that Aboriginal community leader Chicka Dixon recalled that "I went to the government in 1967 and pointed out that there was a need for hostels for Aborigines because of the mass migration of teenagers from the river-banks to Sydney."[36] Like in Seattle, despite this significant growth in Sydney's urban Indigenous population at midcentury, the state government of New South Wales and the Australian federal government either did not acknowledge their presence as a distinct Indigenous community or viewed them as assimilated simply by virtue of their location. Problematically, this meant the government also did not see urban migrants as needing specialized social welfare support.[37] This complete disregard by the state and federal governments would prove to be disastrous for the health of urban Aboriginal migrants in Sydney since their medical problems thus went largely unacknowledged for much of the 1950s and '60s.

As previously noted, historians in both the United States and Australia have typically framed migrants' decisions to move during this period in terms of a choice to pursue upward social mobility and economic opportunities. For example, in two classic accounts of postwar American Indian urbanization published in the 1990s, Joan Weibel-Orlando and Edmund Jefferson Danzinger Jr. wrote respectively about migration to Los Angeles and Detroit, Weibel-Orlando noting that "as with most rural-to-urban migrants in the twentieth century, the Indians' decision to move from traditional homelands was an economic one. Post–World War II Los Angeles was an industrial boom town."[38] While Danzinger Jr. explained that in Detroit "during the [mid-]twentieth century Great Lakes band members traveled by the thousands to Detroit . . . a working man's haven. Millions of laborers from other regions and from other nations followed their dreams to this El Dorado, turning Motor City into one of the most ethnically diverse metropolitan areas in the United States."[39] In Australia, Faye Gale's account of the Aboriginal community that emerged in Adelaide after the war set the tone of scholarly discussions regarding Aboriginal urbanization across the country for a long time.[40] In the 1980s, she considered the reasons for a downturn in urban Aboriginal migration starting in the 1970s. Within her analysis, we see the repetition of the economic story that accounts for not only the postwar boom in urban migration but also the downward turn some twenty years later: "Available data suggest that Aborigines were much better off in the southern cities than in rural communities from the immediate postwar period until the 1970s. However, it is equally apparent that this is no longer the situation. . . . The city, which earlier offered important economic advantages, especially in terms of employment and services, may not claim this lead today."[41]

Accounts like these added up to a fairly generalizable story within the early historiography about the mid-twentieth-century urban Indigenous migrant. In the United States, Donald Fixico, in *Termination and Relocation* (1990), presented this standard, fairly bleak, and seemingly hopeless portrayal: "After leaving their traditional social structures on reservations . . . (relocatees) had nothing. . . . The city's alien environment was unlike anything they had experienced. . . . As members of a small minority attempting to adjust to the urban scene, Indian Americans felt inferior. Loss of morale and pride threatened their personal identity, causing many relocatees to wander and drift in cities, searching for fundamental elements as they knew them traditionally. . . . Some Indians contemplated self-destruction; the more depressed individuals committed suicide."[42]

Presenting Native people as victims of federal policy, Fixico suggested that many were incapable of culturally adapting within urban America. Interestingly, there is not much to tell between this typical story in either the Australian or US case. Gale's account, for example, concluded that urban Aborigines, more so than any other kind of migrant, experienced urban change as "catastrophic": "Traditional Aboriginal society was determined by a more static and much smaller community than that to be found in any Australian city. All of the Aboriginal's concepts of life and of self, his beliefs and his codes of behavior, as well as his whole economic structure, were vastly different from those of the western European's culture, which dominates Australian cities today. While for all people the city tends to break past traditional ties, for the Aboriginal, the enforced change has often been catastrophic."[43]

As these two accounts demonstrate, early scholarly studies focused primarily on the economic motivations for Indigenous urban migration in the postwar period, and they evaluated the formation of these communities in a way that pathologized Indigenous urban community life and cultural loss. Critiquing this historiographical tradition, US historian James LaGrand has more recently written, "Although social-science models for studying urban Indians have proved somewhat unsatisfactory, historians at times have not done much better. Those who have studied American Indians living during the latter half of the twentieth century most often have focused on two major policies of the federal government's Bureau of Indian Affairs (BIA) during that period: termination and relocation."[44] As with much of the American and Australian historical records of Indigenous peoples, these early scholars thus wrote from a colonizing perspective, defining success, failure, levels of assimilation, and lifestyles from the standpoint of the Australian and

American mainstream. Using polarized assessments to evaluate urban Indigenous residents as either American *or* Indian, Australian *or* Aboriginal, scholars generally accepted a maladjustment model where, accordingly, Indigenous people "failed" when they did not fully assimilate or integrate into US or Australian society.[45] As such, most studies of Indigenous postwar urbanization have also focused on the costs of urban life for American Indians and Aboriginal Australians, emphasizing social and economic problems and rarely commenting on positive outcomes or strategies for cultural organization and survival. In effect, this mode of perceiving and studying pan-Indigenous urban culture and society has therefore reproduced the colonial logics of spatial governance, casting these diasporic and pan-Indigenous urban communities as "problematic" and ill-adapted.[46]

By contrast, a closer look at accounts by migrants and their families, and a closer scrutiny of government files that contain traces of migrants' stories in the archives, reveal a subset of health-related experiences that depart from the "typical" economic stories above. People's experiences varied in important ways, but the two representative accounts I shared at the top of this chapter illustrate many of the most significant aspects of these medical migration stories: the predominance of women and children within these narratives, and the significance of high expectations for a better (healthier) life in cities. Interestingly, in the United States, these health-related migration stories seem to correlate in many cases with people who moved of their own volition and not as part of the BIA relocation program. In Australia, since there was no official government relocation program akin to the one sponsored by the BIA, the vast majority of urban relocatees were people who migrated without much official assistance.[47] Whereas in Australia this type of postwar Aboriginal migrant is the norm, in the United States, historians by and large have neglected these kinds of migrants because they are harder to locate in the archive. At the time however, Indigenous community members within US cities had a term for differentiating between these kinds of migrants and the people who came as part of the official relocation program. In the United States, individuals and families who had undergone "self-relocation," or who were "self-relocatees," were known to be an especially vulnerable segment of the community, susceptible to falling through the cracks in cities.[48] Hence, as I was told by many of my informants in Seattle, Native community leaders at the time were especially concerned to look out for these people and to make contact with them as soon as they arrived in the city.[49] The stories of these "self-relocatees" are missing from the vast majority of histories about urban Indians. We come to see some of them through the health stories, however. The neglect of "self-relocatees" in the US historiography is an oversight that needs to be corrected. Since some of these self-relocatees come to light through the health-related experiences of urban migrants, this suggests that more work can be done to find additional cases of self-relocatees.[50] They may have represented an earlier phase of this midcentury migration history, meaning they might speak to the broader social problems and stresses facing Indigenous people on reservations in the United States in the late 1940s and early 1950s.[51]

In both Dot's and Bill's stories, for example, we get a sense of significant factors that both drove and drew Indigenous people (especially families) into the cities in the postwar era. In both national contexts, my informants expressed memories of a belief that health conditions and options for treatment would be better in the city than in the country. And as represented in both Bill's and Dot's personal narratives, the other side of this hope for better things in the cities was also a clear dissatisfaction with the quality of care available to them in their home communities. These two overarching factors—conditions in the country and beliefs about the city—are vital in understanding the history of what drove the postwar medical migration of Indigenous people in both the United States and Australia.

Medical Services and Health Conditions on Reserves and Reservations Pre-1950

In the nineteenth century, government-provided medical services for Indigenous peoples in the United States and Australia were born from the very same impulse. In the very first instance, they grew from the colonists' desires to protect themselves against Indigenous people. In the United States, the beginnings of a health care system for Native Americans might be traced to an authorization by President Thomas Jefferson to supply vaccinations for visiting tribal delegations to Washington, DC.[52] This single act established a practice that soon became incorporated into the work of the US Army; by 1803, troops were being instructed to supply smallpox vaccines to neighboring Indian villages while they were stationed at outposts along the frontier. More an act to protect soldiers than to ensure the survival of Native people, this early work of vaccine supply soon led Congress to appropriate revenue for Indian health care for the stated purposes of preventing "the further decline and final extinction of the Indian tribes."[53] Most of these initial funds were dispensed to missionary organizations for education and "such other duties as may be enjoined" to protect and preserve the American Indians adjoining the frontier settlements of the United States.[54] Finally, in 1824, superintendent of Indian trade Thomas McKenney administered these funds and established an Office of Indian Affairs under the direction of the secretary of war. In a perfect encapsulation of the spirit in which these services had been conceived, the dispensation of medical care to Native Americans was thus first administered through the War Department as an act of defense.[55]

In Australia, reference to colonial practices and policies with respect to Aboriginal health care are scattered, but what is clear from the Australian historical literature is that much like in the United States, particular policies pertaining to Aboriginal health in the nineteenth century were circumscribed and were part and parcel of the wider policies to contain and control Aboriginal people. Indeed, the impetus for the development of specific health policies relating to Aboriginal people came, much like it did in the United States, from the European settlers' desires to protect themselves from the contagious diseases that were having such devastating effect on the Aboriginal population. Venereal diseases, such as syphilis in Queensland, for instance, spread so rapidly in the late nineteenth century that reports in the 1890s referred to more than half the Aboriginal population suffering from the disease in some areas.[56] Taking more drastic measures than the initial US approach of immunizing against the spread of these contagious diseases, in Australia the first solution was to relocate Aboriginal people away from European settlements. In response to the rapid increase in venereal disease in Western Australia, eventually the pressure grew for dedicated hospitals that would isolate but also treat Aboriginal patients. In the early 1900s, the Western Australian government therefore established hospitals on Bernier and Dorre Islands, west of Canarvon, on the northwest coast of Western Australia. These so-called lock hospitals received many of their patients in chains after police had forcibly removed them to the islands.

Regarded as both the sources and carriers of various life-threatening and contagious diseases, Indigenous peoples in the United States and Australia were therefore subjected to a host of similar, questionable health policies and practices in the nineteenth and early twentieth centuries in the name of "protection."[57] The one consistent and significant difference to note between the medical services provided to Indigenous people in the United States and Australia concerns the status of health care for Native Americans as part of their treaty negotiations. In the United States, treaty-making was of course the primary vehicle by which the United States dealt with tribal nations until the late nineteenth century. Treaties were not only a form of recognition by the United Sates of the limited sovereignty of tribal governments, but they were also the method of providing goods and services to tribes in exchange for cessions of land, federal protection, and peace and friendship. Of the 382 ratified Indian treaties, thirty-one, or 12 percent, contained provisions related to medical care. Of these, twenty-eight provided for physicians and nine for hospitals.[58] Despite these treaty provisions for hospitals and medical services, however, the United States often failed to fulfill its obligations, and when it did, it usually did so many years later. However imperfectly the US government met its side of these agreements though, what these treaties meant was that in matters of health, this established a basis of legal obligation and responsibility toward Native Americans on the part of the federal government that was absent in the Australian case, where treaties were never made with the Indigenous population. With the exception of this duty of care that the US treaties established (what some historians have characterized as only a "vague sense of responsibility" in the realm of health), we can say that across much of the nineteenth century, the status, purpose, and mode of delivery of medical care for Indigenous people in both the United States and Australia looked much the same.[59] They were preoccupied with containing the threat of contagion associated with Indigenous peoples' diseases through the methods of isolation or vaccination. And all of this was done in the name of paternalistic policies of "protection," which in truth were designed more to protect the settler population.

By the turn of the twentieth century, in both settler nations, it was becoming increasingly difficult to overlook the deficiencies of these containment and isolation models of "care." What's more, policies and practices of the federal governments were also leading to new health problems. For example, shortly after the turn of the twentieth century, Dr. Laurence W. White, superintendent of the Lac du Flambeau (Wisconsin) Indian School, lamented with participants at the annual Lake Mohonk Conference that the health maladies affecting American Indians were to a large measure the direct responsibility of the US government, which forced changes on Native people without preparing them ahead of time. "The Indian," White reported, "was taken from a domain as large as the continent itself and compelled to occupy very restricted areas before he was taught the proper rules of sanitation." Dietary changes "to which he was not accustomed" were also forced on him before he had "a knowledge of how properly to prepare it." Being "forced into a new world and compelled to live a new life without a rule or law yet learned, by which he might adjust himself to his new surroundings," the American Indians struggled, White argued, "to survive."[60] Across the United States, other avowedly "humanitarian-minded" doctors from the time also recognized that the real "white plague" in Indian Country was not tuberculosis but "the vices of white men" perpetrated on Indian women (i.e., the transmission of venereal diseases) by the "less than scrupulous."[61]

Remarkably, the deteriorating health situation of Aboriginal people in Australia by the turn of the twentieth century was understood in strikingly similar terms. In the period from about 1850 to the early 1930s, the systematic removal of Aboriginal children believed to be of "mixed decent," in order that they would be successfully assimilated into the "lower orders" of Australian society, created generations of dislocated families and the mass institutionalization of Aboriginal children into establishments much like the American Indian boarding schools—though they were not called this in Australia. By the 1920s, a subset of medical practitioners in Australia were starting to recognize the disastrous effect that institutionalization was having on Aboriginal children's health. Much like their counterparts in the United States, doctors in Australia wrote in medical reports that the "change from small, semi-nomadic communities into large aggregations of people from many different areas" was seen to be causing "a rapid increase of both communicable diseases and social tensions" within these institutions.[62] At the same time, much like the condemnation of "white vices" in the US case, Australian missionaries also blamed the spread of venereal diseases and of access to alcohol among the Aboriginal population on "depraved whites" who lived close by, and whose "excesses" brought both social conflict and ill-health into Aboriginal reserve communities.[63]

The rapid push to "civilize" Indigenous peoples in both the United States and Australia by means of interspersing the Indigenous population with white residents and the institutionalization of Indigenous children, therefore took its toll not only in a decreasing land base and displaced political and social structures but also in the further decline of Indigenous people's health. By the 1920s, poor housing and susceptibility to successive waves of disease had created a health crisis on reserves and reservations. In the United States this development was poorly understood by the government, and in Australia the federal government was almost entirely ignorant of the problem. What this looked like in terms of health conditions on the ground was rather stark. While preventative medicine was becoming the norm for the wider settler populace by this time, it was slow to materialize in Indian Country and on Aboriginal reserves in Australia, where the emphasis remained curative. Consequently, in order to reduce the backlog of unmet Indigenous health needs, most of the annual federal budgets that initially went toward Indigenous medical care went toward hospital construction only. Of course, although hospitals were an important part of the campaign against disease, they simply handled daily emergencies. Thus, for example, although there were eighty-seven (generally under resourced) hospitals serving Native people by 1924 in the United States, the wider medical infrastructure was simply too limited to handle the sheer volume of need in Indian Country.[64]

If services were so limited, then what were the main health problems faced, and what minimal care and treatment could the average Native person therefore expect to receive in the first few decades of the twentieth century? The most significant published source on Indian health in this time comes from the 1928 Meriam Report. Led by government technocrat Lewis Meriam and compiled by a staff of nine highly qualified specialists, this 872-page report found that "practically every activity undertaken by the national government for the promotion of the health of Indians is below a reasonable standard of efficiency."[65] In evaluating the health program, the Meriam staff found inadequate health facilities and equipment, unqualified and/or a shortage of health personnel, inadequate salaries and housing for health professionals, and a system of purchasing obsolete and outdated medical supplies and medicines from excess army and navy supplies. The Meriam staff also found a pressing need for keeping accurate medical statistics as a method of combatting the spread of disease and allowing a modern approach to fighting disease. They reported that an overall "lack of vision and real understanding" of what needed to be done precluded the establishment of "a real program of preventative medicine."[66] The campaign against tuberculosis was found to be ineffective, and the approach to treating trachoma "perfunctory at best."[67] Untrained instructors teaching health education and inadequate provisions for establishing working relations with state and local health organizations to attack disease and insanitary conditions were also cited in support of the report's position on the gross inefficiency of medical services for Indians in the late 1920s.[68]

Had the report stopped there, it would have been damning enough. But Meriam also found a lack of attention to environmental matters that not only precluded a preventative health program but also rendered any program of basic health services largely ineffective. An extremely low standard of living and poor housing on reservations were just two of many socioeconomic factors influencing health care that were worsened by a misguided

Indian Service. Improper (or complete lack of) sanitation facilities and an inadequate food supply compounded this even further. Moreover, the Indian Service was found by Meriam's report to be so preoccupied with matters of "real estate" that it ignored basic social and health concerns: "It seems," he wrote, "as if the government assumed that some magic in individual ownership of property [through allotment] would in itself prove an educational factor, but unfortunately this policy has for the most part operated in the opposite direction."[69] Looking ahead to the 1930s and '40s, Meriam thus concluded that the only hope Native people had in their fight against disease was for the Indian Service to expand its medical services beyond the mere utilization of hospitals. To improve health conditions required environmental changes. The construction of sanitation facilities, provision of potable water, and improved housing were all therefore essential. Medical care had to be improved. Additional public health clinics to identify incipient cases of tuberculosis and trachoma were also needed. Furthermore:

> More and better trained doctors and nurses are required. The [plans]
> of hospitals and sanitaria should be brought up at least to the
> recognized minimum standards for such institutions elsewhere.
> The practice of salvaging old buildings and converting them into
> hospitals should be discontinued. . . . Hospitals and sanitaria should be
> administered by persons fitted by training and experience for that class
> of work. . . . Patient labor should be utilized only when the physician
> certifies that it will not injure the patient and retard his cure. . . . The
> salaries and entrance qualifications for cooks in hospitals and sanitaria
> should be raised so that each institution has a good one, competent to
> prepare special diets and to serve well-prepared meals. . . . For the care
> of bed patients the ratio of nurses to patients should be one to seven,
> and for the care of ambulant cases one to thirty.[70]

In short, the details and recommendations of the report give us some idea of the level of care (or lack thereof) that people had been receiving at Indian hospitals until this time. Accordingly, Meriam's report focused on the need to create an effective public health program that could prevent disease rather than wait for it to happen. Public health nurses had to replace untrained nurses and matrons. Physicians trained as public health specialists were also essential. State and local governments also had to assume more responsibility for Indian health care, with the federal government subsidizing such services. Any transfer of responsibility, however, was to be cautiously implemented: "The sooner the States and counties can be brought to the positions where they will render services and the Indians to the point where they will look to the government of the county in which they live, the better," Meriam opined. "But the national government must direct and guide the transition. It must not withdraw until the transition has been completely effected; otherwise the Indians will fall between two stools."[71]

The Meriam report was indeed a catalyst in improving Indian health care from this point onward. As I discuss in the following chapter, many of the recommendations were implemented in subsequent years. Yet, although Indian health conditions showed signs of improvement by the late 1930s and '40s, they remained more than two generations behind the national averages at the time of World War II. Much of this had to do with the fact that despite a growing number of state and country facilities by the 1940s, many Native people were unable to actually avail themselves of such treatment facilities due to the distance such facilities were from their homes. By mid-century, for example, 145 counties provided services for children with disabilities. Yet, this covered just 60 percent of the Native population. Of this number, only one-third of American Indians had access to such treatment. In order to obtain services, it was common for children to travel 100 miles or more. In many cases, especially in the West, the only transportation available was a wagon drawn by a team of horses, making travel slow and arduous.[72] Considering that infant mortality and childhood diseases were among the principle causes of death among American Indians at the time, the lack of pediatricians and nutritionists in the Indian Service was another serious difficulty. The superintendent of the Tohono O'odham Reservation, for example, reported in 1949 that the population curve of the tribe resembled that of "medieval Europe": "Of approximately 260 infants born each year, one-fourth die within twelve months; at the age of 6 there are only 160 left; at the age of eighteen, only 125."[73] The life expectancy of non-Native infants at the time was sixty years in 1949, compared to that of Tohono O'odham infants, which was just seventeen. In the face of such knowledge, medical director Fred Foard concluded in 1949 that "the comparison of the weighted [Tohono O'odham] age curve with that of the US as a whole tells an almost incredible health story. Only a birth rate double that of the country as a whole enables the [Tohono O'odham] to survive at all."[74]

Despite some improvements to infant and early childhood care and treatment, Native American children, by and large, still faced a variety of challenges by midcentury that could be life-threatening due to the almost near absence of available medical care: Chicken pox, impetigo, measles, whooping cough, infant paralysis, and sundry health complications were more prevalent among Native children than among non-Native children. In 1954, Native Americans faced a measles death rate twenty times the non-Native rate. Deaths from pneumonia and influenza were four times the non-Native rate, and infant deaths were three times the comparable non-Native rate.[75] Maternal mortality rates were also substantially higher among Native people.[76] Many of the infant and childhood diseases were exacerbated by dietary changes or poor diets. Physicians frequently commented on the severity of intestinal diseases among Native children, which they attributed to poor diets. Indeed, malnutrition overwhelmed the Indian Service in its efforts to mitigate infant diseases in the 1930s and '40s: the introduction and heavy reliance upon processed white flour, refined sugar, canned goods, and other government commodities, combined with the exclusion of traditional foods, "resulted in poor nutrition, undernourishment, dental defects, and susceptibility to disease," concluded Indian commissioner John Collier in 1944.[77]

Finally, prior to 1940, sanitation efforts in Indian Country extended no further than occasional cleanups, even though the Public Health Service Sanitary Engineering Corps provided assistance in surveying water and sewer systems for Indian Service hospitals and schools.[78] Outside of these activities though, little was done for individual families, making sanitation the most neglected element of the Indian health program. In 1936, BIA officer James Townsend lamented, "There is no regular program of sanitation in the Indian health service" even though the "great need for sanitation exists among the smaller Indian villages (which) usually obtain water in a nearby stream, spring or well which may be open to contamination."[79] Moreover, he reported that most Native homes had "no method of excreta disposal and those that do almost invariably use a privy of the surface type."[80] In Alaska the sanitary conditions were especially bad: "Garbage and refuse disposal," Indian Service agent Thomas Parron wrote in 1954, "generally is very primitive, consisting usually of dumping upon the ground surface or over river embankments."[81] When Fred Foard was assigned by the Public Health Service to oversee the Division of Indian Health in 1948, he viewed the lack of basic sanitation as the single greatest culprit in the campaign to eliminate health hazards in Indian Country. At the time, there were only two sanitary engineers in Indian Country, and only one dedicated his full attention to public health work—and he was assigned exclusively to the Navajo nation. To overcome these deficiencies, Foard relied on the assistance of the Public Health Service, which appointed H. Norman Old to the

Division of Indian Health to serve as its first full-time environmental sanitary engineer. Within the Indian Service, Old conducted forty-five environmental surveys in eighteen states and developed a framework for a servicewide sanitation program. In the process, he concluded the high mortality and morbidity rates among American Indians and Alaska Natives were the result of faulty sanitation. Diseases such as dysentery, diarrhea, and enteritis were prevalent among infants and children, with protozoa infestations common.[82] Nowhere were inadequate sanitation facilities more disturbing than in the American Indian and Alaska Native morbidity and mortality rates, which is significant for my study given that Seattle was the most common urban destination for Alaska Native migrants after World War II. Diseases such as trachoma, tuberculosis, influenza, gastroenteric disorder, meningitis, and others resulted from or were compounded by unsanitary conditions. Improper excreta disposal and other human waste contributed to the spread of microorganisms that precipitated outbreaks of dysentery, hepatitis, and illnesses such as intestinal protozoa. Hence, nothing less than a full-scale assault on environmental and sanitation conditions was needed.[83]

As midcentury drew nigh, the health services available and care provided to American Indians and Alaska Natives remained woefully inadequate. What was necessary to elevate health conditions and care to an adequate level was a new paradigm, one that focused on an Indian Country–wide approach rather than sporadic, emergency-based services. Such an undertaking required, among other things, a medical statistical service to tabulate, correlate, and analyze morbidity, mortality, and other vital statistics. This would encourage research into specific pathogens and challenges facing Native people. By the early 1950s, the Division of Indian Health—while showing improvement over its pre-1930s services—was thus ripe for integration with the Public Health Service. From the perspective of Indian community members on the reservations, however, an easy solution seemed to be to simply move to where health services and conditions might be better. In light of the terrible health conditions on reservations, it is certainly not hard to believe that many Native families and individuals may have taken this option. Moreover, when we consider the later centrality of health issues in the political organizing that erupted in US cities among the urban Indigenous communities in the 1960s and '70s, this would also suggest that health was at the forefront of the concerns and experiences of many relocatees. While such stories are harder to locate in the archive, the oral histories of families and individuals in Seattle confirm the view that health was a significant consideration for many who moved there in the postwar period.

Among the individuals who recalled specific health reasons or incidents that had compelled their own families to move to Seattle, foremost among their memories were the difficulties of accessing health care from the reservation. Many informants described the need to travel great distances in order to see a doctor. This was remembered as an especially arduous undertaking when one was already feeling unwell. Jania Garcia (Haida), the daughter of Seattle Indian Health Board founder Adeline Garcia (Haida), recalled how in later life her mother and other Alaska Native women in Seattle would often reflect back on "the tough times," and particularly how hard it had been for them to take care of their children's health in Alaska given that (a) "outside of our traditional foods, as kids we didn't eat so well because of money but also because it was just harder to get good food"; and (b) "health services and basic sanitation in our community was essentially nonexistent there for my mother's generation, so they often chose to leave."[84] Indeed the vast majority of my informants ranked their mother's concern for the health of her children as being the main driving force behind their family's relocation. In some cases, it was because a child had a specific condition that required specialized or more accessible care. In other cases, the concern for the child's health was described as a more generalized consideration or a preemptive concern. Some informants, like Bill, also remembered that their parents had their own health issues, which they thought would improve in the city.[85] In a few instances, informants associated their family's decision to move with a specific incident, such as one case in which an interviewee recalled that her father's surgical procedure in a city hospital caused her family to move temporarily, "but then we just ended up staying."[86] If people did not recall a specific health reason or incident that had motivated their relocation, then often people would mention "better health conditions" as one of a few key factors ("better jobs," "education," etc.) that had attracted them to the city, proving that even within the more standard "economic" narratives about migration, health conditions were as much a part of people's framework for evaluating their reasons to stay or go. Compared with much of the historical literature on postwar Indian urbanization, these medical migration stories thus widen our perspective on the factors that compelled people to move to cities in this period. Moreover, they underscore both the poor state of health services for reservation communities in the postwar period and the prevalence of assumptions that health conditions would be better in the cities.

In Australia, it is harder to draw a comprehensive picture of Aboriginal health conditions in the early part of the twentieth century since the Aboriginal population in Australia was not regularly enumerated, and because the control of Indigenous affairs was highly particularized under the control of the states until the 1960s. In comparison to the United States, Australian government–provided health services for Indigenous people between 1900 and 1950 largely reflected wider policies to contain and control Aboriginal people. Namely, in the first half of the twentieth century, the vast majority of Aboriginal people gained access to health services only if they were gainfully employed. Hence in Western Australia and in Queensland, where the Aboriginal populations were largest, any Aboriginal person employed under contract was legally entitled to free medical treatment and prescribed rations, although this regulation was not (like the provisions of US treaties in theory) strictly enforced. It was therefore frequently up to resident magistrates to dispense medicines to impoverished, sick, Aboriginal people. Judges also infrequently sent very ill people to the nearest hospital, where as a rule, Aboriginal people were treated off the actual hospital premises, either on the verandah (porch) or in the yard. It should be noted here that medical care for Euro-Australians at the time was also fairly rudimentary, and that treatment at home was the norm until well into the twentieth century.[87] But despite this, it is clear that medical treatment for Aboriginal people in many parts of Australia was crude or nonexistent, even approaching the mid-twentieth century. As late as 1973, for example, the Maryborough Hospital in Queensland refused to admit a seriously wounded Aboriginal woman who subsequently died, on the following grounds: "It has been a rule of the Maryborough Hospital ever since it has been in existence . . . that aboriginals should not be admitted as patients—both from lack of separate accommodation for them and the absolute dislike—we might say almost refusal of the servants to attend upon them."[88] The blatant racism that still pervaded the Australian medical system even as late as the 1970s cannot be understated.

The lack of medical services for Aboriginal people in both Western Australia and Queensland was typical of other parts of Australia too. Eduard J. Beck's widely cited history of European medical services in the Northern Territory, for instance, notes that only in the 1930s, when it was apparent that the Aboriginal population was not dying out as predicted, were health services for Aboriginal people initiated in any systematic way.[89] To illustrate the level of medical inattention Aboriginal populations received under the provision of the states, Beck described how prior to the assumption of responsibility for the Northern Territory by the Commonwealth government in 1911, most legislation pertaining to the Aboriginal population was designed to restrict contact between European and Chinese males and Aboriginal females, thus attempting to isolate Aboriginal disease from the wider population. A short-lived attempt was made in 1911 to establish a health service for Aboriginal people. However, this failed when the three "medical protectors" appointed left their posts and were not replaced. Instead, between 1911 and 1925, medical kits were dispensed widely throughout the Northern Territory, and infrequent visits by medical personnel took place. The Inland Mission Hostel at Stuart, established in 1916, did not treat Aboriginal patients until 1958, even though they would have been by far the most populous group in the region.[90] The appointment of Cecil E. Cook as chief medical officer and chief protector in 1927 saw the establishment of the Northern Territory Medical Service and the gradual upgrading of medical and hospital services for the European and Aboriginal populations. In the decade 1929–39, five hospitals and a leprosarium were established outside Darwin. In the Northern Territory, it was thus not until the 1950s that organized health services for Aboriginal people were established and overseen by the Welfare Branch.[91] Beck's research only described the Northern Territory, but a similar pattern existed in other states, where special provisions for Aboriginal health prior to the 1960s consisted largely of negative policies designed to protect white Australia from possible contagion from infectious diseases. Compulsory examinations and, in some cases, forced isolation, remained in the legislation up until the 1960s.[92]

While Aboriginal hospitals were gradually established across Australia during the 1920s, they were often little more than a tin shed in which Aboriginal people received the most rudimentary treatment. Sometimes communities might be luckier and inherit obsolete hospitals as newer buildings were established for the white populace. Generally though, in many parts of Australia until the 1930s Aboriginal people who were sick had no access to medical care other than these sparse and very basic Aboriginal hospitals. And even then, as in the Australian Inland Mission in Hall's Creek, Western Australia, sometimes these hospitals would only admit Aboriginal patients for treatment after the Aborigines department of that state started paying an annual subsidy of 100 pounds.[93] Slowly, and in piecemeal fashion, public hospitals in Australia started to provide segregated accommodation for Aboriginal patients in the late 1930s. The following comments from an Aboriginal woman who in 1937 was admitted for a postnatal operation indicate how harrowing these experiences could be:

> I was put in the Native Ward and instead of putting me on a macintosh [a bed covering] the Matron put me on some old newspaper. After the operation, the new sister asked Matron if she could give me a wash and Matron shook her head and said, "We don't do that." The new sister seemed startled. So I had to lie in my own mess, until I ran away. . . . I don't know how I managed to get home. There was another native woman in the hospital at the time, also a native boy about ten years of age, who had to empty my pans, and Rose, the other woman, had to attend my baby and sponge her over for me.[94]

Although the period immediately following World War II saw gradual improvements to the health services for Aboriginal people, it was still possible, in 1947, for the Mullewa Aboriginal Hospital in Western Australia to require all patients to do their own laundry, feed themselves, and collect firewood. As late as 1949, it was also possible for the matron of King Edward Memorial Hospital (then as now the major obstetric teaching hospital in Western Australia) to declare without one hint of irony in a letter to her superior that "it's all very well to talk about the rights of natives, but I do not think that people who talk in this way would like to be in the next bed to some of these women."[95] Hospital facilities on many Aboriginal settlements and missions were so poor in this period that they may actually have been a part of the problem. A report made of a visit to Yuendumu in 1966, for example, revealed that milk for infants was prepared in the hospital's dressing room where open buckets containing soiled disposable napkins and used dressings from purulent wounds were also kept.[96]

What did this discriminatory, minimal, or in some cases entirely absent or even damaging medical care imply for Aboriginal health conditions across Australia in the first half of the twentieth century? Though the health data on Aboriginal people is scarce prior to the 1960s, a picture of Aboriginal health on reserves and stations can be stitched together from knowledge about the environmental conditions of reserves, from the scattered writings of missionaries, anthropologists, a few doctors, and the spotted records of welfare officers and hospitals. Mortality data on Aboriginal communities comes from two main sources—the number of deaths recorded for institutionalized or semi-institutionalized Aboriginal communities, and the causes of death as listed in Bureau of Census and Statistics records prior to

1967.[97] A few special surveys undertaken by health departments, usually for limited areas or selected communities, can also be used.

These sources reveal that within the central and northern reserves, the mission and government settlements/reserves clearly proved disastrous for the health of the Aboriginal inhabitants. Living habits suitable for a handful of people who moved camp regularly were totally unsuitable for several hundred settled permanently in one area. Authorities were slow to provide facilities such as piped water and sanitation. Houses built at some settlements were rudimentary and not acceptable to the Aboriginal occupants. Moreover, most of the settlements had poor facilities for dealing with the vast majority of typical health problems that arose, such as tuberculosis, malnutrition, gastrointestinal disorders, anemia, diarrhea, pneumonia, circulatory disease, chronic respiratory diseases such as bronchitis and emphysema, trachoma, and deaths due to accidents.[98]

Attempts to solve the problems were often misguided, to say the least. For example, in an attempt during the late 1940s to address malnutrition, the commonwealth government replaced rations with the provision of meals, and wages were paid partly in the form of meal tickets for all family members. Communal feeding of this kind, apart from the social and family disruption it caused, also had a serious health consequence as it introduced and increased the risk of cross-infection. Much of this had been attributed by the authorities to overcrowding in living quarters, but a survey of infant mortality rates in the southern region of the Northern Territory in the late 1950s showed that overcrowding represented a minimal source of infection compared with the communal dining room.[99] This survey showed that communal dining rooms were a health hazard because it was there that children, whose ages ranged from eight weeks to three-and-a-half years, were exposed to infection when solid foods were introduced to them. As late as 1956, hygiene arrangements in dining rooms and kitchens were very unsatisfactory, as a health inspector's report on the communal dining room facilities at Yuendumu revealed:

a. The hot water system had been defective for six days. This was caused by a shortage of kerosene, which is used in this hot water system.
b. Plates and other utensils remained dirty and greasy after being washed.
c. Shelves in the kitchen were littered with food scraps and dirty utensils.

d. Window ledges in the dining room contained food scraps.
e. The area surrounding the kitchen was littered with tins, bones, and other refuse.
f. All grease traps were dirty and appeared to have not been closed for several days.
g. Garbage drums were not being washed after being emptied.
h. The area under the garbage stand was dirty and covered with food particles. The area was very damp and could provide an attractive breeding area for flies.
i. Food for the children's meals was placed on the table approximately twenty minutes before commencement of the meal.
j. The food supplied for infant feeding was supplied on the plates fifteen minutes before the meal. Flies swarmed over the food.[100]

For those Aboriginal people who had jobs and access to health care through their work, the situation was often no better than for those at institutions. Most pastoralists showed little concern for the health of their Aboriginal workers, as Charles Duguid, a medical practitioner from Adelaide, observed after a journey into central and northern Australia during the late 1930s:

My visits to the cattle station made me depressed and ashamed beyond measure. As I approached one homestead on a cold, cheerless, rainy day, old men, women, and children came running down a hillside. They were all painfully thin and hungry, their clothes were mere rags. Later, over a cup of tea in the homestead, I asked why the Aborigines we had seen did not get more food. They get Government rations, was the reply. At that time official instructions were as follows; the rations or weekly allowance to each person receiving relief must not exceed flour, 5lb, sugar 1lb, tea 1/4lb.[101]

In 1945, anthropologists Catherine and Roland Berndt found no improvement and reported that Aboriginal workers were poorly fed across the country. In their journals they recorded that at Wave Hill "each working man and woman was given three times daily a slice of dry bread, one piece of usually cooked meat (sometimes in the form of a bone), and a dipper of tea."[102] Officially each station set aside a day each week on which rations were distributed to the aged and infirm and the dependents of employees. The Berndts discovered, however, that the weekly ration consisted only of "two to three pounds of flour, sometimes with rising (to those requesting it); one half to one pound of sugar (often less), to which was added a small handful of tea (under one ounce), and one stick of tobacco (to those requesting it)."[103] Moreover, indicating the questionable quality of these rations, at the time of their visit the Berndts also reported that "a slightly larger amount of flour was sometimes issued because it contained weevils. A number of Aborigines refused to use it, complaining that it caused pain and discomfort after eating."[104]

On top of these general conditions of neglect, the plight of pregnant Aboriginal women particularly concerned the Berndts. They found that neither pregnant women nor nursing mothers received any extra food to supplement their diet of bread and cooked beef. They reported that during their visit to Wave Hill, three births took place. In the first case, the mother was a young woman, usually employed in the homestead, who had four surviving children. Her last-born child had died in infancy. The new arrival was stillborn, and the mother was very ill, but nothing was known of this at the homestead until the Berndts supplied the information. The second birth was normal, but in the third case both the mother and child (firstborn) died within a few hours of each other. Shortly after the Berndts left Wave Hill another birth took place. The mother was another young woman normally employed at the homestead. Her infant also died, and although the doctor was summoned from the nearby town of Katherine, this mother reportedly died too.[105] Thus in a two-month period, only one out of four births was healthy. Another study of the living conditions of Aboriginal workers on cattle stations was carried out in the late 1950s by Sydney ethnographer Frank Stevens. His findings revealed little change in conditions since the reports of Duguid and the Berndts. For example, Stevens described the health of the Aboriginal workers he encountered in the following manner: "Our inquiries concerning native health brought many references to sore throats, chest complaints, pussy ears, dysentery, malnutrition, eye complaints, scabies, ringworm, and diarrhea. From a general survey the Aboriginal work force did not look well."[106]

With health conditions such as these, it is not surprising that in 1946 hundreds of Aboriginal employees and their families walked off pastoral stations in the Pilbara district of Western Australia. Nor is it surprising that nearly twenty years later, the occupants of the "blacks camp" deserted the Wave Hill Station in the Northern Territory and moved to Wattle Creek, where they demanded rights of ownership. While Australian historians have given much attention to the mistreatment of Aboriginal labor, they have said little about what these deplorable health and medical conditions implied for the desirability of movement to the cities. The backdrop of these early experiences with negligible health care by hospitals and employers, and the widespread appalling health conditions that most Indigenous people in Australia lived in prior to 1960, shed light on why Aboriginal people might have decided to leave rural and reserve communities.

Like a number of my informants in Seattle, many people in Sydney recalled moving because of the insufficiency of rural medical services. Many people spoke about the inordinate distance of medical services from their homes, and of how rough the conditions had been in facilities set up for Aboriginal patients.[107] Others also recalled that medical providers and doctors were frequently dismissive of Aboriginal patients or could get away with treating them poorly in the country because "there was nobody to tell them not to."[108] The discrimination encountered by one woman when seeking medical care during a particularly serious case of gastroenteritis had been so bad that she recalled "it got me to start thinking seriously about the possibilities for getting away from this bull—–t. I can honestly remember thinking to myself, it just can't get any worse than this."[109] For others, it might not have been their own health issues but those of a family member that had compelled them to move. For instance, David remembered how when his brother got into an accident and ended up being transferred to a hospital in Sydney for treatment, he had decided to join him because "somebody needed to be there with him."[110] Like many Aboriginal patients who came involuntarily to Sydney for hospitalization, Jack and his brother ended up staying on in Sydney. A final group of migration stories concerned those who had moved as children. Much like the cases I encountered in Seattle, these people also cited a strong memory of their mother being concerned for their welfare: "I remember mum said us kids were always getting sick and catching all sorts of bugs on account of the bad water and that, which was one of the reasons I think she thought we'd be better off coming here."[111] Interestingly, though it has been largely ignored by subsequent studies of urban Aboriginal migration, even Gale, in her much-cited 1972 study, had made note of the prevalence of medical reasons compelling the movement of Aboriginal people into cities like Adelaide. She wrote, "A second major group of people who came to the city without option were those who came for medical reasons. The centralized nature of South Australian services means that there are few specialist medical facilities available in the country areas. Furthermore, such services are limited in the Northern Territory, so that any patients who require special treatment or long-term therapy must be sent to Adelaide."[112] Of all the people surveyed in her study, Gale recorded that some "12 percent or 199 persons in the survey had come to Adelaide purely for medical treatment and had remained in the city for at least six consecutive months." She also found that others moved because they required long-term therapy such as "treatment in a mental hospital" or "regular outpatient treatment as a result of such illnesses as poliomyelitis."[113] In these ways, and also because she found that "some came to the city for hospitalisation but, on discharge decided to stay in the city," Gale's findings reflect the stories I encountered in Sydney, and hence her research can be used to draw general conclusions about the centrality of medical reasons within Aboriginal urbanization across Australia. As part of her study, Gale concluded that "medical reasons assume major significance in the movement of Aborigines to the city."[114]

Beliefs About Health Services in the City

On the other side of these stories that attest to the health reasons driving Indigenous migrants into American and Australian cities during the postwar years, there are also a host of factors that account for why migrants were drawn into cities specifically as places of refuge for health. These beliefs and hopes were furnished by the promises and impressions purposefully made by government publications and representatives.

In 1952 the New South Wales Aborigines Protection Board (later the Aborigines Welfare Board) launched an assimilationist propaganda magazine called *Dawn*. In 1969 it was rebranded as *New Dawn*. As illustrated in the publication's title banner (see figure 1.1), the journal imagined itself speaking to an audience of "traditional" Aboriginal people (represented by the man on the left) who were eager to learn about the habits of life that would guarantee their acceptance into Australian society (represented by the modern cityscape on the right). Gazing purposefully into the distance, the man in the masthead is separated from his potential destiny in the city only by the word *Dawn* (from which rays of sunshine emanate), as if to signify that the magazine itself might serve as a bridge to that future world.

Designed for distribution among all New South Wales Aboriginal stations and reserves, where it was hoped that people starved of information about their friends and kin in the cities would avidly read it and hopefully be inspired to follow suit, *Dawn* was in every way a classic government propaganda text. Across its entire lifespan, it was filled with scenes of conviviality: of Christmas fairs and music concerts; sporting events and award presentations; with stories of good workers and resourceful housekeepers; with

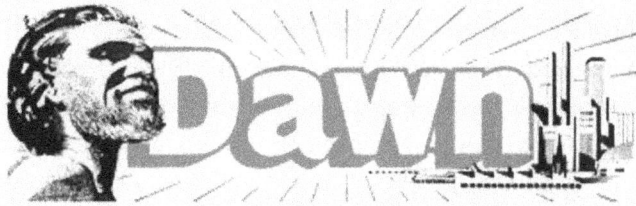

Dawn and New Dawn 1952-1975

FIGURE 1.1 *Dawn* and *New Dawn* magazine logo.

images of wholesome and active youth; and boasting letters of appreciation from readers toward the board's work. Photographs of grateful families standing outside their new urban and suburban homes were common.
As suggested by the testimonies of my interviewees, Aboriginal people who
can recall the sorts of scenes that were depicted on the pages of *Dawn* and
New Dawn are today generally scornful of these images and narratives. One
of the main reasons they recall the publication so contemptuously is precisely because many individuals and families had felt betrayed and deceived
upon arrival in the cities.[115] Whereas the magazine had given the distinct
impression that their lives (especially their health) would be improved by
urbanization, for many migrants, the stark reality of urban life proved to
be quite the opposite.

These assimilationist and propagandist strategies were not unique to the
Australian context. In the 1950s, the Bureau of Indian Affairs in Western
Washington also started to publish its own newsletter, to which it gave a
similarly themed title, *New Horizons*. In his annual "Narrative Summation"
of the "Relocation Operations" of the fiscal year, in 1959 superintendent
C. W. Ringley of the BIA Western Washington Agency explained the significance of the newsletter: "One of our main problems," he wrote in his report, "has been for improved communications between the Agency and the
people." In an effort to increase both the frequency and quality of this communication between the BIA and Native people on reservations, Ringley
explained that the newly renamed *New Horizons* would be "mailed to [re-
location] applicants, tribal officials, and other agencies and organizations
interested in both our program and the welfare of Indian people in general."[116] He made a point of underscoring that the publication would serve
as the main mouthpiece of the government on reservations, informing tribal

communities, their representatives, and any potential relocatees of "any changes in policies, new or additional opportunities being offered, as well as excerpts from letters received from relocatees."[117] With greater transparency about what relocation entailed, and information about what relocatees could expect once they arrived in cities, it was hoped that any potential misgivings and concerns that people might have about the process would be assuaged and in turn, that relocation numbers would grow. To this end, Ringley stressed in his report that *New Horizons* would provide guidance for how "interested persons may obtain further information or arrange for personal interviews" to find out more about the relocation process.[118] He reported that great success had already been achieved after the publication's first year of distribution under the new title of *New Horizons*: "We have mailed an average of 250 to 300 copies of *New Horizons* each month and feel the expense has been justified by the resulting rise in inquiries and applications received." Indeed, this initial response had been so encouraging that Ringley reported, "It is planned to not only continue this publication but to expand on its area coverage [to other parts of Washington State], and on its news coverage."[119]

A close comparative reading of these parallel publications *Dawn* and *New Horizons* therefore provides invaluable perspective on the ways that both the Australian and US governments had attempted to push the idea of urbanization on the Aboriginal and Native American populations in New South Wales and Washington State respectively. By paying close attention to the messages that the two governments were sending about health and health care specifically, we see that it played no small role in these governments' attempts to draw people into cities. Moreover, the very fact that both governments were clearly making an effort to emphasize health matters in almost every issue of these publications is rather telling. It indicates that both governments had reason to believe health was a topic of central importance to their readership. This supports the idea that Indigenous people were leaving rural areas at this time in search of healthier living conditions.

The first observation to make about these publications is that across the 1950s and early 1960s, *Dawn* and *New Horizons* were similarly preoccupied with convincing their readership of two main ideas when it came to health and health care. On the one hand, the two publications obviously wanted their readers to believe that the government would prioritize the health needs of any Indigenous person who was willing to move. On the other hand, these publications were also clearly concerned to convince their readership that Indigenous people would actually have no need for government support in the cities because they would become healthier simply by virtue of their acquiescence to the process of assimilation and urbanization.

In terms of content, across the 1950s and '60s *Dawn* and *New Horizons* contained very similar articles, which explicitly advertised the government's intention to prioritize Indigenous health as a part of the urbanization and relocation process. For example, in its second issue in February 1952, the very first article of *Dawn* was titled "Health is Important." In this editorial, the magazine explicitly stated that the Aborigines Welfare Board "realises that health is perhaps the most important [issue] of all, because unless the aborigine is bodily healthy, he cannot be expected to take a normal part in the community."[120] In a typical expression of its commitment to improving the health of those Aboriginal people willing to assimilate, the article continued to claim that "the Aborigines Welfare Board of New South Wales is determined that the aboriginal people will enjoy every facility for maintaining themselves at a [health] standard equal to that of the white community." It therefore encouraged its readers to take the first step toward assimilation and urbanization by moving onto the government-controlled stations or settlements in New South Wales that served as a gateway to Sydney. As a way of drawing people into the stations, the article underscored the abundant health services they offered:

Each station is under the care of a Manager, assisted by his wife who acts as Matron, and she is usually a trained nurse or has had experience in medical care. A well-equipped medical treatment unit, including a dispensary, is provided on each station, and the Matron is in attendance for a specified time each day. She also visits the people in their homes and watches carefully for any signs of neglect, sickness or malnutrition. On a number of stations, a visiting medical officer is retained and he maintains a very close scrutiny of the aborigines on the Station. When sickness or accidents of a more serious nature occur, patients are conveyed to the nearest public hospital, where they are entitled to, and receive, treatment in the public wards on exactly the same basis as a white person.[121]

This painted a vastly different picture to the situation of medical care on reserves, and what's more, the magazine repeatedly gave the impression that this level of attention and equality of access would be maintained in the cities. For example, in the following year, the February 1953 issue of *Dawn* published a short feature on "Dr. Drew," a physician who had been treating Aboriginal people on stations across New South Wales. Reporting on his transition back into his Sydney-based practice, the article stated, "Dr. Drew has a real and sincere interest in the welfare of the aborigines and is determined that they shall be accorded every modern medical facility in the city."[122] This was obviously intended to offer reassurances that Aboriginal people could expect high levels of medical care in the cities as well. Supporting such claims with real-life stories and testimonies from Indigenous people who had relocated was also a key strategy of both magazines in their efforts to present a picture of the cities as places of refuge for one's health. In the same issue that featured Dr. Drew, for example, *Dawn* published a short piece on Roslyn Sloane, a young Aboriginal girl from Cootamundra who was brought into Sydney by her mother for medical treatment on her eyes. The article boasted that "the little one's case was given immediate consideration by the [hospital] authorities concerned," and after treatment, "the authorities were delighted at the favorable reaction of the child to her new surroundings, and expressed the opinion that she and her mother were a most promising subject for adjustment into city life."[123]

We also see the Bureau of Indian Affairs taking a very similar approach in *New Horizons*. Multiple issues across the late 1950s explicitly referred to the provision of medical services as a part of the "package" that relocatees would receive. Indeed, in a list of ten services included in this "package," item numbers one, three, and seven were related to provisions for health: "1. Cost of required physical examination prior to relocation"; "3. Subsistence (food) allowance while travelling to destination"; and "7. Full hospital and medical insurance coverage not to exceed the first year."[124] In another issue of the newsletter, the exact nature of this health coverage (item 7) was explained in greater detail:

> Health coverage protection: Protection is provided each relocatee and his family for health care during the first year of their relocation. The Bureau of Indian Affairs makes available through Health Services, Incorporated, Chicago Illinois, a company owned by the various Blue Cross and Blue Shield Societies of the various states, health protection that includes: (1) hospitalization; (2) surgical care; and (3) calls by a doctor or a physician at the relocatee's home, or office calls at the doctor's or physician's office by the relocatees. This protection is provided for a period of one year and at the end of the one-year period he has the option of continuing this coverage at his own expense.[125]

Much like in *Dawn*, such claims of reliable health support in the cities were also backed up by personal testimony in *New Horizons*. For example, in the September 1959 issue, the magazine featured the testimony of several employers in Seattle, who all attested to the conditions of equal treatment in the city and painted a view of an environment that was not simply conducive to Native integration into the mainstream but also specifically the improvement of their health. One employer was recorded as saying that "at the present time, the Indians of Seattle live pretty much in the same manner as their non-Indian neighbors do."[126] Another claimed that "the Indian children all attend the public schools with the white youngsters. They use modern dress and associate with the non-Indians in public life. Their health is on par with others."[127] Yet another was reported as saying, "Segregation is not a problem. It is my opinion that the Indians who move to the city are more progressive, more self-reliant, and as a result more healthy than most of the Indians in other parts of the West. I have a high regard for them and enjoy working with them."[128] In sum, the testimonies of these employers not only gave the impression that work conditions would be favorable and that integration into the mainstream culture and society would be easy, but that relocatee's health would be improved as a result of their living in the city and being given the same opportunities and access to resources as non-Indians.

Of course, not all readers of *Dawn* and *New Horizons* fully believed these assimilationist success stories at face value. This became increasingly true after an initial wave of migrants returned to the rural areas with stories of neglect and mistreatment. For example, Peter B. Williams of Nambuca Heads, NSW, wrote to the editor of *Dawn* in 1962, requesting that the publication start to include more articles written by Aboriginal people since in his words, "If an article is written by a white person the dark people are often not interested as they have had too many broken promises and their treatment has not been encouraging."[129]

The March 1959 "Narrative Report" of Western Washington BIA relocation officer Fred H. Claymore revealed the existence of various rumors that were starting to circulate on two reservations in the area, and which were calling into question the reliability of claims being made about health care and other support services provided by the relocation program. According to Claymore's report, what he described as "these stories" were thought to be causing a drop in the number of relocation applications they received that month. He cited various different types of "stories" that were circulating. Most commonly, these included variations of (1) "You will lose your tribal rights to government support as a relocatee"; (2) "You will lose your Indian identity and must call yourself a white man"; (3) "You will be left on your own"; and (4) "You will not be able to return to the reservation."[130] In Claymore's words, "These rumors frightened some applicants."[131] Therefore, to combat these stories, Claymore described in his report how the agency "planned for the holding of tribal community meetings in the near future to not only review but bring up to date the various services offered by Relocation services."[132] It is no coincidence, therefore, that in the very next issue of *New Horizons*, published later that same month, the magazine's editorial went to great lengths to address precisely the doubts that were being voiced in the "stories" specified by Claymore. Directly addressing the various rumors of loss, the editorial was explicit that "you are reminded that if you request assistance to relocate you will not lose any of your rights as an Indian, nor lose any tribal rights."[133] And, "You lose no tribal rights but are entitled to the same privileges as any other citizen."[134] This kind of explicit messaging on the part of the government, which turned out to be patently untrue in the case of health care in cities, became the source of much confusion for urban Indians and meant that many had moved to the cities under the false impression that their health care would be provided for no differently to the way things were on the reservation.

More broadly, *Dawn* and *New Horizons* sought to promote relocation and urbanization by convincing readers that by virtue of assimilating into urban and suburban society they would in fact become healthier and thus be freed from all need for government support in the cities. Interestingly, both publications also promoted this idea in much the same manner. Both tied the causes of Indigenous ill health to Aboriginal and Native American "cultural backwardness." Most notably (and indeed reminiscent of the nineteenth-century concerns about "fringe dwellers" congregating on city streets), both publications frequently pointed to the health risks entailed with living communally, and in ways that did not conform to the strict separation of public and private spaces. In turn, this allowed them to push Indigenous people toward the path of assimilating to white standards of living as a means to achieve good health. Both publications thus ostensibly existed to teach Indigenous people about the habits of life that would guarantee their acceptance into dominant society, and in turn, improve their health. The editors of *New Horizons* emphasized this in one of their early issues, stating that "we want to emphasize that the primary purpose of the Relocation Program, and this publication, is to assist an interested individual in his own effort to better himself and his family, through permanent employment, and better, healthier living habits."[135] Both publications therefore encouraged Indigenous people, especially women, to embrace the idea of homemaking and to take on the health habits of maintaining a clean and tidy abode. For instance, in the April 1953 issue of *Dawn*, chair of the Aborigines Welfare Board C. J. Buttsworth wrote an editorial letter to open that month's issue, in which he emphasized these values: "Aboriginal people would become completely assimilated if they adopted habits and standards of living similar to those of the white community. . . . Home is the cornerstone of our existence and there should be the strongest urge within all people to make their homes comfortable and beautiful happy places in which to live with their families, places to be kept clean and tidy and to be made pretty with paints and flowers."[136]

Buttsworth's tone and his emphasis that homes should be "beautiful" also represents the gendered norms and ideology that underlay many of *Dawn's* regular columns and features, especially during its first decade of publication. Three of these regular columns, "In the Garden," "Home Hints," and "Health Hints," were clearly aimed at women and were illustrative of the central ideological ambition informing Aboriginal Affairs at this time: to encourage Aboriginal people to embrace the domesticated lifestyle of the nuclear family. By providing "tips" such as "how to remove grease spots from working men's clothes,"[137] "how to transplant small flowers or vegetables without disturbing the roots,"[138] and how to manage "the multitude of duties" to which "the modern housewife has to attend,"[139] the government demonstrated its preoccupation with persuading Aboriginal people, particularly women, to take pride in the private space of the nuclear family as an outward symbol of their state of moral and physical well-being. In his editorial for the May 1953 issue of *Dawn*, superintendent of Aboriginal Welfare M. H. Saxby addressed Aboriginal people on the matter of their housekeeping. The deliberate comparisons he drew between the different standards of "progress" achieved by various Aboriginal families he had visited was also typical of the AWB's efforts to foster a degree of competition among readers for AWB praise:

> I have been impressed by the keen interest and pride displayed in many instances. The bright interiors and nice surroundings with colourful flower gardens and vegetable patches are very pleasing, and indicate a desire on the part of many to take full advantage of the opportunities afforded by the Board for better housing and an improved standard of living.

On the other hand, it has been a disappointment to notice that in some instances families are not taking the same pride in their new homes and a number of them are showing neglect.[140]

While perhaps less heavy-handed in its approach, the BIA also employed this tactic of fostering a spirit of "friendly competition" among potential relocatees. In *New Horizons*, the Western Washington Agency published a regular column it called "Relocation News and Notes." In this, the stories of successfully relocated families and individuals were featured alongside cheerful photographs and notable doses of enthusiasm. For instance, in the September 1957 issue, it was reported that "Clarence H. and Margaret E. (Pierre) Hatch, (Snohomish & Lummi), and their four children [moved] to San Francisco the middle of August. . . . They have since obtained permanent housing in a very nice six-room flat chosen by Margaret, one block from shopping center. . . . This family also expresses their happiness and joy with their new location."[141] In the September 1959 issue, the newsletter republished an article from the *Seattle Post-Intelligencer* titled "Happy Indian" and which it introduced in the following way: "The following letter was voluntarily written to the Editor of the Seattle P.I. by James Cook, enrolled member of the Makah Tribe, formerly from Neah Bay, Washington, and now living in Seattle."[142] The contents of Cook's letter attested to how "truly wonderful" his experience of relocation had been, including the fact that "the government also takes care of any hospital care I may need."[143]

In Australia, perhaps the most explicit example of this "friendly competition" that the AWB sought to encourage among its readers was its regular column "Our Real Citizens." In this feature, which usually took up an entire page, the photographs of recently "exempted" Aboriginal men and women were displayed as a means of endorsing and advertising the feasibility of the road toward citizenship. By applying to become "exempt" from the supervision of the AWB (i.e., by opting out of government "wardship" status), Aboriginal people would, so the idea went, become "full citizens" and thereby gain access to equal treatment within the Australian community, as well as all the services and privileges that this status entailed.[144] Moreover, as exemplified in their language, the AWB was much more concerned than the BIA to stress that citizenship and inclusion in the mainstream was a reward for good behavior rather than an entitlement. Aboriginal people would have to "earn" the "privileges of being a citizen" by "continued good conduct," "initiative," and the "expressed willingness" to accept not simply the benefits but also the "responsibilities" of Australian citizenship.[145] As understood at the time, inclusion in the nation entailed more than legal equality, important though that attainment was. It also required Aboriginal people to be treated with respect and dignity and to be welcomed as full participants in the life of the community. Hence references to "equality," "full citizenship," and "inclusion" in the period that actually preceded Aboriginal legal citizenship in 1967 often meant to suggest an appeal to the cultural norms of citizenship without legal status. This is precisely how the editors of *Dawn* sought to use the language of citizenship in a July 1953 article titled "Our Real Citizens: More Exempted Aborigines." In this article, the photographs of two Aboriginal men were accompanied by a short description: "This is the third occasion on which we have published the photographs of those aboriginal men and women who feel justly proud of the fact that they have received their Exemption Certification . . . and have, in fact, become real citizens in every sense of the word." Making it clear that citizenship should be an aspiration for cultural as much as legal acceptance, the article continued: "The certificates are not handed out indiscriminately. . . . They must be earned by continued good conduct, initiative and the expressed willingness to accept not only the privileges of being a citizen, but also the responsibilities."[146]

The magazine's constant emphasis on hygiene, healthy "habits," and home care made clear that a significant part of the "good behavior" demanded by Australian citizenship consisted of letting go of "old" (i.e., Indigenous) ways of living because this was standing in the way, not only of Indigenous peoples' good health, but also their ability to be productive citizens. Throughout its years in print, but especially in the first decade of publication, *Dawn* thus repeatedly referred to the idea that good health was central to the project of Australian citizenship and acculturation. This of course reflected earlier assimilationist and civilizing models in both the United States and Australia, whereby Indigenous children were removed from their families and communities to be placed in government- or missionary-run institutions and boarding schools for the avowed purpose of teaching them, among other things, the domestic habits of white society.[147] The standard curriculum at federal boarding schools in the United States and at institutions in Australia was very comparable, usually consisting of half days in the classroom and the rest at manual labor for boys, and at practicing "domestic arts" for the girls. The rhetoric in *Dawn* and *New Horizons*, such as repeated calls to "become health conscious," was in many ways just an extension of this older model of assimilation applied to potential urban relocatees.

In a 1952 public health announcement published in *Dawn* titled "Are You a Fifth Columnist? Guard Your Country's Heath," the magazine employed its usual cultural shaming tactics to implore its Aboriginal readers to "do something of value to the community" and thereby "perform" the "duties of citizenship." Of course, it did this frequently by pushing people toward gainful employment. But as exemplified in this public health announcement, it also emphasized that by becoming "health conscious," Aboriginal people could in turn become "better workers," "better parents," "better neighbours," and "better citizens."[148] Health, in other words, was seen to be a vital first step on the path toward contentment, citizenship, acceptance, and assimilation. The other side of this message, though often not explicitly stated, was clearly the implication that Aboriginal people had until now been responsible for their own exclusion from Australian society, in part due to their lack of regard for their own health, which limited their utility within society. It was therefore also up to them to make the necessary changes to improve their health and to gain inclusion. And *Dawn* and *New Horizons* supposedly provided a road map for navigating these changes.

Provided they could achieve the standards of hygiene and health, initiative, productivity, and good parenthood set by the Australian and American mainstream, then the AWB and BIA were both clear about the good fortunes that would follow for urban Indigenous people. Their messaging was simple, and it was the same: that assimilation would not entail the loss of any rights or privileges for Indigenous people, but rather, they would finally attain the rights and privileges enjoyed by all American and Australian citizens. In the March 1959 issue of *New Horizons*, the BIA reminded its readers of this. The editors wrote:

> You are reminded that if you request assistance to relocate you will
> not lose any of your rights as an Indian, nor lose any tribal rights.
> Relocation merely extends financial assistance for you and your family
> and assists you to make contact with prospective employees for a job.
> You are also assisted in finding a place to live and, if needed, assisted
> with purchase of furniture, range, refrigerator and other items needed
> for your new home. Relocation is no different than if you move from
> your home or reservation in Bellingham, Everett, Seattle, Tacoma, San
> Francisco or New York City on your own. You lose no tribal rights but
> as long as you are making efforts to join the community, you are
> entitled to the same privileges as any other citizen. On relocation this

same thing is true. You can live as anyone else and have the same freedom to move about that you have here at home.[149]

These two ideas—(1) that health care would be better for Indigenous people in the cities, and (2) that by virtue of assimilating, Indigenous people's health would improve in cities, thereby "freeing" them from the need for government care and "wardship" status—worked together to create much confusion on the part of urban relocatees in both the United States and Australia. Because of the ambiguity these ideas created about the precise nature and extent of the government's commitment toward supporting Indigenous health in the cities, urban relocatees often faced extraordinary confusion, once they arrived in cities, about whether they were eligible for special government health provisions. Many people left reserves and reservations expecting to encounter equal treatment in the mainstream medical system, but (for reasons I will unpack in subsequent chapters) they discovered this was impossible to find once they actually got to the cities.

Health as Connective Tissue between Urban and Rural Communities

The promises of better health care in the cities only resulted in disappointment for most urban Indigenous migrants. Some urban relocatees understood and accepted the prospect that once they moved to cities they were expected to rely on the welfare and social services available to them as regular citizens. But many also held on to the conviction that the government should be responsible for ensuring their welfare, if not due to the historic obligations and agreements entailed as a part of Indigenous land dispossession, then as a matter of new obligations entailed by the firm encouragement they had been given to relocate from rural land bases to the cities. The reality, of course, regardless of whether people actually accepted the assimilationist bargain, was that in both the United States and Australia, it was nearly impossible for Indigenous people to acquire medical care in cities during the 1950s and '60s due to a combination of discrimination, lack of knowledge about services available, and the high cost of care. As I discuss in great detail in the following chapters, in practice, it soon became clear that while assimilation was intended to improve Indigenous people's health and access to health care by turning them into "full citizens," few provisions were actually made by the US and Australian governments for Indigenous people in cities to receive the social services and other trappings of citizenship available to other Australians and Americans.[150]

While both federal governments had seen the elimination of tribal sovereignty (in the United States) and wardship status (in Australia) as the means to create a new kind of Indigenous citizenry—one that would be more in line with the individual liberal citizen-subject of the American and Australian mainstream—the irony was that in doing so, they actually created a highly vulnerable population that had no real means to access medical care to sustain themselves as productive, healthy members of the community. The gap between the stated aims of federal policy and its consequences for urban Indigenous migrants turned on the contradiction between the theory of assimilation and the reality of life in a racist society—that is, changes in federal Indigenous policy in the postwar period, although couched in the language of emancipation, equality, inclusion, and citizenship, were at odds with the views of most Americans and Australians at the time, who were actually positioned to determine whether or not Indigenous people were treated as "full citizens." Indigenous migrants thus came to cities in the postwar period because of their medical reasons, because of reservation unemployment, to pursue an education, or because of policies designed to encourage them into cities. But in practice, because the vast majority of Australians and Americans were not willing to accept them as part of the mainstream, they did not become "full citizens" in the city so much as an urban minority group with few claims to full citizenship. Moreover, because the governments of these nations were committed to a policy of integration, thereby refusing to recognize urban Indigenous communities as distinct (either politically or culturally), these communities were largely invisible from a structural perspective. In the United States, a further irony existed insofar as Indians had been made US citizens in 1924 (by fiat), yet this citizenship did not carry with it the right to health care, like many Indian treaties did. Thus, in practice, for many Native people, urbanization actually meant a *loss* of rights to health care because of residency requirements attached to federal health services; that is, they ended up with fewer, as opposed to more, rights in the city.

As the gap between rhetoric and reality became increasingly clear to urban Indigenous migrants, many wondered what they stood to gain from the "full" citizenship associated with living in the cities. In the realm of health care, the communities in Seattle and Sydney came up with remarkably similar solutions for their lack of access to necessary medical services in these cities. As I discuss in subsequent chapters, each community created their own medical clinic run by and for members of their community. More than just a practical response to their lack of health care access, however, I argue that these clinics were a political symbol and reflection of a developing pan-Indigenous identity grounded in their common histories, current struggles, and an urban politics that sought to expand and reframe the idea of Indigenous sovereignty to be inclusive of nonterritorial and nongovernmental goals as well. Moreover, the politics of these clinics challenged official paradigms of citizenship and identity—the spatial logics of colonial governance—that sought to differentiate Indigenous peoples' identities as American *or* Indian, Australian *or* Aboriginal, on the basis of where they lived. Instead, what the clinics reflected was that urban migrants did not imagine themselves as singular citizens or unitary subjects; rather, they held multiple ideas about their citizenship and belonging, and complicated feelings of belonging.

These complex forms of community and identity were expressed in another significant set of repercussions caused by the lack of health care access in the cities. Many urban migrants ended up moving back and forth between cities and reserves/reservations during the 1950s and '60s in order to be able to access health care at all. We can find evidence of this movement back and forth in BIA case files of individual relocatees, and in the memories of migrants' descendants, who can recall stories of their relatives moving between the reserves and cities in times of illness. These experiences support the view that many had moved in the first place in order to improve their health prospects. Once it became clear that these prospects were slim, however, we find that many people simply preferred to go home. And for many who chose to stay in spite of the poor conditions of health care, this meant that their community's medical needs and rights to health care only grew as a politically charged issue. Moreover, the movement of people back and forth highlights the failure of the government's plans; contrary to the explicit purpose of the assimilation policies, ironically the lack of provisions for Indigenous health care in the cities actually meant that as a matter of necessity, people retained ties and maintained networks of connection with their home communities.

The health-driven process of movement back and forth between urban and rural spaces may be understood in the context of recent scholarly work that has sought to unsettle the strict dichotomy between urban and rural Indigenous communities. In particular, the work of scholars such as Renya K. Ramirez and Myla Vincenti Carpio is instructive. Respectively, these two scholars have written about how "many urban Native Americans maintain connections to tribal communities or assert their tribal identities while living away from a land base," and argue against the assumptions of urban Indigenous cultural dislocation by showing that "many engage in a pattern of constant movement between the reservation and the city, maintaining specific tribal identities despite their urban addresses."[151] These scholars shift the perspective on urban Indigenous communities in the twentieth century away from accounts dramatized by "the image of the drunk on skid row"—a stereotype that continues to shape policy and attitudes.[152] Instead, they focus on illuminating positive outcomes, continuities, and strategies for cultural organizing and survival. In conversation with this scholarship, I suggest that health concerns might be seen as a kind of connective tissue that joined communities and families separated by the (government-imposed) imagined urban/rural divide. As Carpio and Ramirez have shown, and as the fact of medical migration suggests, this should complicate our understanding of what happened to the linkages between city and reserve communities during this period, and also suggests that urban communities were not the culturally disconnected groups that government rhetoric at the time suggested they were. Furthermore, recognizing this continued connection and affiliation with home communities is also significant for being able to understand the specific terms on which urban Indigenous communities thereby went on to press for federally supported health care as a matter of Indigenous rights in the 1970s. Before turning to that part of the history, however, the next chapter explains what the US and Australian federal governments had intended for urban Indigenous people's health care in cities, and we also begin to see the fallout of these plans as they ultimately failed to deliver on their promises.

2 Whose Responsibility?

Federal Government Policy and the (Mis)Management of Indigenous Health Care, 1950–1970

. . . .

An old joke in Indian Country goes simply, "Don't get sick after June."[1] The cartoon shown in figure 2.1, produced in 2005 by Oglala Lakota artist Marty Two Bulls, speaks directly to the unspoken punch line of this joke since it vividly illustrates how one could easily die waiting for care at the Indian Health Service (IHS). While, in its lifetime, this joke has mostly referred to IHS services for reservation communities (where scarce resources are known to run dry in the second half of the calendar year), the gravity of this joke and the underlying truth in the cartoon below have held as much relevance for the state of urban Indian medical services since the middle decades of the twentieth century. Moreover, while no such joke exists in the Australian context, when I related this joke and shared this cartoon with many of my Aboriginal informants in Australia, their response was to knowingly laugh at what these images suggested: "It's been the same for us, you know," is how one of my interviewees reacted.[2]

. . . . . .

It did not take long for postwar Indigenous migrants in cities across the United States and Australia to realize that the better health care they were promised in cities had been a chimera. Speaking before a public forum convened in 1969 by the National Council of Indian Opportunity's Committee on Urban Indians, Vance Tahmahkera of Fort Worth, Texas, voiced the concerns and frustrations felt by many urban Indian relocatees who felt abandoned by the federal government in the cities: "You know, a lot of us came here not even through the Government, we came a long time ago. I've been here since about '48, and there's quite a few Indians in Fort Worth that came the same way. I was wondering if there was some way they could get hospitalization through the government. You know, some of these people don't make enough to pay for hospitalization, it's so high, and it's the responsibility of the government to us as Indians, to take care of this."[3] Two years earlier, in Australia, the *Sydney Morning Herald* ran an exposé on hospitals that were being

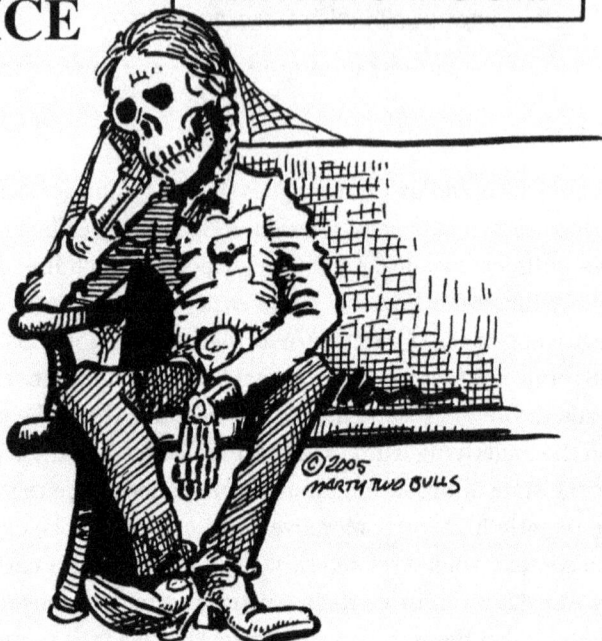

FIGURE 2.1 Cartoon by Marty Two Bulls, 2005. Image courtesy of Marty Two Bulls.

accused of "race discrimination" in the state of New South Wales. A particularly bad case from the article concerned an unnamed Aboriginal patient in Sydney who had pneumonia, and who described to the journalist his experience of waiting in the hospital for treatment from "9 p.m. until 4 a.m. the following day."[4] "Eventually," the patient described how after he "had not even been given a drink of water—he had walked home and was found more dead than alive" by his neighbor the next morning.[5]

As stories like these started to emerge in the US and Australian press during the 1960s, the question of who should bear responsibility for Indigenous health care became a hotly debated issue among national and state government officials, Indigenous communities and their leaders, medical professionals, and public health representatives. Several arguments prevailed. In keeping with a more conservative view of public health, many government policymakers asserted that health was the responsibility of the individual, and thus favored measures that would focus on reforming individual behavior. By contrast, an increasingly liberal line of thinking among many public health officials pointed to the importance of understanding health as part of a broader social context, and thus asserted government responsibility for improving urban Indigenous housing conditions and economic opportunities, and combating discrimination in the medical system. Indigenous communities and their leaders were divided. Many believed that all Indigenous people, regardless of their place of residence, were owed free or subsidized government health care as a part of historic agreements and moral obligations entailed by the dispossession of their lands. Others, who viewed the demands of the urban communities as a threat to the limited government resources set aside for reserve and reservation communities, tended to support the government view that urban relocation signaled a tacit agreement on the part of relocatees to forfeit their rights and claims as Indigenous people in favor of "equal treatment" as regular citizens.[6]

Speaking before a conference of Indian superintendents in Denver, Colorado, on October 16, 1961, commissioner of Indian Affairs Philleo Nash articulated some of the main contours of this debate as it was taking place in the United States. On the one hand, he pointed out that many people felt that "to declare that Indians are entitled to services as Indians or because of their Indianness is clearly not going to lead to equal enjoyment of citizenship rights because other citizens receive the spectrum of services that we call 'Community Services'—welfare, education, and law and order—from local government on a basis of local citizenship and local taxation."[7] On the other hand, Nash also recognized that if conservatives were right in assuming that Indian reservations were, in fact, the isolated and disconnected "preserves" they declared them to be, then this would be a far simpler problem as their care could straightforwardly be a matter of federal responsibility. The problem, as Nash went on to unpack for his colleagues, was that ever since urban Indigenous migration accelerated in the postwar years, reservations were clearly not the isolated communities that many conservatives claimed they were. "The fact is," Nash explained to his counterparts, "Indians, like other citizens, move about freely and are increasingly living under circumstances where the tribal affiliation is so tenuous that it begins to disappear."[8] But at the very same time, Nash also pointed out, with movement off the reservation, "the inclination to turn to the Bureau of Indian Affairs does not disappear and both Indians and their non-Indian neighbors [in cities] assume that welfare, education, health and law and order services ought to be provided by the Federal Government."[9]

This was the core of the problem that was making it so hard for urban Indigenous people in both the United States and Australia to access medical treatment in cities. Discriminatory (or at best uninformed) medical providers often assumed Indigenous people could get free treatment from the government, and thus preferred to send them away rather than treat them. Those urban Indigenous people like Vance Tahmahkera and the unnamed pneumonia patient in Sydney felt the repercussions of this confusion most acutely. Unable to afford mainstream services, or repeatedly turned away from public hospitals by authorities who discriminated against them or mistakenly assumed they could access free government care elsewhere, many urban Indigenous people discovered after turning back to government services that they actually no longer qualified for them since they now lived off the reservation/reserve. Rejected by both the mainstream medical system and the government-provided services, urban Indigenous people thus often went without medical care at all. These on-the-ground repercussions of the government's ill-conceived attempts to assimilate urban Indigenous relocatees via the mainstream health care system are the subject of chapters 3 and 4, where I look in close detail at the experiences and responses of urban Indigenous people in Seattle and Sydney who struggled to access mainstream medical care in these cities during the 1950s and '60s. To set up the full context for their experiences, this chapter focuses on providing a top-down view. It explains precisely how the governments of the United States and Australia had intended the provision of health care for urban pan-Indigenous communities to play out over the course of the 1950s and '60s, and what this had been intended to achieve in terms of the policy objective of Indigenous assimilation.

While there is a very practical side to this story that the chapter tells, I am also preoccupied here with understanding how governmental attempts to foreclose free government health services from the urban communities were yet another expression of the logics of spatial governance.[10] Whether it was couched in the language of promoting and protecting the interests of "equal citizenship," or more blatantly explained as part of a tacit agreement that Indigenous people had supposedly made upon relocating themselves and/or accepting government assistance in moving to the cities, it is clear that the welfare of the urban pan-Indigenous communities raised a philosophically difficult question for the US and Australian federal governments alike: Were these people deserving of continued access to government services like reserve/reservation communities, and if so, on what basis? Answering this question required that these federal governments make a prior determination that harkened back to questions of spatial governance: Did these people still have a legitimate claim to Indigenous status (and thus a right to make claims on the government) outside of the reserve/reservation? In short, did Indigenous rights and identity "hold" off the reserve/reservation, or could migrants effectively be said to have forfeited all this upon movement into the cities? Philleo Nash posed this very difficulty to his colleagues in Denver when he asked them to consider how on the matter of urban Indigenous health care, "some of the States are quick to deny jurisdiction and are unwilling to accept responsibility."[11] Faced with the reality that many urban Indigenous people simply couldn't afford or access mainstream medical services, he thus asked, "Where is the equal protection of the laws then?"[12] Outlining the great difficulty this put before the Bureau of Indian Affairs, Nash closed out his comments with the following remarks, which spelled out the nature of the balancing act that the government was trying to perform: "We in the Central Office are asking you who must make determinations of eligibility almost daily the following questions: How can we provide community services to those who need them without destroying our objective of equal citizenship rights and responsibilities?"[13]

Shifting Ground: Indigenous Health Policy in the United States and Australia, 1950–1970

In July 1953, public health hospital director and veteran cardiologist James Shaw was appointed director of the newly renamed Branch of Indian Health. Shaw quickly made it his priority to integrate Indian medical services with those at the state and local government levels. In a letter to a colleague, he wrote that his main goal as the new director was to "improve American Indian and Alaska Native health status" by overcoming the "backlog of disease and disability accumulated through generations of neglect."[14] In order to do this, Shaw firmly believed it would be necessary to formally transfer the responsibility for Indian health to the Public Health Service (PHS). Years of experience in the PHS had convinced him that its support structures would offer better funding for hospital construction and the provision of important services missing from Indian health facilities, such as dental care.[15] With the aid of surgeon general Leonard A. Scheele, Shaw thus began to press for this transfer soon after his appointment.

Shaw's proposal was by no means an unforeseen or unexpected one. Proposals for an official transfer of Indian medical services to the Public Health Service were in fact made by the House Committee on Indian Affairs as early as 1919. And not even ten years later, as discussed in the previous chapter, the 872-page Meriam Report had also made it abundantly clear by 1928 that medical services for American Indians were woefully underresourced and needed greater support from the broader medical infrastructure.[16] This was not simply the view of the government, either. By the 1950s Native Americans on reservations had also stepped up their demands for more comprehensive health care programs and better health care facilities.[17] Rather than channeling more funds directly into Indian facilities, however, the direction the federal government adopted in the 1950s instead pushed for more integration of Indian medical services with the mainstream. This is not what Native communities and advocates had had in mind. But unsurprisingly, given the broader government commitment (under the banner of termination-era politics) to curtailing its obligations toward Native Americans at this time, the consolidation of the Branch of Indian Health with the PHS went ahead largely unchallenged.[18] Indeed, some eight years prior to Shaw's appointment, the Senate Committee on Indian Affairs had already asked whether it would be beneficial for Indian Health to become "a part of a relief and welfare function appertaining to local government."[19] Such questions had also been entertained as part of the postwar debate over repealing the 1934 Indian Reorganization Act (which commissioner of Indian Affairs John Collier had championed as a means of restoring limited forms of tribal self-rule, the end of land allotment, and the general enhancement of tribes via measures such as better education). In other words, by the time Shaw took over as director of the Branch of Indian Health, Congress had already started moving in the direction he was pushing for because by the 1950s Congress was already looking to codify the cessation, or rather the "termination," of federal responsibilities toward tribes.

While before the 1950s, both the Public Health Service and the Bureau of Indian Affairs rejected the idea of consolidation as being both undesirable and impracticable, the end of World War II had initiated a wave of postwar domestic policies under President Truman's "Fair Deal" that sought the widescale elimination of duplication in government. This undoubtedly lay important groundwork for advancing the case to consolidate Indian health with public health. In particular, the 1948 Commission on the Organization of the Executive Branch of the Government, chaired by former president Herbert Hoover, was created to investigate ways of reducing government waste. It spent considerable time scrutinizing government expenditure in Indian Country in particular and concluded that greater responsibility for public health services should be assumed by state and local health authorities.[20] The Hoover Commission was undoubtedly an important impetus for change, even though other agencies (public and private) by this time had also recommended consolidation.[21]

Among its recommendations, the Hoover Commission identified that Indian service hospitals and physicians needed to begin charging fees. Moreover, until state and local health authorities could assume total responsibility for Indian health services, the commission advocated that Indian patients should increasingly be directed to off-reservation hospitals operated by the federal government, as well as contract physicians who provided services under the authority of the Johnson-O'Malley Act.[22] Giving voice to the cost-saving and assimilative goals of these measures, the secretary of the interior at the time, Oscar Chapman, reasoned that such streamlining would hasten the "gradual liquidation of [Indian service] hospitals and the absorption of Indian patients into other federal or non-Federal systems."[23] In other words, even by the time Shaw was formulating his plans for a formal transfer of Indian medical services to the Public Health Service, the government had already been funneling Indian patients toward state and local health facilities.

Between 1950 and 1953 this approach resulted in the closure of several notable Indian hospitals. For example, the Fort Berthold Indian Hospital (North Dakota) was shut down in August 1951. Commissioner of Indian Affairs Dillon Myer also proposed the closure of seven more Indian hospitals the following year.[24] In the immediate postwar period, the general paucity of hospital services in rural America, along with the recommendations of the 1948 Hoover Commission, prompted both houses of Congress to seriously consider the construction of joint-use facilities. Several measures ensued that blurred the lines between Indian and mainstream services. For example, in 1949 congressman Harold Patten (D-AZ) introduced HR 3635 authorizing non-Indians to use Indian service hospitals.[25] In all, a total of eight Indian hospitals were closed between 1951 and 1955.[26]

One can see the imprint of World War II in the way these changes were justified. Thousands of Native Americans had served in the war, and many left their reservations in the postwar period to participate in the urban relocation program. The federal government used both facts to reason that Native people were prepared to give up their Indian entitlements in favor of equal citizenship as Americans. In 1953, two crucial developments ushered in the so-called termination era in federal Indian policy.[27] First, House Concurrent Resolution 108 called for the official "termination" of federal supervision for Indians "at the earliest possible time" and the abolition of all government facilities "whose primary purpose was to serve any Indian tribe or individual."[28] Second, Public Law 83-280 conferred jurisdiction over criminal and civil offenses involving Indians in Indian Country in several states. While rarely mentioned, one of the most significant next steps in meeting the overall policy objective of "termination" came when President Eisenhower signed Public Law 83-586 (also known as "the Indian Health Transfer Act") into existence in 1954.[29] With this act, Shaw's proposal was finally realized, and the Public Health Service officially became the agency responsible for the federal government's provision of health services to American Indians via the establishment of the IHS. Indicating the significance of this health transfer to the overall objective of termination, Indian commissioner Glenn Emmons called the 1954 Indian Health Transfer Act the "biggest reduction of program responsibilities in the history of the [Indian] Bureau."[30] To be precise, on July 1, 1955, the transfer saw 56 hospitals, 13 school infirmaries, and 970 buildings valued at nearly $40 million, as well as 3,500 health employees change hands to the PHS.[31]

Scholars typically agree that the efficiency and quality of care provided by the Indian Health Division were significantly improved during its first years in the Public Health Service as the newly formed IHS. While problems certainly persisted, initial signs were mostly encouraging. For example, a positive impact on the quality of care was noted on account of the additional medical staff, including specialists from nearly every field of medicine. In all, during the first year of the transfer, the full-time medical staff of the IHS grew 45 percent, surpassing 5,000 people by 1959.[32] Physicians more than doubled to 300 and for the first time included a substantial number of pediatricians, surgeons, and maternal and childhood specialists. Dentists, dental assistants, and technicians almost tripled, reaching 100 in all. Sanitary engineers and sanitarians also increased from just fourteen to sixty-eight. Graduate nurses increased from 783 to 890, with practical nurses increasing from 289 to 486. Pharmacists, medical and social workers, community workers, medical record librarians, dietitians, and nutritionists also increased four or fivefold.[33] Indeed, for the first time, it appeared as though American Indians and Alaska Natives might actually receive comprehensive care. The positive changes reflected in the addition of so many staff were also gradually supported by the introduction of improved and modernized health facilities.

Despite the visible expansion of services, increasing appropriations, growing numbers of medical specialists, and legislatively sanctioned construction projects, the effectiveness of the program ultimately had to be measured by health outcomes. When viewed in this light, the Public Health Service performed better in some areas than others. It made important strides in tuberculosis and infant mortality. But overall, by the 1960s Indian health conditions were still at least a generation behind the national standard. The impact of the transition into public health for Native people living away from reservations is also rarely considered as a means of appraising the success or failure of the program. In part, this is because with the change, Native people who did not reside on reservations were no longer included in the group eligible to receive services. The eligibility rules of the Tacoma (Cushman) Indian Hospital in Washington State were typical of the regulations enforced by public health hospitals in admitting Native patients for free care:

> The evidence of eligibility to be presented:
>
> A. *American Indians* must be able to produce proof that he [*sic*] is regarded as an Indian by the community in which he lives by reason of tribal membership enrollment, residence of tax-exempt land, ownership of restricted property, and active participation in tribal affairs. Referral by a BIA Agency Superintendent or a PHS Officer will usually be considered as evidence of eligibility.
>
> B. *Alaskan Indians, Aleut, Eskimos.* Referral by the Alaska Native Service. Patients applying as Natives of Alaska will be referred to the Alaska Native Service, but if in need of immediate hospitalization, may be admitted pending confirmation of eligibility through our Social Service Department.[34]

As these regulations make clear, any Native person wishing to receive services *as an Indian* at a public health hospital had to prove residence on tax-exempt land. In a certain light then, looking to the repercussions on non-reservation Indian health might seem an irrelevant category for appraising the impact of the switch to the Public Health Service. On the other hand, by excluding this as a factor, one might say this simply reinstates the violence of the exclusionary categories that were imposed on Native people by the government. In the next section of this chapter, I look closely at how these administrative and structural changes impacted urban Indians. But first, I turn to the structure of health services in Australia, and how Aboriginal people were positioned within that system.

Australia has traditionally had a mixture of government-sponsored and private health services and practitioners. While the commonwealth government has always maintained a prominent role in the funding and regulation of health services, the provision of these services has largely been a state matter. With respect to Aboriginal people, as discussed in the previous chapter, there were few systematic attempts to provide medical care to Aboriginal people at all until the mid-nineteenth century. By this time, in many states Aboriginal people employed under contracts had become entitled to free medical treatment and prescribed rations. This regulation, however, was by no means enforced. From the 1860s, resident magistrates could also dispense medicine to sick Aboriginal people who were impoverished, and they could also send them to local hospitals for treatment. Such treatment would usually take place outdoors (external to the medical facilities), or later, in segregated wards. Segregated treatment such as this was the norm for roughly the next 100 years. In other words, until the 1960s, it was not uncommon for Aboriginal people across Australia to be refused medical treatment at mainstream hospitals or to have to wait in segregated rooms to get treated or to see a doctor, which might not even take place inside the medical facilities but in a separate, outdoor space.[35]

As working-class agitation for affordable or free medical care gradually began in Australia around the turn of the twentieth century, the first hospitals (which were privately owned) increasingly came to be subsidized by the government. Public-minded interest groups were largely unsuccessful in their efforts to secure free care until the introduction of the Medibank universal insurance scheme by the Whitlam government in 1975. For the period between World War II and 1975, then, Australia worked on a private but government-subsidized health insurance system. This mixed mode of public and private health care in the twentieth century was intended to provide a wide range of community and public health services that would cater to Aboriginal as well as non-Aboriginal people, even if only under policies of segregated treatment. Until the 1970s, health policy for Aboriginal people was also not separate from the more general policies that contained and controlled most aspects of their everyday lives. In keeping with the rest of the national approach to Aboriginal Affairs, then, the oversight and provision of health services for Aboriginal people was thus maintained at the state level until the late 1960s.

Programs offered by the different states were similar, with emphases on preventative health through education and attempts to persuade Aboriginal people to use existing health care services where possible.[36] This reflected the Australian government's firm commitment to a policy of assimilation in Indigenous Affairs at this time. Much like in the United States during the era of "termination," under Australia's assimilation policy of the 1950s and '60s, the extensive Aboriginal reserves across the country were gradually retracted without compensation to Aboriginal people. Other services and provisions deemed to be blatant relics of the segregative past were also steadily dismantled. In the field of health, this extended toward gradual attempts to do away with segregated hospital wards in the 1960s, meaning Aboriginal people were increasingly expected, from this time, to use mainstream hospital and medical care like the rest of Australian society. However, the determination by the federal government that Aboriginal people should live in the same manner as other Australians did not take into account that many of those other Australians were unwilling to admit Aboriginal people into their society. When Aboriginal people attempted to access mainstream medical services, then, they were often turned away by hospital staff who held the view expressed by the head matron of Perth's King Edward Memorial Hospital in 1949, when she wrote in a memo, "It is all very well to talk about the rights of natives, but I do not think that people who talk in this way would like to be in the next bed to some of these women."[37] As in the United States as well, many Australian providers were under the misconception that Aboriginal people could access free care from the government, and thus preferred to let somebody else treat them rather than introduce Aboriginal patients into their facilities.

Similar to the United States at this time, the period following World War II also saw gradual and mixed improvements to health services for Aboriginal people in Australia, both in public hospitals and the remaining mission hospitals and reserve clinics serving Aboriginal populations who had moved off their traditional territories. In part, the improvements seen during this time were a product of the fact that, as in the United States, some Australian states opted to let Aboriginal health services and hospitals be taken over by the Department of Public Health in 1949. This resulted in a more systematized and better-funded approach to managing Aboriginal health. Moreover, starting in the early 1960s, as Aboriginal people steadily started moving into cities, an increased number of free government health services were also provided to Aboriginal people on reserves and particularly stations, which served as a funnel (and "training ground") for channeling people into the cities.[38]

There was a clear difference between the positive (preventative) public health measures undertaken by these federal services—for example with the successful treatment of leprosy and trachoma in particular—compared to the reluctance and resistance of local (state) hospital authorities to take on the responsibility for treating Aboriginal patients. In the Northern Territory, for example, it was not until the 1950s that the Welfare Branch organized health services for Aboriginal people at all. A similar pattern existed in other states, where special provisions for Aboriginal health, even if they existed prior to the 1960s, consisted largely of negative policies designed to protect white Australia from possible contagion from infectious diseases, and only dealt with Aboriginal health issues as they came up in emergency situations or as threats to the wider populace. In some cases, forced isolation of sick Aboriginal people remained in the legislation in Australia up until the 1960s.[39]

Australia's momentous 1967 referendum, which eliminated the discriminatory sections of the Constitution regarding the inability of the commonwealth to make special laws for Aboriginal people and to count them in the census, was therefore a significant turning point in Aboriginal health care as well. This development provided the constitutional justification for commonwealth responsibility over Aboriginal health policy. This marked a significant change, especially since starting in the early 1960s there had been growing recognition of the poor state of Aboriginal health. High infant mortality rates, low life expectancy and excessive morbidity were documented for Aboriginal people throughout Australia, but with little distinction being made among remote, rural, and urban dwellers.[40] It was about this time, in the late 1960s, that the first concerted attempts by the federal government were made to provide health services to Aboriginal people, which would begin to address these gross inequalities. Urban Aboriginal agitation for these changes had a lot to do with the government's change of heart. The attempts to tackle the situation were fragmented at first. Moreover, by the early 1970s it was becoming clear that this delivery system was not coping with Aboriginal ill-health in the cities at all, as evidenced not only by the persistently poor morbidity and mortality of urban Aboriginal people but also by their underutilization of the mainstream health services.

The government intended that postwar urban Indigenous migrants would be fit into this schema of health care provision in accordance with its commitment to assimilation in the 1950s and '60s. During the middle third of the twentieth century, assimilation was the central ideology followed by the commonwealth and the states. Under the guidance of Paul Hasluck, commonwealth minister for Aboriginal Affairs from 1951 to 1963, the Australian government shifted its approach so that rather than calling for protection, it appealed for Aboriginal "advancement," "progress," or "uplift."[41]

As seen so explicitly on the pages of *Dawn* magazine discussed in the previous chapter, and like elsewhere in the world, it was clear that during midcentury the grip of "experts" and of a modernist approach to public policy was having a powerful influence on government, administration, and public opinion in Australia. It was characterized by an unwavering faith in the ability of humankind to triumph over nature, and by a confidence in experts, planners, and technicians of various stripes to wipe away the encumbrances of traditions, dispel social conflict, and construct an orderly and harmonious society.[42] In Australia, it is worth noting that aspects of modernist discourse had emerged in the nineteenth century in fields of professional practice, but at this time, the state had played only a "night-watch role," intervening very little in the social and economic lives of its citizens beyond the imposition of law and order.[43] It was only with the expansion of the state in Australia during the twentieth century—in welfare, social regulation, and administration—that modernism solidified into institutional political form. As this faith in experts and in human malleability was enacted in Australia in connection to Aboriginal Affairs, policymakers thus enlisted experts of all sorts. Scientists, planners, bureaucrats, doctors, and others devoted their energies to clearing up the messy and dissonant aspects of the past and designing and realizing a set of strategies for assimilating Aboriginal people that would result in conformity. Many such experts became enormously powerful social engineers with little regard for civil liberties, and they tolerated little resistance. Therefore, those who suffered under these policies included ethnic minorities, the "undeserving poor," and other groups whom authorities believed posed a threat to social order and cultural convention.[44]

As seen in the rhetoric of the New South Wales Aborigines Welfare Board (AWB) in *Dawn* magazine, Aboriginal Affairs in the 1950s and '60s, especially in connection to health, had been designed to direct Aboriginal people toward cultural conformity and "respectable" habits.[45] The most violent and coercive of these measures in Australia was enacted through the removal of children from their families and the forced displacement of many Aboriginal people from traditional lands. Less violently, though not without damage, on the pages of *Dawn*, those who lived on government reserves were also taught to be ashamed of their culture. They were also told that their culture was the source of their ill-health and that conformity to white Australian cultural norms would lead to improvements in their health.

Reserve dwellers thus had to endure regular inspections of their homes as officials imposed standards of hygiene, moral probity, and domestic order of the kind that was valorized on the pages on *Dawn*. The humiliation associated with such inspections left lasting scars on many, particularly women.[46] Those who wished to escape state regulation could apply to be "exempt" from the provisions of Aboriginal welfare legislation, but in doing so, they had to be prepared to become estranged from those who remained under the board's control. In effect, Aboriginal people were given an invidious choice. They could remain poor and under the thumb of state regulation, or secure more citizenship rights (and potentially economic benefits), as well as access to federal services like health care, if they were prepared to surrender communal ties, live on government-run stations, seek out employment away from their families, and eventually assimilate into mainstream Australian society.

Much like in the United States, the way in which this effectively forced Aboriginal people into the mainstream health care system in the cities was disastrous. Many Aboriginal people simply found it impossible to access medical care at all in cities like Sydney during the 1950s, '60s, and '70s either because they couldn't afford it, or because medical providers discriminated heavily against them or assumed they could access medical care elsewhere.[47] This notion that all Indigenous people were entitled to free government care was a stigma that followed Indigenous people into cities, even though it failed to hold true in their case. While this misconception had damaging consequences for the ability of Indigenous people in cities to access medical care, it nonetheless reflected a view held by many urban Indigenous migrants: that they *should* be entitled to free care. The confusion and the damaging outcomes resulting from this assumption on the part of medical providers produced an active debate in public forums about whose responsibility urban Indigenous health should be.

Whose Responsibility?

At the National Council of Indian Opportunity's 1969 Public Forum in Dallas, Texas, Vance Tahmahkera's question about the possibility of hospital coverage for urban Indians in Fort Worth was answered by LaDonna Harris, the presiding chair of the meeting and an urban Indian herself: "To my knowledge," she stated, "there are no health services available other than through your county-state health offices."[48] This, of course, was the outcome of arrangements settled through the Public Health Transfer Act. Chairwoman Harris went on to explain that one of the biggest questions consistently asked of her office at the National Council for Indian Opportunity concerned "the lack of financing for health services to Indians in urban areas."[49] "There are no Federal funds specifically for this program," she explained to the forum attendees. And indeed, she clarified, "This is one of the reasons we are here, to find out what kind of services are needed or not available."[50] She then turned to ask Mr. Tahmahkera, "In your opinion, you feel that health services are needed by the low-income Indian families in this area. Is that what you mean?"[51] Mr. Tahmahkera responded affirmatively to her question, describing why such funding was so desperately needed: "Yes, because in the city-county hospitals, you go there and sometimes have a five or six hour wait. If you're very sick—." His comments stopped short. The implication, of course, was that (much like the cartoon suggests at the top of this chapter) death was always a possibility for Indians in the waiting room. After a brief pause, Mr. Tahmahkera continued to state, "I thought if there was some special doctor to go to through the Government, it would be a big benefit for them to get this health service. It looks like there would be some way that we could try to help them through health benefits."[52]

The exchange between Tahmahkera and Harris continued for some time, before taking a turn that highlighted what many urban Indians also felt was highly hypocritical about the way in which the federal government had structured the public health transfer, which all but abandoned Indians once they became urban residents. "There's another thing I want to bring up," Mr. Tahmahkera declared. "I came down here and I wanted to get my son on relocation. You go back to Anadarko [his community in Oklahoma], and they [the BIA] tell you you're not eligible, you're from out-of-state."[53] What Mr. Tahmahkera was describing here was that the BIA in his home state failed to recognize either him or his son, now that he had successfully relocated their family. And so, he put a question to Harris rather pointedly: "So what explanation do you have for that?"[54] Harris's response to this comment was a clear-cut voicing of the government's logic of spatial governance. She admitted, "Well, of course, that's one of the reasons for these hearings. You know, they even made a ruling on health in Oklahoma City and Tulsa, that if you moved to metropolitan areas that you're considered a non-Indian."[55] Being an urban Indian herself, Harris was quick to add, "This is why, really, we're trying to identify these problems, that you lose part of—." Tahmahkera had cut her off, but we can imagine Harris might have said that one loses a part of their identity or rights as an Indian just by virtue of moving to the city. Clearly incensed by this, Mr. Tahmahkera interjected, "Well actually, it looks like you're all working against your own program, there. You're penalizing the people that go out on their own to do this. You're telling them 'Well, you're not eligible for this program because you moved out of the state.' Then you're trying to move people out to take this training somewhere else, so it looks like you are all just being—."[56] This time, Harris interrupted to finish his thought: "Yes, we're penalizing them just by taking advantage of the program. I certainly do agree with you, and, as I say, that's one of my purposes, to focus attention on the fact that through our own programming, it's a disadvantage to the very people we're trying to serve. I think you make a very good point."[57]

After a brief recess, the forum reconvened and other attendees chimed in with their experiences, adding to the evidence that relocation incurred many disadvantages for Indians by leaving them without access to vital welfare services when they were often the ones who needed them the most. Several people described the drastic measures Native people would go to in cities in order to be able to get the much-needed medical care they couldn't otherwise access: "I know this personally from my own observations," one man said, "that people have lied about residency [on reservations] for health services and educational services because of financial reasons and stay with relatives to establish some residency. I know that puts people in a very awkward position in order to take advantage of some of the programs."[58] Another attendee agreed: "I'd like to see those things corrected. I don't know to what extent they can be, but the fact you moved from the farm or from off the reservation does not mean that you're not Indian or a member of the tribe. We have to recognize this."[59]

As the discussion at the forum was starting to make clear, the problem of accessing health services for diasporic urban Indians was really twofold in terms of how their eligibility was being identified, or rather misidentified. On the one hand, as the comments above attest, the government deemed that Indians were no longer Indian as soon as they moved off the reservation. This resulted in their exclusion from services provided by the government. On the other hand, the assumption on the part of many medical providers that all Indians were entitled, by virtue of being Indian, to access free government services, meant that Native people often got turned away from services in the city as well. As a forum attendee, Mrs. Edwards, explained to chairwoman Harris, "I'd like to get the stigma of the BIA off my back. For instance, I went to Parkland Hospital. My husband carries enough insurance for me, but we have a son who is 23 years old. . . . He didn't have money to see a doctor."[60] Mrs. Edwards went on to describe how, upon arrival at the hospital, her family was greeted with the following response almost immediately: "Why don't you go ask the BIA?"[61] "Everywhere I go," she exclaimed, "this is what comes up!"[62] Clearly exasperated, she implored Harris, "I would like for it to be advertised that the BIA doesn't help all Indians."[63] In response, LaDonna Harris offered this woman much sympathy and articulated a key point about the eligibility of urban Indians for care by the state in this capacity. As she put it, "This is a great misunderstanding nationally. If you are an Indian, people think you can receive all the services from BIA, and, as you say, that is not true. As a [US] citizen however, you should receive the services from that institution anyway. This is a very hard thing to get across to non-Indians sometimes and, particularly, to institutions that ought to know better."[64] As the forum's discussion had by now established, misinformation and discriminatory attitudes worked together to preclude urban Indians from accessing medical treatment. Harris continued to spell out the terms of the debate over responsibility. For one, she stressed the importance of urban Indians realizing and acting on the knowledge that "you are a citizen of this community, this state and nation, you're not owned by the BIA. You don't belong solely to them, you are a citizen. This is a very, very hard problem and, hopefully, by these hearings we're awakening communities and other Federal agencies to this fact."[65] According to this line of thinking then, urban Indians themselves could do more to make their case for medical care qua US citizens. Harris even shared with the forum that in her own personal experience, she too had been faced with such dismissive attitudes, and thus she insisted that anyone concerned to address the welfare of urban Indians must "dramatize" this problem to the extent that "people really realize you are a citizen of this town and this is where the responsibility is in this state and you are, of course, first of all a citizen of the United States."[66]

While Harris certainly won over many of the Indian attendees at the forum with her comments and her empathy for their plight, her impulse to solve the issue of health care access by pushing urban Indians toward the arguments of citizenship and equal rights did not resonate with many other urban Indians who insisted that the federal government *should* be the party responsible for meeting their health needs. Many people held this view because they argued that their treaties extended this to them. And moreover, they argued that the treaties never tied their right to health care to any kind of residency clause. This contrasting view came out as a part of the discussion at a two-day Indian conference convened in Washington State in October 1956 at the Hotel Monte Cristo in Everett. In a session on health, welfare, and education, Dr. Ruth Dunham of the Public Health Service said the objective of transferring the responsibility for Indian Health over to the PHS was to help Native Americans improve their health, with two major points: "(1) to prevent illness and (2) taking care of the sick."[67] Dr. Dunham explained that the PHS pays to provide services (i.e., nurses, doctors, and dentists) on the reservations only. She highlighted a few of their focal points, including the prevention of tuberculosis, the prevention of illness and death among babies and small children, and in the field of sanitation, she outlined that the PHS got help from other departments. In addition to mentioning their health education program, Dr. Dunham said she also wanted to emphasize the preventative side of the PHS—"obtaining of good health, rather than treatment of illnesses, many of which are preventable."[68] Outlining the terms of medical and hospital care, she pointed out that under the new PHS regime, people could go to local doctors and hospitals. Moreover, in recognition of the confusion that these new rules were causing, she informed the conference attendees that pamphlets and letters had been mailed out to reservation residents, defining eligibility. In general, she explained for the benefit of attendees that, simply put, "those who can pay, do pay; and those who cannot pay, get assistance."[69] Much as we saw with the eligibility rules of the Tacoma hospital, Dunham outlined that to obtain assistance, "an Indian must be recognized as a tribal member, live on a reservation, cannot pay the bill, and is not eligible for any of the other assistance programs. One meeting these requirements is considered for PHS aid."[70]

In response to these comments, Tandy Wilbur (Swinomish), a resident of Seattle, put a pointed question to Dr. Dunham, which highlighted the dispute many urban Indians had with the idea that they had to be resident on a reservation in order to be considered eligible (i.e., "Indian") by the government: "That is all very well," she said.[71] "But there is a set of principles involved here," Wilbur averred.[72] "The Indian people had a new civilization thrust upon them in exchange for services. No settlement has been made yet." Moreover, she stressed that "we feel justified in requesting the protection of our health whether on the reservation or in cities. Our people are entitled to service wherever they live."[73] In contrast to the position articulated by Harris—that urban Indians should press the federal government on the basis of their US citizenship—Wilbur was making quite a different point, and one that many urban Indians in Seattle and elsewhere also felt. The words of one of my informants rang true for many urban Indians in the 1960s and '70s, just as it does today: "We were promised health services by our treaties," Dr. Walt Hollow (Assiniboine-Sioux) told me unequivocally in 2013.[74] For many urban Indians holding this view, it was therefore the federal government's responsibility to them *as Indians* to ensure the proper provision of their health care needs, irrespective of where they lived. On the basis of this argument, toward the late 1960s and early 1970s, many urban Indians were therefore adamant in pressing for the government provision of health services to their community (or more precisely, for the provision of government funding to run their own services), not as US citizens but as Native Americans.

In Australia, given the absence of treaties and the lack of jurisdiction that the federal government had over Aboriginal Affairs prior to the 1967 referendum, there were considerable differences in the legal position Aboriginal people were in vis-à-vis the federal government. It is important to clarify that this meant Aboriginal Affairs (including Aboriginal health) were in the hands of the states until 1967. This meant that when Aboriginal people moved off reserves, missions, and stations, they did not lose any officially designated rights as Indigenous persons. Nevertheless, Australian federal and state governments recognized their responsibility toward Indigenous people as "wards of the state," and this, in principle, entailed that their basic needs should be met by the government (including their medical needs). On reserves, missions, and stations, living conditions varied greatly and were in many cases appalling; but at least there, if only superficially, the government recognized its obligation toward Aboriginal people. This was not so for urban populations, who were assumed to be on a path toward assimilation. I also explained in chapter 1 how, to encourage Aboriginal people to relocate into cities, state governments purposefully gave the impression that Aboriginal health needs would be better met through mainstream social welfare and medical services. However, this turned out to be untrue in most urban centers due to rampant discrimination. On both scores then—because the government failed to recognize their Aboriginality in cities and because the government failed to deliver on its promises of better conditions in the cities—urban Aboriginal health activists would later claim, much like in the case of Native Americans, that the government was shirking an obligation rightfully owed to them as Indigenous people. In the Aboriginal case the status they lost (or which the government claimed they had "given up") by moving to the city was that of their wardship status rather than any Indigenous rights per se. But despite this difference, the outcome was much the same for Aboriginal people in cities as it was for urban Indians; the government denied any obligation to provide them services on the basis of their Indigenous identity. This effectively worked to enshrine the spatial logics of colonial governance in health policy since it worked to confine indigeneity to specific locales (i.e., the reserve/reservation).

In contrast to the American case, the path toward securing federal oversight of their health care had to come first for Aboriginal people through citizenship.[75] Without pursuing citizenship first—which meant they could be counted as part of the national community in the census, and hence budgeted for—Aboriginal people in Australia had slim hope of securing federal government resources for their health. This made their approach to pressing for government-funded health care services something of a circuitous path as compared to the Native American case, as it meant they had to first press for these services as Australians deserving of equal treatment before they could do so as Aboriginal people. This produced considerable disagreement, even as late as the early 1970s, about who should bear the responsibility for the health needs of urban Indigenous communities in Australia.

As in the United States, policymakers, medical providers, and experts of various stripes debated the question of responsibility. In 1969 an independent association called Aboriginal Affairs, which described its purpose as being to "promote an informed interest in Aboriginal issues," published a booklet for public consumption titled *Answering Your Questions About Aborigines*.[76] In it, the matter of "who is responsible for Aboriginal health" was addressed in the following way: "The various departments of Aboriginal affairs are concerned with hygiene and nutrition at settlements and missions. Some employ female welfare officers who deal with health problems of Aborigines in the community. However, in most places now Aboriginal health is directly the responsibility of the State Departments of Health. The quality of the services provided has improved dramatically since the war, although the staffing of posts in the far outback is not easily accomplished."[77]

Quite apart from the fact that the document was slightly misleading in neglecting to mention that the federal government now (post-1967) had made provisions in the commonwealth budget to fund Aboriginal programs on reserves (including health for the first time), it is telling that this document also said nothing of the Aboriginal populations in cities. This of course reflected both the levels of misinformation and confusion that still circulated in Australian public discourse as late as 1969 regarding where responsibilities lay for the provision of services to Aboriginal communities. While many rural and urban Aboriginal people alike were of a view that the state and national governments owed them such services as a form of compensation for the dispossession of their lands, state authorities like the New South Wales AWB were in a constant effort to dispel all such expectations and also sought to encourage Aboriginal people to opt into a state insurance plan called "The Hospital Fund."[78] Public announcements and advertisements about The Hospital Fund were published repeatedly by the New South Wales AWB in *Dawn* magazine across the 1950s and '60s. In an effort to discourage Aboriginal readers from demanding free treatment at hospitals, these short notices were explicit that "quite a number of aboriginal people have a wrong idea of their responsibilities in regard to hospital treatment, thinking as they do that just because they are aborigines they are entitled to free treatment. This is far from the case."[79] Instead, as part of its program to assimilate Aboriginal people in New South Wales by encouraging good financial planning, the AWB extolled the virtues of "join[ing] your local Hospital fund" so that "payment of your hospital fees and those for your family are assured."[80] Yet only three years earlier, in an article titled "The Aborigine and His Rights: Facts Misunderstood," the AWB had also claimed on the pages of *Dawn* that "the Board can render services in many cases where the residents are not yet ready for full assimilation into the community and where they welcome the guidance and assistance of the Board. Such services include medical attention and housing, either free or at a greatly reduced rental."[81] As a consequence of these mixed messages and the confusion that resulted, the director of Aboriginal Welfare, Child Welfare, and Social Welfare in Sydney, Ian Mitchell, concluded in 1971 that "most Aborigines are at a severe disadvantage when compared with the rest of the community, for they are unaware of the services available to them."[82] Moreover, he added that there seemed to be "remaining confusion among State and Commonwealth agencies as to their responsibilities."[83]

In an effort to clear up this confusion among various stakeholders, a four-day National Seminar on Health Services for Aborigines was held in Melbourne, at Monash University (May 14–17, 1972). Over the course of the four days, seminar attendees and presenters debated and discussed issues pertaining to Aboriginal health services ranging from "Legal Controls on Alcohol" to "A Method for the Delivery of Health and Mental Health in a Small Aboriginal Population Using the Doctor as a Social Change Agent" to "Voluntary Health Services in the Metropolitan Areas."[84] A close reading of the seminar proceedings gives us invaluable insight into the main issues that were seen to be at stake by the authorities in determining who should provide health services to urban as opposed to rural Aboriginal communities.

The spokesperson for the state of Victoria outlined the general approach of the states to health services for Aboriginal people in the cities. It was clearly inflected with the goals of assimilation: "Health Services for Aborigines in Victoria are those available to all citizens."[85] The representative from South Australia repeated almost the very same line: "Aboriginal people living in cities and towns use normal community services."[86] The spokesperson for New South Wales, which had the nation's largest urban Aboriginal population at the time, did not even mention the provision of services to this community, indicating how far they were from the considerations of health care providers in that state. When urban Aboriginal health did come up, many of the state representatives presented a view that placed all responsibility upon the Aboriginal community members themselves, with very little recognition of the fact that Aboriginal people's lack of access to employment and decent housing due to discrimination in the cities were significant contributing factors to their poor health conditions. For instance, on the matter of housing and its connection to high rates of infection among the urban Aboriginal community in South Australia, the state's spokesperson had the following words to share with seminar attendees: "It is the considered opinion of officers of the South Australian Department of Public Health that any housing programme will only be successful if the people are first taught how to live hygienically in a home and then taught to budget. Regular supervision in the way of home visits is essential."[87]

It was also suggested, by more than one state representative, that Aboriginal people's health in the cities might be improved if they took to more regular exercise: "The adult Aboriginal people do not seem to participate in sport to the same extent as most adult non-Aborigines do. The relative lack of exercise may account for many developing disease patterns."[88] This attention to participation in sporting activities was repeated by the representative from Western Australia, who offered the following remarks to the seminar: "The administrative bodies providing health and medical services are cognisant of the lack of sporting activity among the Aboriginal population, which must be contributing to their health conditions."[89] As a potential solution to managing the problem of Aboriginal ill-health in the cities, the idea of encouraging greater participation in sports had indeed been a longtime strategy of the Aborigines Welfare Board. For example, in the 1950s this idea was repeatedly promoted on the pages of *Dawn* magazine, which included photographs and small articles endorsing the sporting achievements of Aboriginal people like Harry Penrith, who was featured on the front cover of the magazine's February 1953 issue for being "one of the most outstanding athletes Kinchela has produced."[90] An article published later that year titled "The Aborigines Must Help Themselves: Laziness Retards Progress" reprimanded Aboriginal people for not being more active, especially in "events outside their own circle."[91] As an example of how Aboriginal people might achieve this in cities, it gave the case of "those men who play football with white teams" as a prime demonstration of how this might be done.[92] This was typical of the moralizing tone and assimilationist rhetoric that inflected the AWB's outlook on Aboriginal health problems.

While the state representatives at the seminar clearly toed the assimilationist line of blaming the individual and blaming Aboriginal "culture," other participants shared different perspectives. There seemed to be a growing understanding among many of the public health representatives in attendance that the individual's social and economic milieu was as much a predictor of health as was individual behavior. For example, this view was represented at the seminar by David P. Bowler, medical superintendent at Townsville Hospital, in his paper titled "Some Problems Facing an Administrator in Improving Health Services for Aborigines."[93] In his paper, Bowler expressed the view that to be effective, a health service had to address the broader social situation of the target population, including even their own conceptions of health: "Health care is not just curative medicine, but is intimately mixed with and part of the social, moral, and economic structure and development of the community. Do we push forward with assimilation, imposing our Western concepts of health—bottle-feeding babies, drug dependence, child developments rules (which are certainly not the only, or even the best, ways of bringing up children), and a hospital based service? Or do we belatedly begin a dialogue with the Aboriginal community, listening to them, finding out what their ideas of health may be, and what they want?"[94]

In relation to the Aboriginal community in Sydney, this new perspective on health as a social phenomenon had been championed a year earlier by Dr. Norelle Lickiss of the school of Public Health and Tropical Medicine at the University of Sydney. In 1971, Lickiss published an influential study on "The Aboriginal People of Sydney with Special Reference to the Health of Their Children: A Study in Human Ecology."[95] In this work, Lickiss advocated for a new approach to understanding the health problems of Sydney's urban Aboriginal community. "Behind a child," Lickiss wrote, "stretches his history with all its aspects: genetic endowment, intrauterine and extrauterine nutrition, cultural inheritance, biological and psychological insults of childhood, and total life experience."[96] "A child, influenced profoundly by all these," Lickiss claimed, "is in continual interaction with his environment in a dialectical relationship. The outcome of this interaction at any point of time is in some aspects measurable in terms of health, considered as the continuing adjustment of an organism to its environment."[97] Lickiss also introduced a forward-looking dimension to the study. In citing well-known microbiologist Rene Dubos, Lickiss suggested that public health practitioners in Australia should consider Aboriginal health as "not a state but a potentiality—the ability of an individual or social group to modify himself or itself continually not only in order to function better in the present but also to prepare for the future."[98] In conclusion, Lickiss referred to all of these contributing factors as "the concept of child ecology," stressing that "it is important to recognize that a child, being human, is not merely a prisoner of his environment but has some capacity to transcend it, to be to some measure his own maker."[99] Rather than seeking to push the urban Aboriginal population down a path of assimilation, however, this new public health perspective, championed by several of the presenters at the seminar, instead advocated for government investment in better housing and greater employment assistance, as well as putting a degree of the control over health services into the hands of the community itself. Bowler put the point succinctly when suggesting the Australian federal government should start throwing its support behind the idea that Aboriginal people should be the ones providing their own communities with care: "It seems to me that before any lasting improvements can be produced in the health of Aborigines, it will be necessary to train Aboriginal health workers to work with their own people, and to develop a health education programme that is specifically designed for them—and developed by them. The 'expatriate' can advise, and demonstrate, but the desire for change must come from within the group, particularly if any lasting improvements are to be made."[100]

D. Wilson, also of the Public Health Service, added that it was important for the government to apply this approach to all Aboriginal people regardless of where they chose to live: "In any health training programme the wishes of the Aborigines must be respected. Aborigines must be allowed to retain their identity and security. They themselves should choose whether or not they remain in the tribal situation, or move into a European society. Health programmes should be designed to provide for both situations."[101]

In a statement that foreshadowed his later efforts to establish the first Aboriginal community-controlled health service in the nation, Aboriginal activist and Aboriginal Medical Service cofounder Gordon Briscoe affirmed this view and also clarified an issue that was proving to be problematic in discussions between administrators and Aboriginal advocates: "It seems that policy-makers assume the demands of the urban Aboriginal community are tantamount to requests for a completely new brand of medicine to be established: Aboriginal medicine," Briscoe reported, when in fact, as Briscoe explained to the seminar participants, "this of course is not the case." All they were asking for, he outlined, is "a degree of Aboriginal control over what our health services are."[102] Moreover, Briscoe emphasized the importance of this being introduced into the cities because "with the proliferation of Aboriginal migration from the rural to urban setting, due to rural recessions, the slum areas of Sydney provide the location for the largest group of Aborigines in Australia that have been and are still being affected by this process of social destruction."[103] According to Briscoe, the federal government's policy of assimilation was itself to blame for many of the health problems experienced by the Aboriginal community in the cities:

If any Australian citizen deludes himself into thinking that the Aboriginal health problem is not in a state of emergency then they are either ignorant, sadistic or naive. It is an emergency brought about mainly by design and in part by accident. The design is in the form of a racist assimilation policy which attempts to crush the Aboriginal life style out of existence, leaving our people without an economic or political base from which to support health and eating habits. The migration of people from the rural areas had transported this chronic health situation to both the "fringe-dwelling settlements" and the "urban slums."[104]

Therefore, according to Briscoe and other Aboriginal advocates at the seminar, since the federal government had instituted the policy of assimilation—with all its attendant effects on Aboriginal health—it should also be their responsibility to address these health problems: "The city area is the place, I believe, where the greatest possibilities and responsibilities exist toward the Aborigines for the government to provide services," Briscoe argued.[105]

Taking a slightly different angle on the question of responsibility, a final set of views at the seminar drew attention to both the role of the physician and the public at large. Dr. R. E. Coolican, a general practitioner who lived in and practiced medicine in Bourke (a New South Wales town with a high density of Aboriginal people) for twenty-two years, and who was now living in Sydney working at the Royal North Shore Hospital, spoke about the responsibilities that lay with the private practitioner. Indeed, he reminded seminar attendees that "the medical care of the rural Aborigines has, in western NSW, ever been the private charity of the general practitioner."[106] But on the question of the growing urban population—which he concurred with Briscoe had been to some measure created by the federal government—he advocated for the need to see the government take on a greater role: "However great the doctor's social and community responsibilities are, ultimately the responsibility of providing services must rest with the Commonwealth government."[107] And finally, public health nurse Pat McPherson also brought up the point that Australians in the general populace bore a measure of responsibility for ensuring the health of Aboriginal people too. In McPherson's view, this was especially true in the cities because of the importance of the tie between good health and acceptance within the community:

> In the long run, it is on these very ordinary, everyday people of the white community in our cities that the final onus lies, in their acceptance of Aborigines, who are willy nilly being swept, (whether they like it or not) along the road to mutual contribution and co-existence in our communities. The acceptance of Aborigines as people, as a total people, and not only individually as a good tennis player, or fighter, or singer, is the often overlooked component in this matter of health. It is at this level, and perhaps only in a small way, that the influence of the Public Health nurse can be used sensitively and wisely.[108]

Gordon Briscoe responded to McPherson's comments with a concise yet powerful rejoinder: "It is the responsibility of every Australian citizen to voice their own protest over this genocide."[109]

As these various viewpoints make clear, the question of who should take on the responsibility of providing for the health care of the newly expanding diasporic and pan-Indigenous urban communities in the United States and Australia was by no means a straightforward issue, even as late as the early 1970s. This is because, wrapped up in all the discussions about services, funding, responsibilities, and rights were fundamental questions about whether urban Indigenous people should still be recognized as Indigenous given their relocation into the cities. In Australia, this situation was complicated further still by the fact that Aboriginal citizenship remained an unanswered question, even as late as the 1960s. Authorities in both cases were also not in agreement about what the geographical distance of Indigenous people from reserves and reservations implied about their identities and rights as Indigenous people. Many held the view that the movement into cities equated to a loss of Indigenous identity and associated rights. Yet, as the public testimonies of many urban Indigenous relocatees revealed, medical providers and the broader Australian and American public still failed to treat Indigenous people as if they were a part of mainstream culture and society. And this came to an especially dangerous head within the health care system, as Vance Tahmahkera's testimony suggested. Moreover, Indigenous people themselves certainly did not regard their ethnic identities as being determined by where they lived. This situation left many diasporic urban Indigenous people trapped between two places of not belonging. And as a result, the very real implications this had on their inability to claim health services, neither as Australians, Americans, Aboriginals, or Native Americans, simply left them without access at all.

Health and Medicine: Forgotten Frontiers of the Twentieth Century?

What can the parallel experiences of urban Indigenous people in the US and Australian medical systems at this time tell us about the project of settler colonialism in the twentieth century and the significance of health and medicine within it? Chapters 1 and 2 of this book have shown that the postwar years in both the United States and Australia saw efforts to terminate government responsibilities toward Indigenous peoples on reserves and reservations in favor of pushing them toward mainstream societal integration via urbanization and assimilation. It is clear in both cases that health policies and the medical system were part and parcel of the colonial attempt to control Indigenous people by curtailing the ways (and places) in which they were able to claim their identities and rights as Indigenous people. This shared technique of colonial control and denial of services to Indigenous peoples in urban areas should be recognized as yet another manifestation of settler colonialism and public health's spatial forms of governance. In the next two chapters, I discuss how the realities of such contested terrain in the mid-to-late twentieth century roused urban Indigenous health activism. Scholars of Indigenous politics in both the United States and Australia have looked closely at how these tensions of urban migration played out in terms of other important issues, such as continuing hunting and fishing rights, or in terms of land rights. By contrast, I focus on these questions of health because, though rarely the subject of historical analysis, they have always been at the forefront of Indigenous activism in the United States and

Australia. Indeed, health has consistently galvanized Indigenous communities into action in both the United States and Australia, and it is certainly at the forefront of Indigenous politics in both nations in the twenty-first century. Health therefore demands closer scrutiny as an agenda of Indigenous activists.

What the denial, through policy, of health services to urban Indigenous peoples *as Indigenous peoples* tells us about the projects of settler colonialism in both the United States and Australia is that these governments have long defined Indigeneity in spatial terms as much as in terms of blood and culture. As the policy history in this chapter has shown, in the postwar period, this fact was brought to the surface most strikingly in the (mis)management of Indigenous health care. In the twenty-five years after the end of World War II, the governments of the United States and Australia and policymakers in the field of health still refused to recognize diasporic urban Indigenous people as a distinct social group with specific problems, needs, and claims. A central assumption behind the policy of assimilation in both the United States and Australia was that those who chose to live in the cities and towns thereby signaled a preparedness to cede their Indigenous identities and become absorbed into the social mainstream. Hence the fields of Aboriginal and American Indian Affairs dealt predominantly with those who lived on reservations/reserves or in rural areas, until well into the 1960s and early 1970s. As I discuss in the chapters to follow, it was not until the late 1960s that urban pan-Indigenous agitation for recognition in the cities led to their presence in public policy at all. Notably, in the case of the United States, urban Indians entered federal legislation for the first time in the arena of health.[110]

Despite government inattention to these communities, some academic and medical researchers began to focus their attentions on those living in cities and towns from the late 1940s. There was an almost universal perception among these researchers, though, that those who moved to cities had experienced cultural loss. In keeping with the dominant functionalism of the time, these studies therefore depicted new Indigenous urban migrants as being in a state of stalled transition between tradition and modernity, and most accorded with the public norms and policy imperatives of the assimilation era. Ethnographic writing in particular generally lamented the decline of traditional knowledge and the lack of regard that young Indigenous people had for their elders. It appeared to the researchers that the loss of attachment to land sounded the death knell of the old ways. Without those ways, it was held, there was no substance to Indigenous culture.

It is remarkable how in both nations, most public representations of Indigenous people in cities during the 1950s, '60s, and '70s therefore cast them as a disruptive and transgressive presence within what was essentially "civilized" space. Behind the moral panics and shocking headlines of the tabloid presses, however, was the emergence of a counter-colonial movement. Those Indigenous people who had moved to the cities had not in fact relinquished everyday contact with their home communities and the lands and cultures that had traditionally grounded their identities. To be sure (and as I discuss in the next two chapters), these newly forming urban and pan-Indigenous communities certainly faced a struggle to anchor their social and political identities. However, rather than giving in to the pressures to assimilate, the diasporic Indigenous communities in cities like Seattle and Sydney formed new networks. They developed a pan-Indigenous culture and politics that made the Aboriginal rights movement and the American Indian movement a subversive and powerful presence in public life in the last three decades of the twentieth century. City dwellers, especially young people, defied both official expectations and the poor, overcrowded living conditions they experienced, to develop a new urban Indigenous political vernacular; and the community health centers they created, I argue, were an embodiment of this new politics.

Far from undergoing a loss of their Indigeneity with the transition from reserve/reservation to city as some urban ethnographers suggested, Indigenous people were therefore involved in an ongoing process of cultural production combining the old and the new, the traditional and the modern. Urban pan-Indigenous peoples did not by any means eschew ties to their communities of origin but built broader forms of association than would have been possible had they remained on the reserve/reservation. In the previous chapter I discussed how health needs were an integral part of fostering this continued connection. In this chapter I have argued that despite these facts of mobility and continuing connection, Indigeneity in both national contexts continued to be publicly defined in the 1950s, '60s, and '70s in dichotomous or binary spatial terms, meaning that once one left the reserve/reservation, by the letter of the law, one was no longer entitled to rights and recognitions as an Indigenous person. In the context of health care, the next chapters discuss how and why this proved to be a matter of life or death for so many people.

The congregation of Indigenous peoples from different regions in high-density population centers produced new solidarities as well as new identities. Those who came from small country towns or remote areas were able to relate their particular localized experiences to those of other Indigenous people who came from similar places. Moreover, new solidarities were built on a doubled-sided realization that (a) what had happened on the reserves/reservations and in remote rural communities was not peculiar but was part of a more generalized set of experiences; and (b) in the cities, the experiences they had in being excluded from medical treatment were a common struggle born of their structural invisibility as Indigenous people in these places. These new experiences and realizations led to the emergence of a radical pan-Indigenous politics that in relation to health produced a set of common ideas and initiatives in the form of community-controlled medical services. Much like the communities themselves, these health clinics blended facets of the traditional and the new and sought to be as inclusive as possible.

What these parallel solutions can tell us about Indigenous politics, communities, and activism in both settler-colonial nations is that as a social and political issue, health has been of greater importance in galvanizing urban Indigenous communities than has thus far been recognized by scholars. Community-controlled health services came to represent the articulation of a new form of Indigenous politics—one that was deterritorialized, or rather, reterritorialized, and which found ways to assert Indigenous sovereignty and self-determination for communities without recourse to land in the pursuit of their sovereign rights. These health clinics also belied the thesis of cultural loss and demonstrated the emergence of a new diasporic pan-Indigenous politics and culture. With time, these clinics, in the ethos of service that they adopted and in the range of services they provided, came to embody the fact that pan-Indigeneity drew on tradition, but it also innovated. Incorporating diverse elements of multiple Indigenous cultures in their physical appearance, approaches to health, and in their policies toward accepting patients, these clinics lent a new face to Indigeneity in the late twentieth century but also, importantly, provided a sense of anchorage for those who were away from their home community and country. Indeed, as the clinics grew exponentially and started appearing all over the United States and Australia, they began to form their own networks of connection—as "health hubs."[111] It is in this sense that I argue these clinics sought nothing less than to make it possible for Indigenous people to feel at home everywhere within the national spaces of the United States and Australia, and to claim their rights as Indigenous peoples in the same manner, wherever they chose to live.

3   The People Speak, Will You Listen?

Indigenous Health Activism in Seattle, 1950–1970

· ·

On November 14, 1970, at a public forum convened by the US federal government's newly formed National Council on Indian Opportunity (NCIO), a young man sat in the audience, waiting for the right moment.[1] Unlike the many other participants in the public forum, Bill Jeffries (Cherokee-Sioux) had not traveled to Spokane to discuss and debate President Nixon's new Indian Legislative Program.[2] Nor was he there as a representative of a tribal community like the vast majority of attendees. For these reasons, he waited until the official proceedings of the forum were more or less over before he rose from his seat to share the following startling comments: "I have been asked by the American Indian Community in Seattle to request your attention and assistance if at all possible with a problem that has come up in Seattle with one of our American Indians in that area."[3] The case he referred to had become so urgent, Jeffries stressed, that it had even made the local news the day before.[4] He proceeded to share the details with the forum's attendees: "There is a young Indian man from Standing Rock Sioux that is in difficulty in Seattle. He has a very serious kidney ailment and is in need of a kidney machine and right at this time the American Indian Center in Seattle, in cooperation with the Indian and Alaskan Indian Services in Alaska, are trying to raise $20,000 to purchase a kidney machine and keep this young man alive for another year."[5]

Jeffries had been sent to Spokane to submit this plea before the NCIO's public forum at the special urging of Pearl Warren (Makah), the director of the American Indian Women's Service League, as well as the board of the Kinatechitapi Indian Council—two of the first and most prominent American Indian social organizations to be established in Seattle after World War II. As Jeffries explained to his attentive listeners, these organizations, their members, the wider American Indian community in Seattle, and even the University of Washington Hospital where the young man was being treated, were at a loss: "They have exhausted all the resources that they have."[6] Jeffries's presence—indeed interruption—at the forum that morning was therefore a sign of some urgency: "We need to get this money as soon as possible. We have six weeks to accumulate $20,000."[7] Showing that his comments were directed as much—if not more—toward the Native American community members of the audience than to the forum's committee, Jeffries went on to say, "I bring this to your attention today and ask if each one of you or your group, your tribe or organization, could assist in any way."[8] After providing full details of where donations could be sent for "the Ernie Crowfeather Fund," Jeffries closed his comments by underscoring that this was a community issue, not simply an effort to support one man: "Indian to Indian, I can say this will be greatly appreciated by all concerned."[9]

Having done what he set out to do, Jeffries promptly sat back down. But several committee members were clearly troubled by what he had to say. Mr. Bob Jim (Yakama) asked a pressing follow-up question: "What if the money is not forthcoming?"[10] Mr. Earl Old Person (Blackfeet), chairman of the forum and president of the National Council of American Indians, chimed in with an observation: "I think these are some of the things that we're going to have to start digging into. . . . I think there should be a ways and means for help of this kind for people, especially where this is a life that is involved, when it means life or death. So I think we're going to have to start doing something other than to have to go to the tribes and have to go to the individuals. I think there should be some type of program to help an individual to save his life."[11]

The committee's concerns reveal several important things. First, it was not entirely obvious what would happen to Ernie Crowfeather should the group fail to raise the money. Second, Mr. Jeffries's recourse to the tribal networks seemed the standard protocol for a situation of this kind. Third, if establishing some sort of program to serve as a safety net seemed necessary and important to Mr. Old Person, this suggests that Ernie Crowfeather's situation was perhaps not unusual. These brief exchanges indicated how desperate circumstances could get for Native people seeking health care in the cities, and they also underscore the very haphazard nature of the systems that were in place to support them.

To make matters worse, there appeared to be a legitimate concern that Ernie Crowfeather's predicament was also a consequence of his Indian identity. Bob Jim brought this to light when he revealed that Pearl Warren (and perhaps other representatives of the community in Seattle) had already contacted the offices of the NCIO to raise awareness about Crowfeather's case. Jim stated for the record that he was recently "called about this" by the groups mentioned in Jeffries's statement, and that "what they say is that because he's Indian they [the medical services] want to let him die because of his past record." Jim went on: "I know it's possible the P.H.S [Public Health Service] does a lot of this to some Indians, the similar treatment you're talking about. Now, what the implication by the group is that they want to let him die because he's an Indian."[12] Unsure of what this really meant, Jim asked Jeffries, "Could you delve into that a little bit for our benefit?"[13] Concerned not to simplify or sensationalize matters, Jeffries gave a candid yet diplomatic response:

> We're not sure whether this is true or not, Mr. Jim. This has been mentioned and the American Indian Women's Service League there in Seattle is concerned about giving out this idea because if it gets back it could hinder Mr. Crowfeather. . . . This is the impression that the secretary had, Mr. Jim, but she doesn't have it—she can't quote them exactly in saying that "because he's an Indian if we don't have the funds he's just going to die—we're going to turn him out"—but this is a feeling some of the people have and we're trying to evaluate the situation to clarify this thing whether it is or not.[14]

Setting aside the question of discrimination for now, Pearl Warren's phone calls and Bill Jeffries's appearance at the public forum provide a good indication of the methods, strategies, and resources that were available to, and commonly utilized by, urban Indian health activists at this time. By 1970, Jeffries's strategic presence at the public forum to raise funds and to reach out directly to other Native people—especially those in positions of power—was representative of what many activists were doing by this time to marshal support and awareness for the health struggles of Native people living in cities. But the health advocacy of Seattle's urban Indian community was not always so directly targeted at networks of authority, nor was it particularly well-coordinated before the 1970s. Indeed, Jeffries's appearance in Spokane came after at least twenty years of incremental political action that was often disparate, and at times, not even explicitly nor only about health. These early forms of political behavior were nonetheless needed before urban Indian health issues could be taken seriously later as a focal point of much more coordinated community action, particularly in the 1970s, when Seattle's urban Indian health movement arguably reached its zenith.

While the fundraising campaign for Ernie Crowfeather undoubtedly represented something of a pinnacle and galvanizing moment for Seattle's urban Indian health activists, it was only because less dramatic forms of community action around health care access had been ongoing in Seattle for some time by 1970 that Crowfeather's case reached such heights of public attention. Beyond the local news report that Jeffries mentioned in his statement to the public forum, Crowfeather's case received coverage in several publications over the course of the following year and even made the front page of the *New York Times* on October 24, 1971.[15] In 1972, Congress also referred to Crowfeather's case in their debates on amending laws that dealt with end-stage renal failure patients.[16] Indeed, there can be no doubt that Seattle's urban Indian health activists had self-consciously turned Crowfeather's case into a symbol of the larger health inequalities faced by urban Indians, not only in Seattle but across the nation. This, along with other strategic efforts in the 1970s, was eventually influential in discussions that led to both the formal establishment of the Seattle Indian Health Board in 1970, and to the implementation of the Indian Health Care Improvement Act in 1976.

In this chapter, I show the historical developments that built toward these two significant landmarks of urban Indian health activism in Seattle. To do this, I focus on highlighting the stories of numerous groups and individuals who acted—often in less public ways than Bill Jeffries—to improve the status of Native health in Seattle during the 1950s and '60s. In doing so, I bring our attention to forms of politically meaningful behavior and toward a period that is often overlooked in histories of American Indian political activism. I also recount the experiences of people like Ernie Crowfeather, whose personal stories bring the health struggles of postwar urban Indian communities to light. Though individual names are oftentimes obscured in the historical record, in the aggregate, firsthand accounts of Native people's experiences of medical care in the city, along with dire statistical data on the comparatively high rates of disease and morbidity within the urban Indigenous populace, reveals a collective struggle against significant health inequalities.

Visibility

Long before there was a Seattle Indian Health Board, and long before Bill Jeffries traveled to Spokane to speak before the NCIO, a small group of American Indian and Alaska Native women in Seattle served as the de facto social welfare providers for their community in the city. To be sure, American Indians and Alaska Natives who lived in Seattle at this time were eligible for social welfare benefits just like any other American citizen, but the reality was that these services rarely reached them in the postwar years. There was a great deal of uncertainty on the part of newly relocated Native people about exactly what was available to them in the cities, and as established in chapter 2, within the channels of government itself there was an equal amount of confusion over who was responsible for providing services to urban Indians. All this, on top of the cultural barriers and discrimination that oftentimes got in the way of access, meant that in times of need many Native families and individuals in Seattle drew on their community for support rather than the established social welfare infrastructure.

The important role that Native women played in providing this support in Seattle during the 1950s and 1960s was not atypical of the central role that Native women have long played, across rural and urban contexts throughout the United States, in generating and sustaining their communities' cultural and social lives.[17] Despite a wider (and growing) body of literature that centers Native women as historical and political actors, only a fraction of this scholarship has examined Native women's activism in the twentieth century, and it is virtually silent on activism in an urban context.[18] The editors of *Keeping the Campfires Going: Native Women's Activism in Urban Communities*—a short book published in 2009—made a notable intervention into this scholarly space.[19] The essays in this book did much to highlight Native women's activism in urban settings across the United States and Canada, and underscored the vital point that Indigenous women have not only been key political actors through direct participation in political and social movements, but also as keepers of tradition, educators of children, and leaders in city life. Additionally, contributors to this volume showed that Native women were often responsible for creating the networks and organizations that commonly became the backbones of urban Indigenous communities. The examples abound: women's activism and the Indian Community School of Milwaukee; women vendors, market art, and incipient political activism in Anchorage, Alaska; and the urban leadership of Native American women in Chicago and its American Indian Center.[20] More recently, scholars like Sarah Nickel and Sasha Maria Suarez, in their respective research on Indigenous women's political work in British Columbia, Canada, and the Twin Cities (Minneapolis-St. Paul), have gone further in deepening our understanding of just how central Indigenous women's activism has been in the course of twentieth-century Indigenous history in both the Canadian and US contexts.[21] Across these examples, we see that Native women were instrumental in shaping and sustaining their communities in cities, in mobilizing resources to benefit their communities, and in fighting the poverty and discrimination that too often afflicted urban Native peoples. The work of health activism, as both Brianna Theobald and Christine Taitano DeLisle have shown, has long been dominated by Indigenous women.[22] Whether it has been in the service of reproductive justice, health care access, child health, community nutrition, or even the most recent example of fighting COVID-19, Indigenous women have long been the caretakers of their communities' health.[23]

In Seattle, the actions and efforts of the American Indian Women's Service League (hereafter the Service League or AIWSL) during the 1950s and '60s precisely fit this mold. The Service League was initially a casual social group comprising American Indian and Alaska Native women living in Seattle. Most of the women had moved to the city shortly after World War II as part of a generation of American Indian veteran families who followed new economic opportunities in the cities. A few of the women had also come as young students, independent of their families, to pursue better educational opportunities in the city. Under the initiative of Pearl Warren, the women began meeting socially sometime in the early 1950s.

Although no official institutional history of the organization exists in publication, its storied past and community memories of its important work are still very much alive in the recorded oral histories of its founders, former members, and in the memories of scores of Native people in Seattle today. In an interview in 2001, Mary Jo Butterfield, daughter of Pearl Warren, recalled how her mother began the social club:

> When we first moved to Seattle I was in the 6th grade at the time and mom would get really lonesome for Indian people in the city. And so way back even then, she would go out and seek out Indian people. And when you're walking down the street you know when you're looking eye-to-eye to an Indian, and she'd say "Hi," and that's how she met [many of the women]. And it was through such hard times that many of them clung to each other. And the intimacy was there right from the beginning, just from a desire to have something of a family, more than anything else. They missed that.[24]

In the early days, these women (many of whom are pictured in figure 3.1)—Pearl Warren (Makah), Zena DeLorm (Clallam), Adeline Garcia (Haida), Dorothy Lombard (Clallam), Ella Aquino (Lummi), Meredith Mumey (Makah), and others—would meet for social activities in one another's homes.[25] According to Butterfield, by the mid-1950s, all the women in this initial circle of fast friends were married with children, and none worked outside the home.[26] Several of the founders were neighbors and lived in the same defense housing project, which made meeting up easy. At first, their gatherings were mostly an occasion to share news, cook together, and provide mutual support in difficult times. Among a few, friendships even dated back to boarding school days or were formed as young children when their families visited back and forth between neighboring reservations. But as Butterfield recalled, the women "were never a clique, they invited everyone."[27] And as their numbers quickly grew, the women started to view themselves more self-consciously as a group who volunteered their time and labor to helping their fellow Indians across the city "adjust themselves to urban living."[28] This volunteer work may have been as simple as waiting at the Greyhound bus station to greet new arrivals coming in from the reservations.[29] Oftentimes, it meant helping to familiarize these newly arrived individuals and families with the mainstream educational, social welfare, and health agencies that were meant to be at their disposal in the city.[30] As the group expanded and their work increased, the status of these early women as homemakers soon became an asset, as more and more of their activities centered on organizing events that would draw on skills they regularly exercised around the home—cooking and bookkeeping, and making ends meet.

According to Butterfield, by the mid-1950s the organization had organically found its primary social-service purpose. It started to function as a food bank and outreach organization—acquiring donations of food, clothing, eyeglasses, and other essentials from local churches, charities, and individuals, which the women then redistributed to Native people in need throughout Seattle. "And the more they did projects like this, the more they could see the need," Butterfield remembered.[31] Crucially though, community members didn't only benefit from the outreach and charity work that the Service League did. They also contributed to it, and in the process of volunteering their time or donating material items, they too forged the bonds of community among themselves, across the city. According to Butterfield, even "the men from the street" would often come along to sober up and keep themselves busy by helping out with collection and distribution services, and in return, they would get "a meal, a clean pair of pants and a shirt, a new pair of shoes, and even a box of groceries to take with them."[32] The vital effect of "all of this connection in the beginning," as Butterfield put it, was essential, not only to the basic sustenance and survival of the community but to its self-awareness.

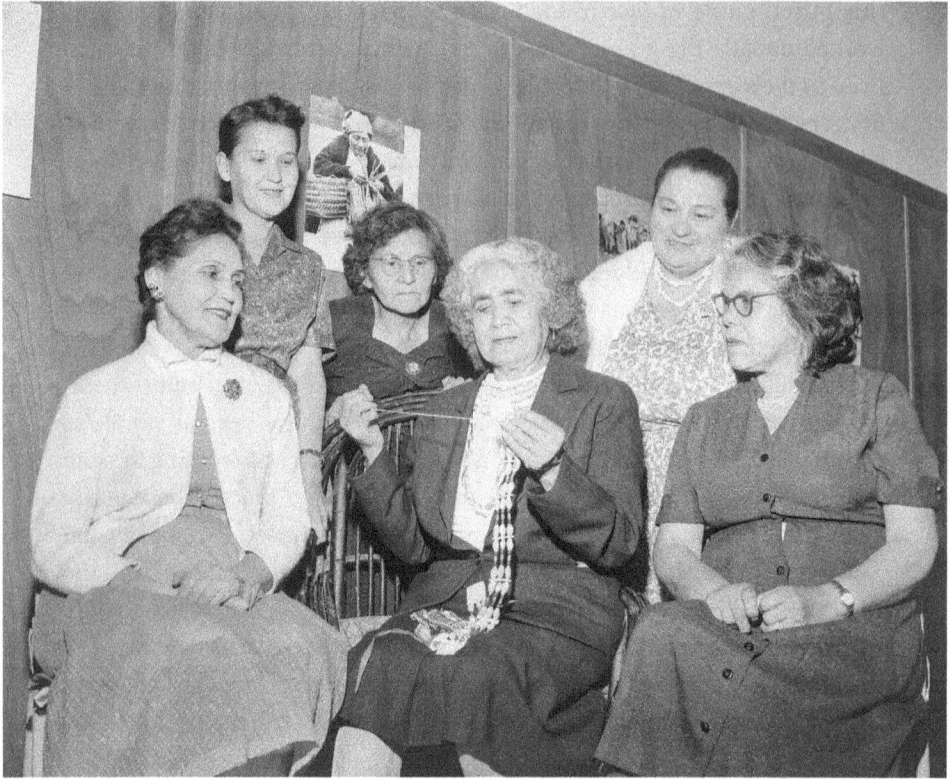

FIGURE 3.1 Martha John demonstrating Native American crafts, Seattle, August 16, 1960. In this image Martha John (*center*) demonstrates how to make a traditional shell-and-bead headband to five other women of the American Indian Women's Service League (*identified from left*): Leona Lyness, Dorothy Lombard, Ella Aquino, Pearl Warren, and Hazel Duarte. Photo courtesy of Museum of History and Industry, Seattle.

By 1958 the membership of the AIWSL had grown to about fifty, and it was around this time that the group decided to officially incorporate. What began as just a volunteer service among a growing circle of friends thus officially became a voluntary social service association with a formal charter. In the words of Pearl Warren, who served as the organization's director until 1971, the official mission of the AIWSL was "to make Indians part of the community they live in and to get non-Indians to recognize us as an Indian group."[33] In Seattle, where the problem of Indian "invisibility" was especially acute in the postwar period, many of the Service League's earliest acts of political advocacy for their community therefore amounted to what was essentially a politics of visibility: actions to simply show the presence of Native people in Seattle, and the creation of opportunities for this community to thrive and achieve a sense of self-awareness. As the rest of this chapter shows, many forms of urban Indian health activism between 1950 and 1970—by the AIWSL but also other organizations and individuals in the city—worked toward these ends. In terms of securing access to health care, establishing this visibility was indispensable as a first step on the road to substantiating their claims that the growing pan-Indian urban community in Seattle both deserved and needed specialized services and funding for an Indian health clinic.

Starting in the 1950s, many urban Indians in Seattle used various means to draw attention to the medical discrimination they faced as a cultural and ethnic group. Some of the earliest examples of this in the historical record come in the form of reports by Bureau of Indian Affairs (BIA) officials. Numerous reports by BIA officers referred to Native people who were returning to their reservations from the city because of health problems and an inability to access services in Seattle. The Urban Indian Relocation Program required "returnees" to file exit reports if they wanted to quit the relocation program and return home for any reason. A survey of the case files reveals a notable number of returnees who cited a medical or health-related cause in their exit reports. For example, on December 8, 1958, Samuel E. Miller reported that he and his entire family were returning to their reservation due to his "shoulder injury."[34] The reporting officer noted that Miller had been unsuccessful in getting treatment for his injury and that it was interfering with his employment. Another example was Gerald R. Edwards, who in May 1962 filed an exit report with the agency to return his entire family to the reservation because of "illness in the family." He "lacked the funds" to pay for his spouse and children to receive care, and thus they had decided to "return to destination."[35] Other cases reflected a preference for medical care at home on the reservation: for example, Joan M. Finkbonner, a single female relocatee, filed her report to return to her reservation because she had "developed an allergy" and had "preferred to return home for required skin treatments."[36] Other times, the reports contained very little information other than simply the words "sickness" or "illness" in the description. In these cases, we can assume that had the returnees been able to get adequate care for their health issues in the cities, they would likely have stayed.

In 1957, BIA relocation officer Fred H. Claymore therefore reported to C. W. Ringley, the superintendent of the Western Washington Agency, that "several families have contacted me over the last few months to provide notification of their return."[37] The reasons they cited, he reported, "include an alarming number of illnesses."[38] In some cases, it appeared that Indian families reported to Claymore that they simply preferred to receive treatment "at home."[39] But for others, there seemed to be a subtext of neglect or mistreatment by mainstream medical services: "Others apparently cannot access medical care without significant trouble."[40] Similar issues were hinted at in a report by the relocation officer at the BIA office in Portland when he made note of several inquiries from Indian families in Seattle, Spokane, and other neighboring cities, about the availability of BIA funds to support travel back to their reservations for "medical reasons."[41]

These subtle references in the BIA reports suggest not only the BIA's disinclination toward controversy but also Native peoples' reluctance at the time to make direct accusations about health discrimination—which we also saw in Jeffries's diplomatic language about Crowfeather's case—especially in official settings. As we saw, Jeffries was very particular about noting that although the American Indian community in Seattle had the "impression" that Crowfeather was being discriminated against by the medical system, they couldn't offer any evidence of this: "This is the impression that the secretary had, Mr. Jim, but she doesn't have it—she can't quote them exactly in saying that 'because he's an Indian if we don't have the funds he's just going to die—we're going to turn him out.'"[42] By comparison, we can contrast this to the much more unequivocal personal memories of community members who recall learning about Crowfeather's case from other community members in the 1970s: "There was no question among us, we Indians in the community felt that Ernie Crowfeather was being discriminated against," remembered Dr. Walt Hollow (Assiniboine-Sioux).[43]

Second, if we take into account that people may have feared potential costs in speaking up about mistreatment, then this also makes a certain amount of discretion understandable in official settings. In writing about the widespread experiences of Native American women who endured unauthorized sterilization practices in the 1970s, Jane Lawrence takes up this issue of reticence when explaining why so few Native women spoke up about their experiences at the time.[44] Lawrence found that women were often fearful their recriminations might jeopardize their receipt of government benefits; hence they were particularly reluctant to speak up about their experiences in more formal or official settings. A hint of this kind of worry is also evident in Jeffries's comments to Mr. Jim: he mentioned at one point that "the American Indian Women's Service League there in Seattle is concerned about giving out this idea because if it gets back it could hinder Mr. Crowfeather."[45]

If people were reticent with government officials, they were often far more forthright with journalists about the prevalence of medical discrimination against Native people. In an investigative report written for the *Seattle Times*, journalist Shelby Gilie exposed the gravity of medical discrimination that was still being faced by Native people in Seattle as late as 1971. She conducted numerous "off the record" interviews with medical providers and also spoke with members of the Muckleshoot tribe living in the city. Her article revealed a spectrum of medical discrimination faced by Native people in the city, including outright refusals to treat them on the part of doctors, and racist assumptions about the causes of their health problems. On the one hand, many doctors reportedly declined to serve Native people at all because—for reasons that were unclear in Gilie's report—they claimed this often entailed more work: "The Muckleshoots say doctors do not want them as patients because it often means extra work in filling out [BIA] forms."[46] On the other hand, the medical personnel whom Gilie spoke with on a "don't quote me basis" often revealed more blatant prejudice: "The fact is that some doctors just don't want Indians sitting around their waiting rooms. They don't want that type of clientele."[47] As this statement might suggest, a great deal of discrimination and mistreatment also came from stereotyped attitudes about the causes of Native health problems. One medical professional shared the following remarks with Gilie: "And lets [sic] say an Indian comes in for a checkup with liquor on his breath. Right away everybody sees the stereotype of 'those drunken Indians,' if they'd just leave the bottle alone they wouldn't have medical problems."[48] Discriminatory attitudes on the part of medical providers, if ever expressed so openly, rarely made their way into the historical record in such explicit terms. More often, as was the case with Ernie Crowfeather, the lines between outright discrimination, insufficient resources, and bureaucratic confusion were frequently—and often strategically—blurred. As one of Gilie's interviewees revealed, doctors would often mask their prejudice behind the excuse of insufficient resources: "Many doctors do not want them [Indians] as patients, but instead health-care professionals say there is a shortage of physicians in the area, and that many doctors are refusing all new patients."[49] Hence the written record is replete with examples of Native patients suspecting that they had encountered discrimination and neglect in the medical system but never quite being sure. One woman wrote into the *Indian Center News* in 1967 and asked fellow readers from the community to share their experiences about "finding a doctor." As she put it, she was "having some difficulty in finding a doctor that would be willing to see me as they all decline to take on new clients." And so she wondered, "Are other Indians out there finding similar difficulties?"[50] While such forms of evidence might suggest that the primary form of Native health advocacy was to speak up in quite public ways about the medical discrimination they faced in cities (alerting relevant authorities in the BIA, or speaking to the press), private forms of awareness-raising—even simple conversations between friends—conceivably did more to increase the visibility of urban Indian health struggles.

When community members encountered discriminatory attitudes or found themselves in circumstances of severe medical neglect, often the first thing they did was speak to each other about these experiences. In doing so, they began to create patterns of community behavior and acts of resistance that eventually became visible to the government and to medical authorities. For instance, community members might tell each other about which doctors to avoid at the hospital, or else they might simply warn each other about issues to be wary of within mainstream medical services to avoid reproach. Common warnings included caution about the enforcement of certain restrictions against visitors and visiting hours, or rules against the performance of cultural ceremonies in the hospital. In an interview in 2000, founding AIWSL member Adeline Garcia recalled how the women of the Service League would "hear about bad stories at the hospital, and we would know to tell others to be prepared."[51] The reverse was also true: if people had good experiences with certain doctors, they would also share this information with each other, and so this, according to Garcia, was how certain doctors got reputations for being "friendly to the Indians."[52]

Although such conversations were private for the most part, thus leaving few traces in the written record, they nonetheless produced an observable effect that did leave a mark: By the late 1960s, it was commonly reported in government hearings, medical studies, and in newspapers that urban Indians were "reluctant to seek medical care" in the cities.[53] During the 1968–69 Urban Indian Hearings held by the NCIO, one Native woman from Phoenix, who was a nurse, noted this reluctance: "Indians are a little bit apprehensive about coming to our hospital because they are a little bit afraid of how they will be treated."[54] In 1968, Don Hannula of the *Seattle Times* reported on the reluctant care-seeking behaviors of Native people in Seattle, attributing this to the prevalence of discrimination in the medical system: "There is a growing but still small number of Indian activists who are beginning to equate many of their problems with Negroes: as one of color."[55] Numerous medical reports from the 1960s also noted how "the Indians seem to avoid seeking medical care unless absolutely necessary because many are wary of the lack of respect their people seem to meet in the medical services."[56] Just below the surface of these observations about the hesitant care-seeking behavior of Native people was, of course, a suggestion that the community was already highly wary at the outset about the use of mainstream health services. This wariness was the result of private acts of information-sharing and awareness-raising within their own community, mostly taking place out of view of the historical record, but which nonetheless produced forms of resistance that would become visible to outsiders in the recognition of this "hesitance" or "reluctance." By the late 1960s, these quieter forms of health advocacy, perhaps more so than public statements about medical mistreatment, had laid the basis for making the health struggles of urban Indians visible to the wider community of Seattle.

Individuals who spoke up both publicly and privately about medical discrimination left an important imprint on their community in the short term by empowering others with the information to engage in protective forms of behavior, such as only seeking out "friendly doctors." Important as this was, as a strategy for creating long-lasting and communitywide change, there was only so much that such disparate and uncoordinated efforts could do. Much more effective in the long term was the kind of visibility and momentum for change that publicity about a case like Ernie Crowfeather's created—not only for the health struggles of urban Indians in Seattle but across the nation. Indeed, insofar as Seattle's Native community was instrumental in agitating for the Indian Health Care Improvement Act in 1976, one might also say that by politicizing the Seattle community, Crowfeather's case was of paramount importance to the advancement of urban Indian health nationwide.

As discussed at the start of this chapter, Crowfeather's case certainly received a lot of public and media attention across the nation in 1970 and 1971. In the end, Pearl Warren and the Kinatechitapi Indian Council took on the task of raising money to pay for Crowfeather's dialysis, using publicity and drawing on help wherever they could find it. In one of their most public campaigns they called on Sonny Sixkiller (Cherokee), then a University of Washington quarterback, who dedicated a game to Crowfeather, and during which he made a heartfelt speech at halftime to solicit donations for the "Ernie Crowfeather Fund."[57] Other publicity and fundraising drives initiated by the community included a partnership with Seattle's Sterling Theater chain, which agreed to donate a "substantial portion of proceeds" from the new movie *Flap* to the Ernie Crowfeather Fund; the AIWSL also formed a committee to go around the city with "coffee cans, collecting nickels and dimes"; the community coordinated with schools to host fundraising events like concerts and craft fairs; and they also targeted the press by writing into various newspapers, appealing directly to readers.[58] As we saw through Bill Jeffries's appearance at the NCIO forum, the community also reached out to national tribal leaders and community members on Crowfeather's behalf and used these dialogues to initiate a broader conversation about the generally poor state of Native health in cities and the dearth of resources to address their problems.[59]

This kind of public attention continued after Crowfeather died in 1971—sadly, though the community managed to raise the $20,000 to keep him alive for a year, after this money ran out, Ernie Crowfeather took his own life by refusing further life-supporting therapy. In the wake of his death, it was reported on the front page of the *New York Times* that "during his two years on the artificial kidney, Ernie's case raised virtually every awesome question that could come up in the application of such costly sophisticated medical care for a person with a devastating illness— questions, basically, of who can be saved and who must die."[60] Even today, Crowfeather's struggle is commonly remembered in Seattle as *the* turning point that put the health struggles of the city's Native community on the map. For instance, Dr. Walt Hollow recalled how for him and many other community members at the time, "we felt that Ernie Crowfeather was being discriminated against. . . . I think the key is that the Indian community felt that, and when they looked at Indian health problems and issues not being properly funded, it was just the fuel at the right time to bring political pressure on the fact that there was an Indian health care need that needed to be met. Something needed to be done about it, and I think Ernie Crowfeather's health issues helped at the time."[61]

Yet even within the community itself, Crowfeather's case could not have garnered the kind of attention it did without several essential preconditions that primed the community—both Indigenous and non-Indigenous—in Seattle to rally around his cause. First, as discussed above—the early public and private reporting, which highlighted the prevalence of medical discrimination and neglect afflicting Seattle's Native community in the 1950s and 1960s. Without these early cases of people speaking up and the community knowledge about medical mistreatment that this behavior created, when Crowfeather's case came along in 1970, it might have appeared, even to Seattle's Indian community, to be an anomaly. As it was, when knowledge of Crowfeather's case started to circulate within the community in the late 1960s, this appeared as only the latest and most egregious case in a long line of problematic encounters with mainstream medical services.

A second factor that allowed Seattle's Indian community to come together over Crowfeather's case was simply a sense of community in and of itself— something that was largely absent in 1950 but which by 1970 had been created by the purposeful actions of early community advocates like the AIWSL. And finally, a third element that was crucial in elevating Crowfeather's case, and in galvanizing the community over health issues in general, was the community-driven amassing of health data. By 1970, this information could serve as evidence that Crowfeather's case was representative of a larger problem, and it also proved vital in later attempts to set up an Indian clinic.

As discussed above, prominent community advocates like Adeline Garcia spearheaded efforts to gather information that would be useful for community members, particularly newcomers to the city, so they would know what to be wary of (prohibitions on certain ceremonies in hospitals, etc.) and where to go for reliable help—medical and otherwise ("friendly doctors," the AIWSL, etc.).[62] This form of fact-collecting, primarily aimed at community members, was also accompanied by efforts to collect information about the community itself and its various needs, so that Seattle's urban Indian leaders could be empowered to pursue specific goals and make informed decisions about precisely what was needed to help their people. This latter practice—information-gathering about the community itself— was a form of political activity that would become especially instrumental as a tool of health activism once the community decided to work toward the creation of an Indian clinic. For example, knowing which doctors were "friendly" to Indians proved to be highly valuable information once the community sought volunteer doctors to work at the Indian clinic. Having the knowledge about what health issues disproportionately afflicted their people also allowed representatives of the community to speak authoritatively to journalists, potential funders, or government representatives about the state of their community's health. This was vital as the community began more actively pursuing permanent sources of funding to support their Indian health clinic in the early 1970s, given that the writing of grant proposals and reports required this data.[63]

The techniques of information-gathering that community leaders eventually used for the purposes of establishing their health clinic began with work that the Service League women had started in the 1950s. Many of the Service League women recalled the experience of going door-to-door "looking for Indians."[64] Sometimes, as Butterfield remembered, her mother would just walk up to people on the street and ask them if they knew any Indians, "and then she'd go find them to see what they needed."[65] From this fairly basic practice of fact-gathering at a face-to-face and informal level, ever more sophisticated and organized channels grew for acquiring information about their community. One of the Service League's best instruments for soliciting information was their monthly newspaper, the *Indian Center News*. As its inaugural issue revealed in 1960, the publication fancied itself almost as a community message board, hence it underscored the role it sought to play as both a collector and disseminator of information about Natives in the Pacific Northwest: "We want you, we ask you, we invite you to submit to us your thoughts and opinions on issues, relating to Indian affairs. We want you to feel that this paper is yours."[66] And crucially, it also expressed a hope that this information would reach readers far and wide: "Our purpose will be to keep all interested persons informed of Indian affairs both on and off the reservations."[67] While not all information that was sought concerned health, it was nonetheless a common topic: a survey of all its publications in the first year of circulation reveals that the *Indian Center News* included stories on health-related topics in every single issue.[68]

In addition to seeking information in these ways, starting in the early 1960s, and as the community became more self-aware, it also began drawing on existing information networks, particularly parent-teacher associations and local school boards, in order to find out about problems that were affecting their community.[69] As I discuss later, it was through such education-based information networks that the community eventually came to learn about the disproportionately high rates of absenteeism among Native school children across Seattle due to "untreated illness."[70] As numerous community members recalled during oral history interviews in 2000 and 2013, this information highlighted the medical neglect of their children and ultimately fueled the movement to establish an Indian clinic in the late 1960s.[71]

Finally, in areas where informational networks did not already exist, the AIWSL increasingly sought to create their own channels for data collection by establishing specific subgroups, or "committees," within their organization, whose specific role was to find important data about their people. Prominent health-related subgroups within the AIWSL included the Hospital Committee, which worked to locate Native patients in hospitals and to organize an Indian Blood Bank Drive; and the Health and Welfare

Committee, whose job it was to "find and help any Indian family in need of temporary help."[72] Other subgroups within the organization included the Clothing Committee, the Indian Education Committee, the Civic Unity Committee, and the Youth Activities Committee; but it is worth noting here that among all the subgroups, the health-related committees became most active in this period, perhaps indicating a singular importance of health issues within the community at this time. These groups tapped into informal and formal networks ranging from the friends and family of hospital patients to the hospital staff themselves in order to keep a running list of Indians who were ill or in hospital in the city, and who might need care in the form of visitors, financial assistance, or donated blood. They then published this information in the *Indian Center News*. For example, in February 1963, the *Indian Center News* announced that "the following patients are at the US Public Health Hospital, Seattle Washington, and would love to be visited by you: Frances Bowechop (Quinault), Mason Pickernell (Quinault), Edward Edwards (Skagit), Paul Smith (Lapwai), Lawrence Sampson (Warm Springs)."[73] Later that year, the newspaper also made an appeal based on their findings about a continued shortage of blood donors: "The AIWSL is continuing to sponsor a blood bank for Indian patients in local hospitals. Anyone eligible to donate blood may do so at Perry Avenue and Madison Street Blood Bank in Seattle. Be sure to stipulate that the blood you give is to be accredited to the Indian Women's Service League Pool. Your donation will sincerely be appreciated by many people."[74]

Over time, the importance of community-led fact-gathering became amplified as Seattle's urban Indians sought to gain increasing visibility and support for their health goals from the municipal and federal governments. By 1970, as the mantle of community leadership was passing from the Service League women to a younger cohort of leaders comprised of people like Bernie Whitebear, Luana Reyes, and Elizabeth Morris, an important initiative was launched by these new leaders to count their own population numbers in the city. Since community members knew that official government census numbers could never reflect the true size of their population, issuing their own demographic data was seen to be a crucial project if their community was to successfully negotiate with the government.[75] As Ralph Forquera (Juaneño Band of California Mission Indians), former executive director of the Seattle Indian Health Board, explained it to me, "The early community leaders knew that something as critical as census numbers could not be left to the government. Whatever they found was not going to be reflective of the true facts on the ground."[76] Attesting to the difficulties of accurately "counting Indians" even today, Forquera explained how the lasting impact of the boarding school experiences still affects people's willingness to disclose their heritage: "Today, many Americans who carry Indian blood often carry scars from past experiences. It is not uncommon to hear Indian people say their parents or grandparents discouraged them from talking about their Indian heritage. We recognize the reluctance many have to accept their Indianness today."[77] In addition to the issue of people misrepresenting their ethnicity to census officers, there was also the matter of their population being indigent and transitory. A proposal brief submitted for funding to support the Indian health clinic in 1971 explained this difficulty of counting their exact population numbers, and thus underscored the importance of having Native people be responsible for collecting information about their own community: "It has been estimated that there are approximately 12,000 American Indians and Alaskan Natives residing in the metropolitan area of Seattle. The precise number is elusive because of the widely distributed and often times reluctant population. Some of Seattle's most economically deprived people are found in this population. Some are migrant workers who live in Seattle for short periods of time, many are disenfranchised Indians who are relocated by the Bureau of Indian Affairs and lost their Indian Health benefits as a result of being off the reservation."[78]

Taking these considerations into account, by the late 1960s, community leaders therefore made a point of collecting and publishing their own data. Sometimes, they cited these data in interviews with the press: in 1970 Pearl Warren related to the *Seattle Post-Intelligencer* that "3,917 Indians" were offered emergency medical care by the community in 1969.[79] Most commonly, the data they collected concerned the health, legal, or educational status of their people. For example, in March 1970 the *Indian Center News* announced the publication of the AIWSL's "legal pamphlets" and advertised that "members of the legal committee will be available to speak to groups in the Seattle area concerning the pamphlet information."[80] Crucial for their funding appeals to support better Indian health care in the city, we can also note that by the time of the 1970 census, while the Seattle-King County Indian population was officially estimated at 7,391 by the US Census Bureau, the community was citing a figure closer to 20,000.[81] Such huge discrepancies could translate into very different outcomes as far as funding was concerned, and so the importance of fact-collecting as an act of political empowerment and creating visibility only increased for Seattle's urban Indians as time wore on and as they increasingly sought federal funds. Confirming the importance of having these facts on hand, Marilyn

Bentz of the AIWSL encountered the following advice from Edmund J. Wood, special assistant to Seattle's mayor, Wes Uhlman, in 1971: "I guess what I was really trying to get across the other night was that the battle for funding of Indian programs is much more likely to be productive if waged with facts, figures, and proposals. As you know, this is the language of administrators. If the ability to communicate in that language can be created from the Indian point of view, I think the Indian community will be far ahead."[82]

These practices of fact-gathering meant that by the time Ernie Crowfeather's case presented itself to the community, his advocates also had strategic use for a face and a name that could lend their raw data a human element and make the community's attempts at visibility that much more successful in the 1970s. Crowfeather's Indian heritage thus became the fulcrum of the public fundraising campaign launched by Pearl Warren and the Kinatechitapi Indian Council. When seeking the support of other Native people—whether on or off reservations—and when trying to engage the sympathies of the wider non-Native community, Crowfeather's supporters made his Indian identity the dominant theme of their campaigns and used the attention they drew through Crowfeather's case to highlight the broader health inequalities afflicting their community. As one of Crowfeather's supporters recalled, "I think the Ernie Crowfeather campaign probably did more to solidify the urban Indian community than any other single incident I can remember. . . . And I think the public, in general, learned something that most of them didn't know, which was that Indians all over the city were suffering."[83]

As critical as these facts and data became, perhaps the most obvious way in which Seattle's Indian community made itself visible to outsiders and forged the bonds of community was through various forms of community-building. Essentially, all of the work done by the AIWSL served this purpose—the very act of forming the AIWSL, and the connections the women created through their food and clothing donations, were some of the earliest activities that helped Seattle's urban Indians to know and to find each other.[84] Yet even their practice of door-knocking, in which the women essentially acted as early "surveyors" and informal census takers of their own community, marked the contours of their community in the city and worked to make the community self-aware and hence visible to itself as well as others. Community newspapers like the *Indian Center News* and the *Northwest Indian News* were critical in this respect as well, allowing urban Indians to develop a sense of their "imagined community" and to directly communicate with each other through the monthly community news and contributor column, "From the Teepees."[85] Indeed, as the community started to become more self-aware, it increasingly organized events that not only drew the attention of the wider population to the active and distinctive presence of an urban pan-Indigenous community in Seattle, but which also increasingly sought to include non-Indians too. This underscores that most Native people, if nothing else, drew attention to the presence of their community in Seattle by participating in cultural events such as powwows and potlatches. A key example of such an event was the annual salmon bake held at Alki Point and organized by the AIWSL, which started it in the late 1950s as a way of bringing the community together over a meal; eventually it opened up to the wider public as a means of raising funds for their organization and other community events and causes.[86]

By providing opportunities for Seattle's wider community to see the vibrancy and diversity of the city's Native community, public cultural events did so much more than just increase the visibility of the city's growing pan-Indian community. Crucially, these events also helped to break the kind of stereotypes that were behind much of the medical discrimination that Natives received in the city. Moreover, these events gave lie to the false premises of assimilationist government policies because they showed how invested members of this growing diasporic community were in maintaining both their distinct individual cultures and in taking on newer forms of shared pan-Indian identity that grew from their urban context. For example, cultural gatherings like powwows and the AIWSL's annual salmon bake provided an occasion for families and communities that were "biresidential" (families that were split between reservation and the city) to come together; that is, relations from reservations would often come into the city to attend cultural events like the salmon bake and connect with friends and family. For the wider community who perhaps knew little about the urban Indigenous community in Seattle, this highlighted what was possibly the least observable—yet not the least important—way in which many urban Indian Seattleites acted politically, on a daily basis, to contest the idea that by moving to the cities they had somehow abandoned their Native culture and identities and all ties to reservation life. Not all, but many diasporic urban Indians lived then (as now) in ways that constantly connected and cut across the boundaries of city and reservation economic, cultural, and political life. A key example of this was hinted at in Bill Jeffries's comments before the NCIO's public forum. As both he and Mr. Old Person suggested, there was nothing unusual about the fact that Jeffries was there to appeal to the tribal communities for help. Indeed, Mr. Old Person's remarks would seem to suggest that in the absence of a formal system to cater specifically to urban Indian health, funding from tribal networks served as a de facto support system for Indian health in the cities.[87] By simply continuing to live in ways that blurred the distinction between reservation and city life, diasporic urban Indians on a daily basis acted politically by giving lie to the government's insistence that because they resided in the city, they should be completely assimilated and hence could be regarded and treated just like any other citizen—or minority, for that matter.

Understanding how the Indigenous community in Seattle engaged in these early forms of health activism through a politics of visibility is essential for any attempt to understand how this community was eventually able to push for the establishment of a dedicated Indian health clinic in the city that drew on federal funds. In the context of the US federal government's "termination" policies, which actively sought to erase all lines of cultural, social, and political distinction between Native people who opted into an urban lifestyle and the many other residents of major cities across the United Sates, Indigenous people in Seattle faced an uphill battle in any attempt to assert their distinctiveness as a community. Part of that challenge involved resisting forces—requirements attached to government funding streams, for instance—that threatened to fold them into the institutional and political spaces of other minority groups. Public cultural events such as the AIWSL's salmon bake and other acts of community-building like their newsletters and food collection work were thus indispensable steps in the avowal of their existence and distinctive identity as a community. And in their struggles to access health care in particular, it is clear that by speaking up about mistreatment and neglect—even if only to each other— and by actively collecting data about their experiences in mainstream health services, urban Indigenous people in Seattle armed themselves with evidence and knowledge that would later prove essential. This was especially true as the goal to establish a dedicated Indian health clinic moved more firmly into the sights of a younger generation of activists.

Space

One of the earliest occurrences that made it clear to Seattle's urban Indian leaders that their community required a clinic of their own came from the repeated experiences that their people had in being rejected from mainstream medical clinics and hospitals. In large part, these rejections were due to health providers either falsely assuming that all Native people could access health care from the government-run Indian Health Service (IHS) facilities, or else claiming such ignorance as a mask for their bigotry. In the 1950s and '60s, countless stories and frustrations were shared, in public and in private, by urban Indians who went to seek medical assistance from mainstream providers, only to get turned away because the doctors and medical staff said they were entitled to care on their reservations through the IHS. Speaking to a reporter from the *Seattle Times* in 1967, Pearl Warren explained the difficulty: "When a nonreservation Indian goes to an agency for assistance, they see that he is an Indian and send him to the BIA. At the BIA, he is told that since he does not live on the reservation, he cannot be helped. In addition, not living on the reservation, he has no spokesman or organization he can talk to like the tribal council."[88] This experience was such a common occurrence, it was referred to colloquially within the community as the phenomenon of being "ping-ponged," and it also became the subject of a well-known joke that circulated in the 1960s about an urban Indian seeking a room at a hospital: "Did you hear the one about the Indian who couldn't get a room? He didn't have a reservation."[89] In 1973, the authors of *The People Speak, Will You Listen?* summed up the problem in their report to the State of Washington: "Most non-Indian health agency personnel mistakenly believe that Indian people are provided with health care through the BIA or Indian Health Service (IHS) even after they leave the reservations and on that basis have denied Indians the health care they were seeking."[90] This was not a problem unique to Seattle's urban Indian community. Reports from almost every state represented at the NCIO's public hearings on urban Indian issues in the late 1960s made mention of this problem.[91]

These experiences, and the problematic fact that Native people had nowhere to congregate socially in the city, lead Pearl Warren and the AIWSL to pursue the establishment of a multipurpose Indian center in 1960. Early proposals for funding to get the center off the ground described the political significance of creating such a space for Seattle's Indian community in one of two ways. On the one hand, community advocates stressed that this was a matter of preventing social isolation: "Probably no white American can feel the real force of the reason behind an Indian Center. There was no place the Indian could go in Seattle. Bars yes; friends [*sic*] homes, maybe. But no club, no meeting place, nowhere a newcomer could go to be with his own people and his own culture."[92] Implicit within this demand for a social space was also a critique of the federal government's expectation that Native people would benefit from the existing infrastructure to which they were, at least in principle, free to draw on for support and services. For instance, it was often expected that schools and employment would allow Native people to integrate socially and economically in the cities. But often these were the spaces where Native people most actively encountered exclusion: Speaking to the *Seattle Post-Intelligencer* a year after the Seattle Indian Center was established, Native student George Abbott explained that "he began going to the Indian Center to meet friends because of the social cliques in high school and the ego-hang-up of so many white students."[93] In the same article, another man reported that although he was a high school graduate and spent eleven months in the air force, "he could only get clean-up jobs in Seattle."[94]

In addition to combatting the issue of social isolation, community advocates also explained the significance of the Seattle Indian Center by drawing attention to the high social and health costs of their community members not having any places to go in the city. Most visibly, as members of the Service League explained, this problem manifested in a widespread practice of congregating on the streets:

> From before the time of the white man the area around Pioneer Square was a gathering place for Indians. As civilization advanced, they continued to gather there . . . once in the heart of Seattle's busy, growing business community, and as the years passed, in a decaying area that until recently supported little more than pawn shops and taverns. This STREET-SIDE gathering place has for years been a festering sore in this community, for often it has not only been a meeting place of the habitués of such spots, but the ONLY place for a young Indian, a family with small children, an elderly Indian needing physical help or hunting a job, to find people of his own race.[95]

When talks about an Indian center began, it was therefore initially conceived of as "an Indian Hospitality and Referral Center."[96] As Pearl Warren clarified to a reporter at the *Seattle Post-Intelligencer*, it was never intended to be "a reservation right in the middle of town."[97] Its ambitions were never meant to be radically separatist in a political sense, but rather as she explained, "we just wanted a place to call our own," to provide a space where Indians could "feel free and proud to be themselves" since there was no real venue for this in the city.[98] Unsurprisingly therefore, recollections of the center's initial location at 2604 1st Avenue, and then when it moved in 1964 to a converted church at 1900 Boren Avenue, portrayed a warm and inviting atmosphere and a space that was always populated with children due to the preschool program and tutoring service for high school students.[99] The presence of children at the center was always an important goal, Warren explained, because of the Service League's ambition to "make Indians part of the community they live in." The center was therefore created with the intention that it would "let our children grow to have pride in the fact they are Indian."[100]

From a practical standpoint, the center also served as a base of operations for the Service League's growing line of charity and outreach work. Indeed, the multipurpose nature of the center was taken as a hallmark of its "unique position": early AIWSL funding applications described it as "a center for social, educational, cultural and recreational activities; to collect and distribute clothing and other supplies in emergency situations; and to educate the white community in regard to Indian problems."[101] All at once, the Indian center thus functioned as a vital community social space, a place to access basic welfare services provided by the community, and it also acted as a vehicle for making others in the city more aware, more knowledgeable, and more accepting about the existence of Seattle's Native community. Without question, it therefore represented a political space: its primary purpose was to enable Seattle's growing pan-Indian community to develop in ways that facilitated their aspirations for self-determination. Pearl Warren encapsulated the essence of this aspiration in a lengthy message on the center's fifth-year anniversary in 1965:

> For too long we have depended upon the non-Indians to do for us, the time has come when we must start doing more for ourselves and each other. Especially since we are all the same, all North American Indians, no matter where we go or what we do our heritage will not change. A most pitiful person is one who doesn't want to acknowledge his Indian ancestry because he is afraid of not being accepted by society. Our Indian teachings say if someone cannot accept you as you then they are not worth knowing. By trying to hide their Indian ancestry, some Indians cheat themselves of a wonderful proud feeling for something that is not worthwhile and that doesn't bring true happiness.[102]

Having an Indian center that served multiple purposes was indeed not unusual in cities with a sizable Native population: cities such as Los Angeles, Minneapolis, and Chicago were known for having substantial and successful Indian centers that served as both a central meeting place and a source of cultural as well as socioeconomic support.[103] The significance of these Indian centers across the nation was stressed in 1969 by Jess Sixkiller of the American Indians United (a group established to represent all urban Indians): Sixkiller pointed out that "at this time, there are over sixty-five [Indian centers] in forty-one states," and sometimes, these represent the only place an Indian can go "just to be Indian."[104]

Two things made the center in Seattle stand out, however. For one, when it first opened in 1960, the Service League women proudly proclaimed that "the Seattle Indian Center occupies a unique position not only in our community, but in the United States—the only organization of its kind, run not only for Indians, but entirely by Indians."[105] Also, the memories of the early Service League women attest to the important "healing and recovery" function that the center soon started to provide for the more disadvantaged members of their community. For instance, Mary Jo Butterfield recalled how "that's what the downstairs was for—the men would come in and sober up and sleep and get some rest from living on the street."[106] In other words, within months of opening its doors, the center found that one of its main roles was to provide shelter and a basic meal for community members in desperate need. The natural extension of this sheltering role, which materialized within months, was a rudimentary health service providing basic care, referrals, and first aid. When combined with the ethic of self-help—"services by and for Indians"—that was so central to the ethos of the Indian center and which had been the modus operandi for the AIWSL all along, we can see the seeds of the Indian health clinic that were sown in these early experiences. Creating a community space like the multipurpose center—which although not owned by the community, was under their exclusive control and direction—was an important first step in the political work of redefining Native sovereignty as a nonterritorial goal; that is, the demand for a comprehensive Indian clinic in later years can be viewed as a more developed iteration of this early aspiration to foster self-determination for diasporic Native peoples through the Indian Center—a place that their community controlled but that was not governed by any one tribal nation.[107]

While first aid, referral, and emergency services were assets to the community for many years, the urgent need for a more comprehensive health service soon became apparent when this makeshift, basic clinic started receiving cases more serious than it could handle, and when it also became clear from the people coming in for this more serious care that they were unable to get their health needs met elsewhere in the city. In 2000, Adeline Garcia recalled one particular case, that prompted her and Pearl Warren to pursue the idea of an Indian clinic:

Then one day, we had a boy who came in and he was cut real bad. Down to the bone. Gives me chills still now. And he was getting real bad. His fingers were getting green, gangrene you know? So I told Pearl, and she called someone, who came to look at it, and cleaned up the wound and gave him antibiotics. I don't know where he stayed, but he told us he couldn't get medicine anywhere else. He would come in, you know he said he had an aunt, but I don't think he did. He would come in the mornings when we opened up, and he slept in the basement. And that was the first time we had to deal with that you know? So Pearl and I were talking about it, and we sort of thought, well we have to do something about it. We should really have a clinic. Just a walk-in clinic.[108]

The early experiences of the AIWSL's simple health service therefore revealed that generic "poverty" programs established as part of the War on Poverty, though intended to meet the needs of Native people in the city, were falling far short. This reflected the experiences of urban Indians across the nation, as a 1970 report by the National American Indian Council revealed: "Federal anti-poverty funds are available for the poor, not for one or two specific poor ethnic groups. We are the poorest, the most neglected, the most destitute of all minority groups. These programs are not enough for our people. We feel that the federal government owes us more than our fair share now, so that it can make up for its years of neglect and indifference."[109] Moreover, Native leaders across the nation drew attention to the problems of access that their people faced within poverty programs due to their small numbers: "The Poor Peoples' Campaign is an example of what happens to Indian people—they get pushed aside because there are too few of them."[110] Speaking about this problem at a press conference in Seattle, Bernie Whitebear (Colville) made the following statement in 1971: "We're at the bottom of the minority totem pole. We have no programs to solve our problems."[111] In part, the insufficiency of mainstream services was due to the problems described above—confusion or misunderstanding on the part of medical providers about the eligibility of all Indians for IHS care, discrimination against Indians seeking care, competition with "larger" minority groups, or lack of knowledge among Indians about the availability of mainstream services. The other part of this equation was cultural, however: Native people reported feeling alienated by the clinical and impersonal settings provided by mainstream services and were put off by the fact that their cultural needs—such as for certain ceremonies to be performed before medical procedures—were not accommodated by mainstream facilities. A leaflet introducing the Seattle Indian Center in later years would make reference to this issue: "Although there may be sources for help, the Indians often have no way to know about them, or they are reluctant or unable to tell their troubles to strangers not of their own race or culture."[112] Crucial to the community's engagements with what I call a "politics of space" was therefore a critique of assimilationist policies that assumed Indian health needs *could* be met by services, funds, and institutional bodies set aside for either low-income groups or other minority groups in the city.

As we saw, the solutions many people came up with to combat these problems included simply avoiding mainstream medical services altogether—people only used them in emergency cases, or else as the BIA reports showed, they might return to their reservations. In the face of all these individual responses, community leaders sought to campaign for the establishment of a dedicated Indian health clinic that would not only provide free services for their people but that would carry over the ethic of "self-help." When discussions were first held about establishing an Indian clinic, it was of central importance that this clinic should be run "by Indians for Indians." Pearl Warren explained the importance of this, in 1965: "We need to help each other—we have depended on others for too long, and must learn to stand on our own feet."[113]

In developing their concept for a Native-run, Native-controlled, free health clinic for Native people, those involved with the Indian center worked closely with a number of allies to create a pilot program with the limited resources they had. The Kinatechitapi Indian Council had been focused on education and employment issues up until the late 1960s, but they proved to be a key player in the establishment of the pilot Indian clinic that opened in 1970. Indeed, before the Seattle Indian Health Board was officially incorporated in 1971 as a private, nonprofit 501(c)3 organization, it functioned more informally from 1970 to 1971 as a pilot program, which the organizing committee decided to call "the Kinatechitapi Indian Clinic." (Not insignificantly, *kinatechitapi* means "Indians of all tribes," or "all our people," in the Blackfeet language).[114]

Through their work with schools, the Kinatechitapi Indian Council came to learn about the high rate of absences among Native children across schools in Seattle. In 1969 it had been discovered by the American Indian Fine Arts and Heritage Program that "Indian children were consistently missing school due to illness."[115] In conjunction with school boards across the city, representatives from the Kinatechitapi Indian Council, the AIWSL, and the Indian center therefore began discussions about the possibility of establishing a medical clinic for Native people that would be staffed by volunteers. The idea was to expand on the emergency and first-aid service offered at the Indian center and find a separate location that could offer more comprehensive care. Without clinical facilities and a fixed location, the committee realized it would be impossible to develop reliable services, hence their first priority was to secure a space from which they would be able to run their health program for free. The committee hoped to find a suitable location that would allow them to borrow a space at no charge. After approaching several health care institutions for help, the committee finally had success with Dr. Willard Johnson, then the director of the US Public Health Service (PHS) hospital in Seattle. In 1970, Johnson offered physical space within the hospital, allowing the organizers to use the second-floor orthopedic clinic of the PHS to run their volunteer pilot program in the evenings.[116]

In February 1970, the Kinatechitapi Indian Clinic therefore opened for services at the PHS hospital. The *Indian Center News* announced its opening to the community: "An Indian Medical Clinic will open on February 2, at the Public Health Hospital (Marine) and will be free to all Indians. There will be no charge for prescriptions, x-rays or doctor calls. The clinic will be open three nights a week: Monday, Wednesday, and Friday from 5 p.m. to 9 p.m. Signs will direct you to the clinic which will be on the 2nd floor. The Clinic will be staffed by Indian volunteers. For more information call the Kinatechitapi Office."[117]

As the authors of an early community history of the SIHB have described, the clinic at first depended entirely on volunteers and operated "on a shoestring budget, using donated supplies, drug samples, and a few purchased pharmaceuticals."[118] One of the clinic's earliest volunteer doctors, Dr. Walt Hollow (Assiniboine-Sioux), recalled how in effect it was an "invisible clinic": "Since the space was used by the orthopedic clinic during the day, all the operations of the Indian clinic had to be stored out of sight when it wasn't in operation. Shopping carts were used to store and transport medical records, and a section of the women's bathroom was walled off to provide space for the shopping cart and the drug samples and supplies. When the Indian clinic was in operation, the carts were wheeled out to the reception desk and exam rooms."[119]

While this was still in many ways a "makeshift operation," it represented a huge step up from the basic clinic at the Indian center, and more than anything, it provided the community with a space that was just for them, run exclusively by their community, for their community. And because of the collaboration with the PHS, the Kinatechitapi Indian Clinic was in a position to offer Seattle's Native population a greater depth of services, including "immediate backup from the hospital emergency room as well as linkage to other services, and PHS doctors and nurses were also a valuable source of volunteers for the Indian clinic."[120] Reportedly, the positive impact of the clinic was felt very quickly within the community: speaking to a reporter for the *Seattle Post-Intelligencer*, Pearl Warren related that within its first few months, the clinic had already "solved immediate and urgent problems of 3,917 Indians."[121]

As vital as its role was, the pilot clinic still lacked the kind of permanence and autonomy that many community members had initially imagined for their dedicated Indian clinic. It took a timely (and seemingly disconnected) feat of political activism to get the clinic the kind of publicity it needed to draw the support that would provide the permanence and autonomy it sought. In the month following the opening of the Kinatechitapi Indian Clinic, a group of Indian activists led by Bernie Whitebear (Colville) and Bob Satiacum (Puyallup) invaded the Fort Lawton military installation to reclaim this land for Seattle's urban Indian community. This event unified the strategies of the politics of visibility with the rationale behind the politics of space, and it was to have a significant impact on the fight for Indian health care that was already underway.

Fort Lawton was a military installation in Seattle that was no longer needed by the Department of Defense. In the late 1960s, the city of Seattle submitted a proposal for this site to be repurposed for a public park. Community members recall that when the news broke that the land, originally ceded as part of the Point Elliott Treaty of 1855, was to be given to the city without its original inhabitants—the Duwamish—having the opportunity to reclaim it, "this immediately galvanized the city's Native community into action," both in solidarity with the sovereignty claims of the Duwamish, and to highlight the needs of a growing Native diaspora in Seattle.[122] Led by Bernie Whitebear, Seattle's Indian community first attempted to negotiate with the city but made little progress. According to the testimonies of those involved in these early negotiations, these initial setbacks compelled the city's Native community to take inspiration from the more militant activism of other urban Indian communities, in particular, the recent occupation of Alcatraz Island by Native activists in San Francisco only months before. Bernie Whitebear and others therefore planned a similar takeover of Fort Lawton.[123] On March 8, 1970, the operation was launched.

Activists occupied the fort from all sides, some scaling the western bluff overlooking Puget Sound, some climbing over fences, some attempting to enter through two heavily guarded gates using diversionary tactics. When some of the activists were first discovered by a roving military police patrol after setting up a tepee and a small campsite inside the fort, Satiacum attempted to read a statement explaining the protestors' actions. The statement read, in part, "We, the Native Americans, reclaim the land known as Fort Lawton in the name of all American Indians by the right of discovery. We feel that this land of Fort Lawton is more suitable to pursue an Indian way of life, as determined by our own standards. By this we mean 'this place does not resemble most Indian reservations.' It has potential for modern facilities, adequate sanitation facilities, health care facilities, fresh running water, educational facilities, fisheries research facilities and transportation facilities."[124] The resonances between the Fort Lawton Proclamation and the Alcatraz Proclamation are striking. At Fort Lawton, however, activists were met with a forty-man MP platoon that had been dispatched from nearby Fort Lewis onto the scene. Officers were ordered to "move in and take them away" and then began holding any activists they could catch within the Fort Lawton stockade. In all, eighty-five persons were detained, questioned, and released that evening with letters of expulsion. The symbolic "invasion" was thus repelled, and the activists' removal from the fort appeared at the time to be a defeat. However, the activists continued to confront the federal and Seattle city governments concerning Native claims to the land at Fort Lawton, immediately calling for demonstrations the next morning at both the fort (where many of the activists involved in the invasion remained camped outside the front gates) and the US federal courthouse in downtown Seattle. Allegations of brutality by officers inside the stockade on the first day of the invasion were quickly reported and would remain a point of contention among protesters as the story unfolded.[125]

The protesters remained outside Fort Lawton for three weeks, and the presence they maintained became known as "Resurrection City." In this time, local community members, particularly the women of the Service League, kept the activists supplied with food, clothing, and moral support. Another attempt to invade the fort occurred on March 15. While seventy-seven were arrested that day, the protesters agreed not to resist arrest, and so unlike the first attempt, this incident was relatively peaceful. On April 2, the protestors agreed to break down Resurrection City and to shift their strategy from occupation to negotiation. One final, unsuccessful attempt to occupy the fort was made, more as a symbolic gesture. At the conclusion of the Fort Lawton invasion, though many of the activists had been arrested, their efforts undoubtedly paid off, as from this point on, we see evidence of the city starting to take urban Indian claims and the community seriously. In particular, it was the Seattle Indian community's insistence on moving things to the negotiating table that was credited for the successful impact of the Fort Lawton invasion. One newspaper reported on this effective result as follows: "Senator Jackson, who sponsored the city's application for the fort land for park use, had words of praise for Whitebear for being willing to take the dispute over the land beyond confrontation to the bargaining table. Whitebear led several assaults on Ft. Lawton and directed a prolonged siege in which a stubborn group of Indians encamped at the gate to dramatize the Indian claim to the surplus land. Jackson said yesterday, 'Unlike Alcatraz, which resulted in nothing, Bernie moved the discussion to the negotiation table.'"[126]

The Fort Lawton invasion was hugely significant as far as the strategies of the activists were concerned. It represented both a culmination and marriage of many political goals, including their concerns for both visibility and space. It also demonstrated a shifting and strengthening determination on the part of the community's leadership to hold the authorities accountable to their political demands. As Satiacum's statement revealed, the ambitions of the community were also growing. Fort Lawton was intended to solve the issue of a permanent location for the health clinic, but the community also envisaged that this space would allow for the development of a comprehensive cultural center, social, education, and legal services, childcare, and orientation for newly arrived Native people in the city. A "negotiating team" of community members and allies was formed by Joyce Reyes, president of the AIWSL after Pearl Warren, and Bernie Whitebear, who represented a group later incorporated as the United Indians of All Tribes Foundation (UIATF). Together, they urged the city to recognize the social and political significance of acquiring this land for Native people in Seattle, to develop their multipurpose center, and placed special emphasis on its role as a health and healing center.[127]

Signaling another shift in the community's activist strategies, in late 1970 Whitebear also applied to the Department of Health, Education, and Welfare (HEW) to request the land on behalf of the community. According to an early history of the SIHB,

(The breadth of the vision, and the inclusion of education and welfare and health services, made HEW the appropriate federal agency to act for the Indian community.) With HEW's application, the Native community's claim to the land was now on an equal basis with the city's claims. The General Services Administration, charged with transferring the land, required the city to negotiate with UIATF and AIWSL to reach an equitable solution before the land would pass from the federal government to the city. Senator Henry Jackson, then chairman of the Interior Committee, played a key role in the transfer of Fort Lawton due to his jurisdiction over Indian Affairs and national parks.[128]

Jackson was sympathetic to the community's claim on the land, and so in November 1971, a historic agreement was forged between the city, the AIWSL, and the UIATF.[129]

While the occupation of Fort Lawton looms large in the history of Native American activism in Seattle, community members recall the significance of the "synergy" among the actions of the UIATF, AIWSL, and the Kinatechitapi Clinic as being critical for understanding the advancement of their health agenda. The national and international press coverage that the occupation of Fort Lawton attracted greatly "enhanced the profile of the Kinatechitapi Clinic." In turn, "the success of the clinic in developing a health delivery system to meet the needs of urban Indians," including the unrecognized tribes of the region, enhanced the credibility of Seattle's urban Indian leadership.[130] In a series of strategic moves that worked synergistically, Bernie Whitebear also "neatly linked the two movements in the public eye by holding a news conference at the clinic after the first clash at Fort Lawton. He asked one of the volunteer doctors to open the clinic to treat those injured during the invasion, and he invited the press to cover the event."[131] This single act simultaneously brought attention both to the success of the pilot Indian health program and the importance for the community of establishing a more permanent location for a more stable and comprehensive clinic.

The takeover of Fort Lawton and the establishment of the Kinatechitapi Indian Clinic were thus critical achievements for Native health activists in Seattle. In each case, the community articulated a clear message about the importance of securing a dedicated multi-tribal and pan-Indigenous space in the city so that their diverse and growing community could exist and flourish in ways that granted them the social, cultural, and political autonomy to ensure their community's needs were met, and to keep their many cultures and traditions alive. By advocating for, and demonstrating the need for these dedicated Native spaces, activists also made a strong case for why existing social support structures and institutions were inadequate to meet the needs of their community. Having taken decisive measures to establish their visibility as a distinct cultural group in the city, and then by taking steps to protect the viability of this culture in the city (by having spaces to just freely "be" Indian, as Jess Sixkiller put it), the community was laying the foundations for itself to exist as a self-determining pan-Indian community within the city. Moreover, these Indigenous spaces provided a model of social services that ran against the grain of the federal government's dominant assimilationist termination and relocation policies, making it clear that diasporic urban Indians in Seattle were not content to "give up" their Indian status and identities just because they lived in the city. The spaces they fought to create were also inclusive of, and in solidarity with, the sovereignty of the unrecognized Duwamish people whose tribal lands they were on. Crucially then, I propose that we might see these pan-Indian spaces as representing the social production of a new kind of political space: not a tribal homeland nor even a mosaic of different homelands that might be seen to displace or challenge the territorial claims of the Indigenous peoples whose lands they were on, but a genuinely inclusive pan-Indian space in the city that actualized a new form of nonterritorial, or "deterritorialized sovereignty"; that is, at Fort Lawton, and in the Kinatechitapi Indian Clinic, Seattle's urban Indian community enacted their right to simply exist as diasporic Indigenous people and to have the resources to function as a community. At work in their efforts was therefore an idea of a portable Indigenous status that was meant to allow Indigenous people to live in cities or, indeed, wherever they chose, without giving up their identity or legal status as Native American and their ability and right to practice Indigenous cultures or to make claims on the government on the basis of this identity. Indeed, the final strand of health activism that remains to be addressed concerns this important issue of making claims against the government. While it was the source of some division within the community, a significant number of urban Indians in Seattle also advocated for their community's right to health care and pursued the creation of an Indian clinic on the basis of their treaty rights. It is to these efforts that I now turn.

Obligation

As the Kinatechitapi Indian Clinic was coming to fruition in late 1969, ideas about an urban Indian "right" to health care increasingly circulated within the community. This represented a significant departure from earlier forms of health activism, since the invocation of treaty rights shifted the focus of the conversation about urban Indian health from a needs-based framework to one that became rights-based. Up until this point, the driving force behind much of the health advocacy of individual community members and organizations like the AIWSL and the Kinatechitapi Indian Council had been to draw attention to the immediate, urgent, and distinctive health needs of their people. The strategy for rallying community support and action was successful such that, by the late 1960s, Seattle's urban Indian community was both vocal and visible enough to raise $20,000 for Ernie Crowfeather, and through strategic alliances with tribes, hospital staff, and local donors, they had secured enough support to recruit volunteers and secure funding to establish basic facilities that could meet their community's immediate problems of health care access in the city. Yet, as a younger generation of activists became more central to the American Indian political scene in Seattle—Bernie Whitebear, Luana Reyes, and Elizabeth Morris—this ethic of self-help started to be viewed as an inherently limited (or limiting) form of activism since the community's demands would thereby always hinge on the identification and substantiation of needs as opposed to an insistence on obligations they were owed as Native peoples. With the initial achievement of the Kinatechitapi Indian Clinic under their belt, and in the context of wider political changes ongoing in the United States and abroad, starting in 1970, a new generation emerged among Seattle's Indian health activists, repositioning themselves and their demands to reflect longer-term goals and adding an insistence on an urban Indian right to health care to their demonstrated need for it.

In their turn toward a rights-based framework, we can see the connections being drawn by Native health activists between their movement and other concurrent political movements of the time. Reflecting back on his days as a medical student at the University of Washington, Dr. Walt Hollow (Assiniboine-Sioux) recalled the way in which he and others in the younger community of activists shifted their arguments toward an invocation of rights: "During the early and mid-60s, we were able to ride on that political pressure and show that Indians were treated just as equally bad as the Blacks were, and that our health care has suffered partly because of all of that, and due to lack of funding by the federal government to meet the obligations that we felt they should be meeting."[132] Describing the strategies they used to pressure the federal government, he said, "And so, it was a combination of documenting the health problems and then bringing up the treaty obligations and putting pressure on the federal government in that civil rights era that the federal government needed to correct a wrong."[133] For Hollow and other activists, the significance of historical ob-ligations became paramount: "And so, we would go back to history here on many of the treaty rights that were not upheld—there are numerous docu-mentations of the federal government promising Indians in various parts of the country certain things and then not fulfilling those obligations. . . . There are hundreds of them—and so we were able to bring those back to light along with the horrible health care problems that we could document, and it made a nice package in retrospect."[134]

This reorientation toward a rights-based framework was most visible in the community's efforts to secure stable sources of funding to expand the Kinatechitapi Indian Clinic into something more permanent and compre-hensive. Dr. Hollow also recalled that at the point younger activists like Bernie Whitebear and Luana Reyes (Colville) started to take over the man-tle of leadership from Pearl Warren and the AIWSL, they decided to ac-tively pursue permanent sources of funding. At the same time, there was a growing dialog within the community about how "these things [health care] were promised to us by our treaties."[135] Throughout the 1970s, in their engagements with the press and in publications circulated within the community itself, there were increasing references to the fact that the fed-eral government had made treaty commitments to provide doctors and medicines for the health care of Indian peoples in exchange for Indigenous lands.[136] By seeking federal funds to support the expansion of their Indian clinic, activists like Whitebear and Reyes thus argued that they were sim-ply seeking what their community was rightfully owed.

Treaties between the United States and tribal nations provide the origi-nal legal foundation for the federal government's obligation to provide health care for Native Americans.[137] Through treaties, the seizure of tribal nations' land and resources by the United States was to be compensated by the federal government's promise to provide payments and services—including the promise to provide health care to tribal citizens.[138] The mod-ern authorization for the provision of health services to Native Americans is the Indian Health Care Improvement Act of 1976 (which the Seattle activists helped usher in), while the primary authorization to pay for federal services for their general welfare remains the Snyder Act of 1921.[139] Congress has also passed additional statutes directing the Indian Health Service to pro-vide health care to Native Americans.[140] Where medical provisions were not specifically listed, most treaties asserted federal protection of tribes in ex-change for land or a pledge by tribes to not engage in political intercourse with other foreign states. This has generally been interpreted to mean that the United States would provide the means to preserve the health of Native people. This fiduciary responsibility is supported by federal court rulings and legislation and is the basis of the federal Indian trust responsibility, which the IHS describes as follows: "The trust relationship establishes a responsibility for a variety of services and benefits to Indian people, including health care. This relationship has been defined in case law and statute as a political relationship. . . . Treaties between the United States government and Indian tribes frequently call for the provision of medical services, the services of physicians, or the provision of hospitals for the care of Indian people."[141]

To be sure, while not all treaties imposed specific health care obligations on the federal government, activists in Seattle frequently pointed out that many of the treaties signed in the Pacific Northwest before 1871 *did*: Article 10 of the 1854 Medicine Creek Treaty with the Nisqually, Puyallup, and Squaxin Tribes was commonly cited for stipulating that "the United States further agree to employ a physician to reside at the said central agency, who shall furnish medicine and advice to their sick, and shall vaccinate them; the expenses of the said school, shops, employees, and medical attendance, to be defrayed by the United States, and not deducted from the annuities."[142] This promise was not unlike similar statements found in Article 14 of the Point Elliott Treaty with the Duwamish and Suquamish, Article 11 of the 1855 Point No Point Treaty with the S'Klallam, and Article 10 of the 1855 Quinault River Treaty with the Quinault.

While reservation communities commonly and uncontroversially referred to such treaties in order to claim their rights to federally funded health care, pan-Indian health activists in Seattle faced a challenge in asserting that this contractual right to health care had not been limited by time or location, and hence applied to diasporic urban Indians as much as it did to reservation communities. The arguments of Seattle's new generation of Indian activists were expressed in their correspondence with one another, in statements to the press, and in meetings to discuss the future of the Kinatechitapi Indian Clinic. Their claims essentially fell along three lines. First, community health advocates were adamant about finding ways to hold the federal government "accountable" to treaty obligations that "provided health care to Indian people wherever they lived."[143] The goal therefore became one of convincing sympathetic legislators that health care promises in treaties were not limited by place or time. Starting in 1970 or 1971, we see Whitebear forging strategic relationships with lawyers and legislators in an effort to get their case across. Second, the community's leaders also argued that it was incorrect and unfair of the federal government to insist that all urban Indians forfeit their Indian identity and rights just by virtue of moving to the city. This led to outcomes that were patently unjust and inconsistent, as Whitebear explained to the *Seattle Times*: "In some instances BIA officials have winked at regulations and helped an off-reservation Indian student with a scholarship. However, the system makes it possible for one brother living at home on the reservation to get a BIA scholarship while another, living with relatives in a nearby city, to get no BIA help."[144] In cases of health, where life and death might be involved, community leaders sought to emphasize how egregious and damaging these seemingly arbitrary restrictions could be, when to all intents and purposes, the only difference between an Indian who qualifies for help and one who doesn't is their residential address. Third, community leaders stressed that economic conditions on reservations were so bad that many Indians had little choice but to move to cities. Therefore, if the alternative was chronic unemployment, the decision to leave the reservation could not, in fairness, be treated as a form of consent or indication that a person was willing to forfeit their rightful claims on the federal government. Moreover, as Reyes remarked in one of her exasperated correspondences, due to the lack of options for social mobility on many reservations, by insisting on such a dichotomy between reservation privileges and the lack of such privileges in an urban context, the federal government's policies were effectively working to root "Indianness" in "poverty."[145]

By pushing the federal government on these three points, community leaders like Whitebear and Reyes sought to compel the federal government into recognizing that they held a genuine obligation to diasporic urban Indians. In pursuing this politics of obligation, urban Indian health advocates did much more than simply make a case for federal funding to support the expansion of their Indian health clinic in Seattle. They also suggested a complete reorienting of the relationship between the federal government and Native people. By asserting that federal obligations to provide health care to Native people still held up in the cities, urban Indian health advocates rejected the tenets of termination, asserted the need to rethink geographies that separated urban and rural communities, and crucially, they also implied the mobility of Native American rights and sovereignty.

While the ultimate goal was to obtain federal IHS funds for urban Indian health programs, the community initially focused on state and local funds, which were more readily attainable. The clinic's first successful grant was obtained in early 1971, from the State Office of Economic Opportunity, and it provided funding for four months with the understanding that further funds from the State Department of Social and Health Services would be available. With this initial funding, the clinic hired Bernie Whitebear as its first executive director. Under Whitebear's leadership, however, the Kinatechitapi Indian Clinic no longer held any close affiliation with the Kinatechitapi Indian Council; thus in early 1971, it was decided that the clinic would become formally incorporated under a different name. On March 18, 1971, the Seattle Indian Health Board (SIHB) was thus born, and under this new name it aggressively pursued its goal of federal funding. In a most deft political move, the SIHB first pursued an application for National Health Service Corps (NHSC) personnel. This application effectively brought the issue of federal policy toward urban Indians into the national spotlight for the first time.

The NHSC application represented such a momentous political maneuver because in 1970 this legislation had allowed for federal personnel to be assigned to provide health care services only in areas that were "medically underserved."[146] In other words, the application process required that the service area be certified by the local medical societies, dental societies, and health planning agencies to be areas where "health personnel and services are inadequate to meet the health need of the residents."[147] The SIHB's NHSC application therefore broke important new ground. Seattle was of course well supplied with physicians, dentists, and nurses; however, the SIHB nonetheless managed to obtain the local certifications needed because there was an established and general acknowledgment that the Native community in the city lacked access to these critical health care services and resources. The dividends of all the community's earlier work in awareness-raising, fact-gathering, and in speaking up about their medical mistreatment finally paid up, in other words, when in December 1971, NHSC administers approved the SIHB's application. Although this was not yet equivalent to establishing a federal obligation to provide health care for all urban Indians, it was undoubtedly a critical first step in convincing the federal government to recognize the legitimacy of urban Indian demands for health care provisions in the cities.

It would not be until the Indian Health Care Improvement Act was passed in 1976 that this political objective of federal recognition was reached. Part of what proved to be so problematic for urban Indians in Seattle was that in making their claims against the federal government, and in seeking to hold it accountable for providing health services to urban Indians, they encountered pushback from tribal communities who saw these efforts to extend free health care to urban Indians as a direct threat to the limited pool of funding set aside for health care on reservations. Between 1971 and 1976, Indian health activists in Seattle therefore brokered strategic alliances with tribal communities.[148]

Though they still had some way to go before they would meet their goal of federal government support, by the time the SIHB was officially incorporated in 1971, it was clear that Seattle's urban Indian health activists had turned their determination to hold the federal government accountable for treaty obligations into one of the most powerful driving forces behind the growth of the clinic. In their efforts to pursue federal funding, the SIHB founders realized there was a unique opportunity for them to radically alter the relationship between the federal government and Native people. A good deal of the inspiration came from an awareness of wider political events and movements unfolding around the same time. These included the influence of other American Indian political groups in other cities, as well as the opposition to the Vietnam War and the civil rights movement. Speaking to a reporter from the *Seattle Post-Intelligencer* about the community's various political efforts, activist and former US commissioner of Indian Affairs Robert L. Bennett (Oneida) said, "There is no doubt about the boost the Indian concept of self-determination has been given by the black revolution."[149]

To be sure, Native American health activism developed against the backdrop of the civil rights movement, but it was the particular confluence of civil rights politics in a health and medical setting that helps us best fit the efforts of Native health activists into a broader story about a changing health care landscape in the United States at this time. As Jenna M. Loyd has shown, the 1960s and '70s in America saw a number of people's health projects emerge that sought to reclaim the clinic by challenging exclusionary racist and sexist relations of medicine: "The free clinic; women's, lesbian, and gay health movements; and the Third World Left's 'serve the people' programs were radical self-help projects designed to meet immediate needs and simultaneously to democratize health knowledge and power, in part through fostering egalitarian, collaborative relationships between health professionals and 'lay' people."[150] The Black Panther Party's People's Free Medical Clinics are perhaps the best known example that emerged from this political moment in health care reform. Alondra Nelson's study of the Black Panther Party's health activism discusses how their efforts included providing basic medical care to the poor, working with lay community members, and engaging trusted health professionals in alternative facilities established by the activists. Nelson asserts that the party's clinics cannot be understood without the context of the "community clinics" movement that was also taking place during this time, and that in addition to the Panthers, the radical health movement of the 1970s included "feminist groups," "hippie counter culturalists," "politicized medical professionals and students," and "the Party's allies in the 'rainbow coalition,' most notably the Young Lords Party."[151] Community health projects whose interventions included lead testing, neighborhood cleanups, food movements, job creation, and community reinvestment also broadened a social understanding of health. Key aims, common to the activists in these other health movements, included exposing egregious medical abuses; democratizing health knowledge and power; democratizing access to health care; and fundamentally reshaping the power of patients, lay people, and consumers over the institutions of health and medicine, as well as a very strong self-help thread that probably became most visible in the women's health movement. Women's collective self-care politics resulted in such innovative and well-known self-help projects as the Boston Women's Health Book Collective's *Our Bodies, Ourselves* and the Feminist Women's Health Centers in Los Angeles. All these people's health projects would hold medicine accountable to its professed humanitarian commitments and simultaneously challenge medicine's grip on the meaning of health. The influence of these broader political currents is unmistakable in the work of Native American health activists at this time; hence we must understand their struggles and their solutions, not simply in the context of these broader health movements but as a part of them. What distinguishes Native American health activists from these other contemporaneous health movements, however, is the historical dimension central to their health politics, which grounded their claims against the federal government in the politics of Indigenous sovereignty and the historic obligations owed to them as a matter of treaty rights and the federal government's trust responsibility.

Much as I have already suggested in relation to the Seattle Indian community's engagement with the politics of space, by pressing the idea that the federal government was duty-bound to provide health care to Native people *wherever they lived*, Seattle's urban Indian health activists made a powerful paradigm-altering claim about the meaning of Native American sovereignty in a new age of urban pan-Indian identity and biresidential (cross rural-urban) living. They sought to show that for Native American sovereignty to continue to have relevance for many Native people who were now moving into cities or living in ways that increasingly defied strict rural-urban boundaries, that sovereignty as a political concept could not continue to be limited by or tied to strict geographic/territorial or tribal boundaries. In essence, urban Indian health activists made a case that American Indian sovereignty needed to be de- (or rather, *re-*) territorialized.

· · · · · ·

By the end of the 1970s, urban Indians living in Seattle could point to two landmark achievements that their community had attained in the area of health. The first was the establishment of the SIHB in 1971. As one of the earliest free clinics in the nation run exclusively by and for urban Native people, this represented a huge step in providing urban Indians in the Pacific Northwest with reliable, "culturally appropriate" access to health care.[152] Moreover, this clinic, due to its grounding in a "self-help" ethic that was so vital to the community starting with the work of the AIWSL in the 1950s, represented a perfect realization of this community's determination to exercise its sovereignty against federal expectations of assimilation in the cities.

The second outcome was the enactment of the Indian Health Care Improvement Act (PL 94-437) in September 1976. Title V of this act, Health Services for Urban Indians, secured provisions for clinics like the SIHB to access federal money as well as community funding and grants, and was the first instance in which urban Indians were written into federal legislation.[153] Soon after it was signed into law, the significance of this act of recognition was neatly expressed by one of Title V's most prominent advocates: "We often speak of Indian Country, it's an old legal term. Well, the Indian Health Care Improvement Act applied Indian Country to urban Indians living in metropolitan centers."[154] The fact that this form of recognition happened first in the field of health is remarkable and seldom discussed by historians, but it is a crucial development within Native American politics and policy, demonstrating the central role of health politics in the broader evolution of Indigenous sovereignty.

4 An Indictment of This Country

Advocating for Aboriginal Health in Sydney, 1960–1980

During the 1960s and 1970s, events at home and overseas awakened the Australian medical community, its politicians, and the broader public to the abysmal state of Aboriginal health across the nation. In 1968, E. Gough Whitlam (soon-to-be Australian prime minister but then leader of Australia's opposition party) encapsulated this moment of national awakening when he criticized the current government for being indifferent to the reality that "the health of Aboriginals is an indictment of this country."[1] In his speech, Whitlam drew attention to a 1963 survey carried out under the auspices of the Australian National University and the Australian Institute of Aboriginal Studies, which showed a death rate of 296 per 1,000 live births among Aboriginal people in central Australia. In the face of such staggering figures, Whitlam opined that this figure "must be among the highest in the world."[2] While this came as shocking news to many of Australia's politicians and the general public, Whitlam's speech was by no means the first time such claims were made. In 1960, doctors found that in the Northern Territory, "leprosy is considered endemic."[3] In 1964, a survey of Aboriginal health conducted in Sydney showed that half of all Aboriginal children born in the South Coast region of New South Wales died within their first year of life.[4] Aboriginal rights activist Roberta (Bobbi) Sykes would later refer to this 1964 survey, saying, "This report was kept 'secret'—but <u>we</u> knew, it was our babies who were dying."[5] While for much of the twentieth century the Aboriginal communities at the center of this suffering lacked the resources to make their circumstances widely known, by the 1970s, Aboriginal health had become a politicized and urgent issue across Australia thanks to the actions of doctors, activists, and allies of the Aboriginal community in Sydney who launched a nascent Aboriginal health movement in the late 1960s and early 1970s.

Foremost among their accomplishments was the creation of the Aboriginal Medical Service (AMS) in Sydney in 1971. The AMS represented a huge practical intervention in the delivery of health care to Aboriginal people in Sydney and beyond.[6] But it also represented a landmark political intervention in the course of Aboriginal politics by giving practical form to new ideas about how Aboriginal self-determination might take shape in the cities. This was a different kind of self-determination politics to that of the highly visible land rights movement in Australia at the time. However, as this chapter shows, the "deterritorialized" politics of Australia's Aboriginal health activists did not detract from, nor run counter to the goals of the broader Aboriginal rights movement of the time. The urban Aboriginal health movement turned on the ability of activists and allies to challenge pervasive racist beliefs about Aboriginal people, and it also required convincing those in power or in a position to help improve Aboriginal health outcomes that they had a social and moral responsibility to do so. By shifting the political discourse around Aboriginal health from one that blamed the victim to one that recognized the social and historical determinants of health, activists moved the needle on many fronts for Aboriginal politics as a whole and demonstrated why good health outcomes were inextricably tied to other political goals, not the least of which included the recognition that Australian cities were Aboriginal sovereign homelands.

Igniting a Health Movement: Nancy Young and the Question of Blame

Physicians who worked with Aboriginal communities in rural Australia during the late 1950s and early 1960s were among the first to speak extensively with Aboriginal communities about their health problems. Well before government officials, these doctors started to realize that the nation had a spiraling health crisis on its hands. Although a few had tried to draw attention to this in the 1950s by publishing research (especially on the alarmingly high rates of Aboriginal infant morbidity and mortality), little serious regard was paid to this looming crisis, even within the medical community, until in 1968 a dramatic court ruling thrust the issue into the national spotlight and cleared a path for doctors and activists alike to lobby for Aboriginal health reform.

The case concerned the trial, conviction, and incarceration of Nancy Young, a 29-year-old Aboriginal woman and single mother of eight. In 1968, the Young family, plus three other adults, lived at the Cunnamulla Reserve (one of the poorest Aboriginal reserves in Queensland) in a single corrugated iron shack measuring just ten by fifteen feet. Their overcrowded home, typical of those on the reserve, was located close to the Cunnamulla town sewerage outlet, and yet there was no sewerage system on the reserve itself.[7] Like many others in her community, Nancy Young lived on next to no income; in the year she was convicted, she told activist Daisy Marchisotti, who visited her in jail, that she had been striving to get by on just six dollars a week, her payment from child endowment and a little part-time waitressing.[8]

Things had started to go terribly wrong for Nancy Young in July 1968, when her youngest child, a five-week-old girl named Evelyn, became sick with what seemed like gastroenteritis. Having no other means of getting her daughter to the closest hospital, Nancy Young carried Evelyn the full three kilometers to get there. The infant was immediately admitted and kept under observation for eight days, until she was sent home because she "looked better."[9] In the inquiry later conducted as part of Nancy Young's trial, it was reported that "no tests were carried out on [Evelyn], and Ms. Nancy Young was given no instructions about feeding or check-ups, nor any vitamins or medicines."[10] Several months later, when Evelyn was four and a half months old, she started displaying the same symptoms. Nancy Young once again carried her daughter the three kilometers to Cunnamulla Hospital. This time, Evelyn was given glucose and water but little else in the way of medical attention.[11] The following day, the duty doctor began what a specialist later called "entirely incorrect treatment."[12] Two days later, Evelyn passed away in the hospital.

A standard inquest and a couple of interviews by the police were conducted immediately after the infant's death, but nothing more happened until approximately three months later, when Nancy Young again came to the hospital. This time, her eldest daughter had fallen ill with all the same symptoms. The very next day, while her eldest daughter was still under observation, Nancy Young was approached by the local police and charged with Evelyn's manslaughter. They arrested her on the grounds that she had failed to provide adequate food to her baby and had not sought medical treatment for her soon enough.[13] Bail was set at $1,000, which neither Nancy, nor anyone she knew, could afford.[14] She spent the next three months in jail awaiting trial.

For the duration of her early arrest, Nancy Young's story did not break into the mainstream press. The Australian public only started to hear about it through news reportage on the eventual outcome of her trial in 1969. Both the controversial conduct and conclusion of the trial provoked widespread coverage across national publications and television alike. Many articles speculated about the potential biasing influence of comments made to the jury by the judge at the outset of the proceedings. A key factor in Nancy Young's conviction, some reporters contended, was that her counsel had decided to keep her from the witness box because in their experience and estimation, many uneducated Aboriginal defendants tended to just say what they believed authority figures expected from them.[15] Yet in response to this decision, the judge advised the all-white, all-male jury that "it is legitimate for you to take this failure [to appear before the jury] into account as a consideration, which makes it less unsafe to infer guilt than it otherwise would have been."[16] The jury heard key medical witnesses from both sides but in the end ruled as the judge appeared to expect of them. Therefore, early in 1969, Nancy Young was found guilty of her daughter Evelyn's manslaughter, for which she received three years of hard labor in jail.

It was the severity of this ruling that made headlines across national newspapers.[17] The outraged response of the Australian public was evident in the calls that streamed into radio stations and in the dozens of letters received by newspaper editors. A main issue under contention was the unreasonable dismissal of the evidence given by the defense's key medical witness, Dr. Archie Kalokerinos. At the time, Dr. Kalokerinos was regarded as a leading expert on Aboriginal child health. He testified that he believed scurvy to be the primary cause of Evelyn's death, with pneumonia a secondary cause.[18] His view was based on research he had been conducting with Aboriginal children since 1957, which indicated that, because of the inadequate diet of their mothers, many Aboriginal children were born with an inbuilt vitamin C deficiency, which, if not remedied, led to scurvy, severe weight loss, dehydration, and death—all symptoms that might be mistaken for gastroenteritis.[19] He argued that the failure of the hospital to administer or recommend vitamin C, and Nancy Young's inability to buy fresh fruit at the inflated Cunnamulla prices, made the onset of scurvy in Evelyn inevitable. Whether or not the hospital might be found negligent, Dr. Kalokerinos certainly believed Nancy Young was blameless in the situation.[20]

This question of Nancy Young's "blameworthiness" clearly stirred the Australian public. In 1969, prominent Aboriginal rights activist Jack Horner—who at the time was serving as the general secretary of the nation's most vocal national Aboriginal rights advocacy group, the Federal Council for the Advancement of Aborigines and Torres Strait Islanders (FCAATSI)—issued a press statement that encapsulated much of the public response to her trial:

The blame lies much more with the inhuman system of hopeless and futureless Aboriginal reserves and settlements, imposed by authority. There are thousands of Aboriginal mothers in exactly the similar situation as Mrs. Young. They cannot possibly feed their children adequately. This is because poverty, isolation and ignorance surround them on reserves. Their own malnutrition combines with these social factors to inhibit good mothercraft under the most pressing and extreme conditions. The Federal Council for the Advancement of Aborigines and Torres Strait Islanders is not at all satisfied that in this case the blame for the death of the 4 month old baby can be properly laid with the mother.[21]

Countless letters sent to local newspapers and to organizations petitioning for Nancy Young's release echoed Horner's comments. For example, on April 28, 1969, concerned citizen Mr. C. Leabeater of Coogee (Sydney) addressed a letter to the "chairman" of FCAATSI and shared intimate details of his own infant daughter's brush with death due to scurvy, hoping that her example might be used to bolster the Young case: "Just 20 years ago my daughter, then 10 months old was very ill and continually retched. . . . After several days and many tests, Dr. Geike diagnosed scurvy and had reason to believe the baby was lucky to be saved. . . . If our experience can be mentioned, I do hope in some way it may make an impression on those people who considered Mrs. Young guilty."[22] In another expression of support, on April 30, 1969, P. Foster of Double Bay (Sydney) contacted the Sydney University Law Society and included a small monetary contribution with his letter: "Dear Sir: Herewith my small donation towards Mrs. Young's defence [sic]. Not that I think it would take a very brilliant lawyer to get her off."[23] The more expressive and outraged among the general public tended to write in to newspapers, such as Ms. Erica Parker, whose letter to the editor of the *Sydney Morning Herald* on April 30, 1969, ended with an exasperated assertion that "this is stock-taking time in State Parliament."[24] Letters such as these suggested that most Australians were convinced by Dr. Kalokerinos's testimony, as well as his conclusion that Nancy Young could not be held accountable. Indeed, the double injustice of a dubious trial and the sheer hopelessness of the Young family's circumstances raised the political resonance of this case and very quickly turned Nancy Young and her children into symbols of the grave structural inequalities that Aboriginal Australians faced in small-town Australia. It also awakened the nation, for the first time, to the endemic problems of Aboriginal health and especially the vulnerability of Aboriginal infants and children.

By galvanizing disparate groups into a more identifiable "movement," Nancy Young's case brought together medical experts, Aboriginal activists, and allies from within government and the media, who would eventually help build the AMS. Moreover, the case instantly politicized the issue of Aboriginal health by focusing squarely on the question of blame. On the evening of the trial, protest meetings were held in Sydney, led by students Chris Owens and Geoff Robertson from the Sydney University Law Society.[25] That same night, the Australian Broadcasting Commission (ABC), one of Australia's largest television networks at the time, ran a television news program *This Day Tonight*, which screened a damning ten-minute account of the case. For weeks and months following Nancy Young's conviction, Aboriginal activists and advocates lead by FCAATSI also sprang into action, writing countless letters of appeal to lawyers, medical and political organizations, individual doctors, government representatives, and various political newsletters, calling for an urgent public response to the injustice of the case and the wider problems of medical discrimination and Aboriginal mortality it highlighted.[26]

Within months of Nancy Young's conviction, another ABC television program, *Four Corners*, aired an in-depth study of Cunnamulla and its Aboriginal community. Titled *Out of Sight, Out of Mind*, the program revealed the abject squalor of the reserve where Nancy Young and her children lived and exposed the town's racism in a series of interviews with local white residents.[27] The report showed that at the time of Evelyn's death, Cunnamulla's bowling club, two of its three hotels, and the best seats in the theater were off-limits to Aboriginal people. The exposé also revealed that more money was being spent by the local shire on the maintenance and upkeep of the local cemetery than on the Aboriginal reserve where the Youngs and other Aboriginal families lived in overcrowded and unsanitary conditions. Nancy Young's crime, according to the program's narrator, "was not that she did not look after her children, but that she upset Cunnamulla's whites by bringing her sick children to *their* hospital."[28] The closing shot of the television report was indicative of the significant role emergent new data was playing in making Aboriginal health problems apparent to Australians. Overlaid on top of a close-up of Evelyn's grave, a simple sentence lingered in bold text across the screen. It reiterated the very same statistic and sentiment that were a focal point of Whitlam's speech the year before: "The Aboriginal figure of 296 deaths per 1000 births is the highest in the world."[29] Indeed, in conjunction with Whitlam's speech, the airing of *Out of Sight, Out of Mind* is still remembered by many who became involved in the Aboriginal health activism of the era as "the moment" when the nation truly woke up to the terrible reality of Aboriginal health conditions across Australia.[30]

Why did it fall on this particular case to rouse the sympathies of the general public and to rally the efforts of activists into coordinated action? After all, as Jack Horner's press statement had intimated in the wake of the court ruling, Nancy Young was not alone in her struggles: "There are thousands of Aboriginal mothers in exactly the similar situation as Mrs. Young."[31] Part of the reason the Young case drew so much attention is simply an issue of timing. By 1967 (the year before Young was initially arrested), the political mood around Aboriginal Affairs in Australia was electric: In May 1967, campaigners for Aboriginal rights won the most decisive referendum victory in Australian history. Led by a coalition of white and Black activists joined through FCAATSI, campaigners sought the deletion of the two references to Aboriginal people in the Australian Constitution. The repeal of section 127 provided for Aboriginal people to finally be counted in the national census.[32] The amendment of section 51 (xxvi) furthermore enabled the commonwealth to enact "special laws" for Aboriginal people in particular circumstances, paving the way for the federal government (rather than states) to assume a greater role in Aboriginal Affairs.[33] The removal of these sections from the Constitution would, campaigners claimed, inaugurate a new era of acceptance and equality for Aboriginal people. This argument struck a chord with the wider populace to such an extent that, on referendum day, 90.77 percent of the Australian electorate voted to get rid of the two constitutional references. Ever since, the 1967 referendum has been popularly memorialized as the moment when Aboriginal people gained equal rights with other Australians.[34] In truth, the actionable progress made by the referendum was modest. As Australian historians have increasingly acknowledged, the real significance of the 1967 referendum lay not in any actual expansion of legal rights but in the symbolic affirmation of Aboriginal people's acceptance into the national community.[35]

Interestingly, the strategy of the referendum campaign bore similarity to the movement around Nancy Young's case. In both instances, campaigners had rallied support for their causes by framing their initiatives (respectively, constitutional change and social reform) as vital to Australia's national reputation and self-esteem. As one historian put it, the activists thereby converted what could have been a mundane, legalistic tinkering with the Constitution into "a plebiscite on Australian nationhood."[36] Physicians and

Aboriginal activists also deployed this rhetorical strategy of calling Australia's moral standing into question. We saw hints of this in the way activists and members of the public responded to the critical question of Nancy Young's blameworthiness. The powerful resonance of this aspect of the case was expressed in an open letter to the Australian medical community written by Dr. Barry Christophers, a politically minded physician who had joined as the secretary of FCAATSI's Equal Wages Committee in 1963. He got to the heart of the matter when he wrote that "to blame parental neglect where the cause is chronic unemployment and under employment, low wages, lack of property, lack of savings, absence of food reserves in the house, and chronic shortage of cash is to punish Aborigines for our discrimination against them."[37] Indeed, Nancy Young's conviction seemed to turn the Aboriginal health crisis into an issue that brought Australia's moral standing into question and into the spotlight. It was this, I argue, that moved so many people to pay attention to Aboriginal health in a way they had not before.[38]

The significance of the referendum as a backdrop to the Nancy Young case and to the consequent attention that was paid to Aboriginal health problems can also be measured in terms of how it politicized those who responded most vocally to the Young case. It is notable, for example, that FCAATSI—who led the way with the referendum—was also at the helm of efforts to rally support for Nancy Young.[39] In a similar vein, it is also significant that the referendum (with its language of "equality," "inclusion," and "rights") seemed to highlight the injustices of Aboriginal health problems all the more. Nancy and Evelyn Young caught the attention of the nation because there was something especially disquieting about the realities of Aboriginal infant mortality rates coming to light during such a celebratory moment in Aboriginal politics.

Bolstering the initial protests and concerted efforts to get Nancy Young's conviction removed, more far-reaching attempts were soon launched by concerned doctors and activists, who quickly seized the opportunity presented by the Young case to bring attention to the dire conditions of Aboriginal health more generally, and the discrimination Aboriginal people faced within Australia's medical system. In other words, the political momentum generated by the Young case was harnessed by Aboriginal health advocates and put to use in subsequent efforts to build the Aboriginal Medical Service.

In tracing how doctors, activists, and allies contributed to the founding of the AMS the ensuing discussion pivots backward and forward from the Young case. I pay special attention to the activism that targeted the invisibility of urban Aboriginal health problems since this was the primary population to be served by the AMS. That said, it is still worth noting that much of the activism in Sydney around Aboriginal health at this time actually aimed to benefit both rural and urban populations in equal measure. This is an important difference to underscore between the Indigenous health activism in Sydney and Seattle as it reflects the very different political position that Indigenous people in Australia negotiated from. Unlike in the United States, Indigenous people in Australia did not have treaties or other forms of federal recognition on which to base their arguments that the government owed them health care. Instead, Aboriginal people pushed for federal oversight of their health care first through their claims to citizenship, arguing that they were owed "equal treatment," and later, as they became steeped in ideas of Black Power and self-determination, as a matter of government obligations to them *as Aboriginal people*, on the basis of structural and historic mistreatment and neglect. Reflecting on their political position, activist Naomi Mayers (Yorta Yorta) later wrote that "in setting up our own [health] organization, we were saying [to the federal government], 'You were responsible for handling Aboriginal health and you have made an absolute mess of it. You have never listened, and we being Aborigines know what we want, know what causes the problems, and we know what has to be done to fix it, and we are going to make these decisions ourselves.' And we did."[40] With little differentiation between the government's neglect of rural and urban Aboriginal health prior to this, activists therefore treated a gain for rural communities as a gain for urban communities, and vice versa. Once attention was paid to Aboriginal health starting in the 1960s, however, rural health issues seemed to dominate medical research, the popular imagination, and government policies. In examining the efforts that led to the establishment of the AMS, I therefore pay particular attention to the way in which Sydney's Aboriginal health activists had to work to combat the invisibility of their urban community and its health problems, even as Australians were becoming increasingly conscious of (and indeed, perhaps self-conscious about) the realities of poor Aboriginal health across the nation.

Doctors and Data

Beginning in the late 1950s, a collection of concerned physicians who worked closely with Aboriginal communities across Australia started to speak up about the severity and ubiquity of the health problems they were seeing in their patients. At first, reports about their experiences and findings were limited to medical journals and related publications.[41] Such articles mostly addressed Aboriginal health problems in rural settings, rarely touching upon the health issues affecting urban populations. Yet, as Sydney-based medical researcher Dr. Peter Moodie would later point out, even though the collection of Aboriginal health data was showing marked growth by the mid-1960s, relatively little of this new information was published by the services or departments directly involved with the provision of care or funding for Aboriginal health. Rather, most of the new studies and even basic descriptive statistics on Aboriginal health were emanating from universities, research institutes, or individuals within or outside the public service who published their findings in medical or other academic journals. Apart from the limited reach such information could have, as Moodie pointed out, such independent or semi-independent inquiries (valuable as they might be for their independence) were often "severely handicapped where access to raw data had been denied or restricted for accredited researchers." Moreover, Moodie drew attention to the political dimensions of this knowledge and its dissemination, noting that data on Aboriginal health "may be seen as reflecting adversely on past and present policies and practices [and thus] may be used as political ammunition."[42] In other words, Moodie recognized the inherently political nature of health research. Yet, like many other resolute medical practitioners and researchers dedicated to improving Aboriginal health in the 1960s, he also saw an opportunity in this: "But if 'politics' were to be kept out of 'health,' the latter could not be discussed openly at all. If health was not a political issue, very little would be done about it at the community level and 'public health' would not be an effective force."[43]

Doctors and researchers like Moodie put the politics of health to effective use by generating "buzz" around their research. For example, Dr. Archie Kalokerinos (the chief medical witness for the defense in Nancy Young's trial) drummed up public and media attention to generate public pressure in favor of freeing the young Aboriginal mother. His instrumental role in "breaking" Nancy Young's story to the press is revealed in a private letter sent in 1972 by prominent Aboriginal activist Faith Bandler to Sir Robert Madgwick, chairman of the ABC:

That story did not break in the Press: southern newspapers depended on the Brisbane "Courier-Mail" for their Queensland copy, but either the "Mail" had a policy of rejecting news adverse to Queensland interests, or it felt it was not interesting. At any rate, they heard nothing.

But the late Frank Bennett, in a brilliant piece of reporting, both honest and sincere, on *This Day Tonight* related this story from Sydney (because he had heard of it independently, from Dr. A. Kalokerinos). Had it not been for Dr. Kalokerinos and for Mr. Bennett, Mrs. Nancy Young, who was later pardoned by the Queensland government, under pressure of public opinion informed by this organization [FCAATSI], would still be in a Brisbane gaol.[44]

Kalokerinos was not alone in utilizing the press in this way. Many other savvy doctors and medical researchers took their health data to the popular media to generate public interest and concern for issues that might otherwise have "lain untouched, gathering dust," as Moodie had put it. For example, in 1957, Dr. Barry Christophers, then also president of the Victorian Council for Aboriginal Rights, made a public appeal through the *Sydney Morning Herald* for the health needs of Aboriginal people to be taken more seriously.[45] In a short article reporting on the latest research into Aboriginal malnutrition, Christophers alluded to a racial double standard in Australia's treatment of white and Black health issues: "If the life of a white citizen is threatened by fire, flood, starvation or thirst, then the Army and Air Force are called to his aid within hours—and quite rightly so. But, the starving natives under similar circumstances depend upon inadequate charity."[46] Foretelling the work that many other doctors would later do via the AMS, Christophers also used this article to appeal directly to the moral conscience of his colleagues: "I feel sure that if any doctor in Australia were brought face to face with these suffering natives he would offer his services free and willingly to help them. Our profession should not content itself with such a passive role. It should urgently seek out ill-health wherever it be and treat it."[47] These efforts to publicize and politicize Aboriginal health research succeeded in exposing the public to the severity of Aboriginal health problems, and thus by the early 1970s many newspaper articles had started to describe the "rampant malnutrition" among Aboriginal children as "an Australian health scandal."[48]

Researchers like Kalokerinos and Christophers also appealed directly to government officials through letter-writing campaigns or by sending "letters to the editor" to mainstream newspapers. For example, Dr. L. Lazarus, director of the Garavan Institute of Medical Research at St. Vincent's Hospital in Sydney, sent a series of identical letters to multiple newspaper editors in 1972. His letter of March 2 to the *Sydney Morning Herald* read:

SIR, — I am writing in support of the plea by Dr. Coombs ("Herald," February 26) for an increase in spending on Aborigines. The infant and maternal malnutrition to which he refers results not only in physical handicaps but also in irreversible mental handicaps. . . .

The malnourished child born to a malnourished mother is less able to learn the complex skills needed to deal with modern society; he forever remains handicapped and his children ultimately will be restricted in society by the same set of conditions. Active intervention is required to break this self-perpetuating system, from which the unfortunate victims cannot themselves escape.[49]

Lazarus sent the same letter to the *Australian* and the *Canberra Times*.[50] These letters (and many others like them) were occasions to publicly shame government representatives for their neglect of Aboriginal health, to appeal to the better natures of individual government personnel, or else to implore them to see a political opportunity in championing the cause of Aboriginal health.[51] In 1970, Dr. Dick Armstrong of the University of Sydney and the FCAATSI Health Committee appealed directly to a known Aboriginal champion in the House of Representatives, Mr. Gordon Bryant, imploring him to support the idea of "seeking a meeting with Princess Anne [of Great Britain] in connection with the health of Aboriginal children."[52] Suggesting what might be gained for Bryant, Armstrong wrote, "Look upon it as a good exercise in public relations, if nothing else."[53]

A more common rhetorical strategy used by doctors, researchers, reporters, and activists involved simultaneously stirring up a sense of shame and moral duty. This was done most effectively through the idea that Aboriginal health statistics were "the worst in the world." Dr. Kalokerinos invoked this idea repeatedly in media interviews and in research articles, such as "Aboriginal Infant Mortality and Ascorbic Acid Deficiency Patterns," in which he wrote, "It has now been established beyond doubt that the Australian Aboriginal Infant Mortality Rate is one of the highest in the world."[54] Notably, we saw this turn of phrase in Whitlam's 1968 speech, but it is also worth remembering that by the time he used these very words ("the highest in the world"), this expression had been used over and over by doctors in their efforts to stir politicians to action. Whitlam's use of this phrase in 1968 might therefore be taken as evidence of their success in this regard.

Medical practitioners and researchers were also instrumental in changing some fundamental (and racist) social attitudes about Aboriginal health. Even into the late 1960s, it was commonly held that Aboriginal health problems were the result of behaviors, choices, or a "culture" that invited poor health. The 1960 *Report of the Aborigines Welfare Board of New South Wales* encapsulated this view. Taking a tone reminiscent of the board's rhetoric in *Dawn* magazine, this report stated, "It is a matter for regret, however, that numbers of aborigines, particularly those living off Stations and Reserves, appear content to reside in sub-standard dwellings and make no effort to improve their living conditions. Many also seem incapable of, or unwilling to shoulder responsibility and face up to their obligations, particularly in meeting their rental liabilities and medical expenses."[55] More than their alleged "unwillingness" to improve their living standards or meet various living expenses, the report also blamed Aboriginal people for the discrimination they faced from non-Aboriginal people in cities: "Such arises from social and hygiene reasons rather than because of colour."[56] The report entirely dismissed charges of unequal treatment and discrimination as "extravagant" and actually criticized such claims for worsening interracial hostilities. Instead, the report blamed many of the aforementioned problems—failed payments, discrimination—on the irresponsible way in which Aboriginal city-dwellers "squandered" what little money they had on alcohol and related activities: "A much stronger emphasis should be placed on the fact that many aborigines and persons with an admixture of aboriginal blood, can do more to improve their living standards by applying money to the necessities of their families and homes instead of squandering it in gambling and other useless and wasteful avenues, including drink."[57]

Pushing back against these entrenched views was a mammoth task. Doctors and other health workers made an important contribution by encouraging a discourse about the social, economic, and environmental determinants of health. In numerous articles, public statements, and soundbites in the popular press, medical experts stressed "cycles of causation" that interwove the main problems afflicting both rural and urban Aboriginal communities: inadequate or impermanent housing; racial discrimination in education, employment, housing, and health contexts; cultural isolation; and mistreatment by law enforcement were all emphasized alongside the problems of ill-health and lack of access to medical services. For example, in 1970 and 1971, Gloria Bainikolo and Don Williams, both field officers for the New South Wales Health Commission, described the "vicious circle" of poor housing and poor health to journalists from the *Australian Women's Weekly* and the *Sydney Morning Herald*: "They more often than not come up against the racist attitudes of potential landlords. What do they do? They move in with fortunate relatives in commission homes and live 20 to 30 to a house in defiance of the regulations. In appalling conditions like this, it's not long before white neighbours react and the friction starts—the husband drinks excessively and then every one gets sick. There's no way out—it's a vicious circle."[58]

Describing the same phenomenon, but underscoring the added problem of this community's invisibility (in medical research and in the public conscience), Williams referred to these families as "Sydney's forgotten blacks."[59] After years in the field ("an experience which really opened my eyes to the plight of Aborigines"), Williams told *Sydney Morning Herald* reporter Colin Allison that "usually unemployed, on the dole [social welfare], in and out of hospital, and often without permanent housing, they huddle with relatives or friends in Housing Commission homes, dodging commission inspectors on the lookout for breaches of the one-family one-home regulation. It's a hell of a life."[60] In another case in 1970, speaking about the problem of brain damage among Aboriginal children resulting from poverty and inadequate diets, Dr. B. Nurcombe (pediatric psychiatrist at the University of New South Wales) told a reporter from the *Australian* that a "complex network of vicious circles" meant that Aboriginal people in the city were more likely to "fall prey to diseases from living in an overcrowded, insanitary environment."[61] Dr. Ross Macleod, the first doctor hired by the AMS, also vividly described to me how he and his colleagues attempted to advocate for better Aboriginal housing in Redfern after they "discovered" that the root cause of ear infections and parasites encountered in Aboriginal children at the clinic could be traced back to the overcrowded and unsanitary conditions of their city housing, which made it very easy for infections to spread.[62]

By stressing these "circles" or "cycles" of causation, doctors and health workers did much to shift public discourse away from blaming Aboriginal people for "bad choices," and toward focusing attention more directly on the social and economic conditions that characterized Aboriginal life in Australia. Indeed, it was not long before this language of "cycles" and "circles" was echoed in public letters written by activists and members of the public. For example, in 1971 activist Daisy Marchisotti wrote into *FCAATSI News* about the problem of Aboriginal infant mortality, stating, "A nurse, or sending a doctor cannot solve this problem, which is one of insufficient food to eat, insufficient money to buy food, insufficient work and insufficient wages when you do get work—a circle from which there is no escape for the Aborigine."[63] This kind of growing public response, typical of letters sent in to newspapers by the early 1970s, reflected the language, ideas, and advocacy work of doctors and health workers like Christophers, Moodie, Kalokerinos, Bainikolo, and Williams.

Importantly, by shifting the discussion toward social, economic, and environmental causes, doctors and health workers turned Aboriginal health conditions into a moral issue in which questions of blame and responsibility were paramount. In this regard, the Nancy Young case was especially significant given the connection between Evelyn Young's illnesses and the appalling living conditions in Cunnamulla. Not long after Nancy Young's conviction, doctors actively used the legal case to question the way in which causes of Aboriginal ill-health were being discussed, even within their profession. In October 1969, Dr. James Kalokerinos (brother of Dr. Archie Kalokerinos) contacted Dr. Barry Christophers and commended him on a recent comment in the *Medical Journal of Australia*, in which he was able to "put down the essence of the problem."[64] The "essence of the problem" referred back to the question of Nancy Young's blameworthiness and the extent to which, as Christophers put it, "to blame parental neglect where the cause is chronic unemployment and under employment, low wages, lack of property, lack of savings, absence of food reserves in the house, and chronic shortage of cash is to punish Aborigines for our discrimination against them."[65] Christophers further underscored the need to reframe the social, political, and medical discourses regarding the causes of Aboriginal ill-health when he wrote, "Infant death rates are a direct measure of poverty. To blame parental neglect for the high Aboriginal infant mortality rates is a dangerous attempt to divert attention from the truth."[66]

Doctors were also instrumental in challenging the invisibility of urban Aboriginal health issues, which flew under the radar for several reasons. First, even when Aboriginal health research was conducted, it tended to focus on the rural areas. Ironically then, the common and damaging misconception that all Aboriginal health problems in Australia were confined to rural areas was encouraged by the media attention to Nancy Young's trial. Second, as I unpack in further detail later in this chapter, most urban Aboriginal people simply avoided mainstream medical care altogether, meaning that very little was known by the medical community about this population. What little data was collected about urban Aboriginal health was also often subsumed by the larger policy goal of assimilation, meaning that instead of being recorded in ways that might identify them as Aboriginal health issues, the problems afflicting these communities were often categorized in ways that absorbed them into other population groups ("the urban poor" for example). In this last dimension, urban Aboriginal people were effectively erased from health data.

By conducting new research that singled out urban populations, doctors therefore played a critical role in combatting this lack of knowledge about urban Aboriginal health. Dr. J. Norelle Lickiss, a researcher in the Department of Tropical Medicine at the School of Public Health at Sydney University, focused on the health of urban Aboriginal children. In 1968, Lickiss conducted an environmental assessment of 120 Aboriginal child residents of Sydney to determine connections between their health status and socioeconomic environmental factors. The publications from this study alone attest to just how little the medical community knew about urban Aboriginal health. For instance, Lickiss underscored that "beyond impressions that all is not well, very little is known about the health of the Aboriginal children in Sydney," and "it is not known whether the high mortality and morbidity trends in Aboriginal children prevailing elsewhere in Australia are echoed in the Sydney scene."[67] Lickiss's studies revealed that while slightly better in certain respects, the situation of Aboriginal children's health on the whole was much the same in cities as it was across the country. In particular, it was found that "morbidity and mortality patterns appear to resemble those of Aboriginal children elsewhere, though the rates are probably not quite as high."[68]

Another physician drawn to urban Aboriginal health problems was Dr. David Smith (who would later volunteer his medical expertise to the AMS). In the late 1960s, Smith often spoke to the press about Aboriginal health in Sydney in order to bring attention to what he described as "serious health problems that parallel those of the world's most deprived and dispossessed minorities."[69] For instance, he described Aboriginal poverty as "deeper than that of America's ghetto blacks," and he compared the Aboriginal health problems he saw in Sydney to those of "the dispossessed North American Indians."[70] Smith was also determined to shift the discussion around Aboriginal health from that of "purely the crisis role" to "the curative work—to preventative medicine." From his perspective, this required addressing broader social and environmental factors; hence he linked the "grave health problems" of Sydney's Aboriginal population to their "shocking slum housing." Like Dr. Ross Macleod had described to me, Dr. Smith also blamed Aboriginal health problems in Sydney on their "overcrowded" and "damp" living conditions.[71]

Other studies emerging around this time took a similarly broad interest in issues affecting "urban Aborigines." In Sydney, anthropologist and

Aboriginal rights advocate Pamela Beasley conducted a demographic study of the Aboriginal population in Sydney during 1964–66. She recorded details such as geographic dispersal of the community; age distribution; reasons for relocation to Sydney from other origin points; employment and unemployment information; marriage data; educational level; and housing status.[72] In addition to this broad survey, she also published a report in 1967 that focused on the problem of "City Aborigines and Overcrowding."[73] Notably, Beasley was also in correspondence with Eugene D. Stockton, a chaplain to the Aboriginal population in Sydney, who acted as her informant and authored a detailed research paper on "The Domestic Situation of Aborigines in Sydney."[74] Emblematic of this growing social-scientific interest in the urban populations, the Department of Adult Education at the University of Adelaide devised a ten-week radio course for the general public advertised as "a course that looks at some of the main concerns of Aboriginal people living in Adelaide, such as identity, special social and educational needs, Aborigines and the law, and land rights."[75] Operating as part of a program called *Radio University*, "The Urban Aborigine" aired twice a week over the ten-week duration of the course. It was oriented around a series of interviews with people working on the front lines of Aboriginal social welfare in Adelaide. These interviews provided Australians a rare glimpse into what urban life was like for Aboriginal people living in Australian cities at this time.

One of the more highly publicized interviews featured prominent Aboriginal activist and poet Oodgeroo Noonuccal, who spoke at length about the health conditions of the urban Aboriginal community in Adelaide.[76] After quoting some key data from an address by prominent Australian economist and public servant Dr. H. C. Coombs, Noonuccal turned her attention to the political dimensions of these health problems, excoriating the government for grossly underfunding programs for Aboriginal health: "When you sense the extent of the health problem and then read that the Federal Government in the coming year is allocating only 3/4 million dollars for Aboriginal health, you realize that the situation is not likely to improve in the near future—rather the reverse."[77] Noonuccal also singled out specific government personnel, criticizing them for being dishonest about the facts on hand: "I also feel that if Mr. Wentworth was honest with Parliament and the nation, he would, in speaking to the recent States Grants (Aboriginal Advancement) Bill 1969, have given some of the pertinent facts I have spoken about tonight and which he must know well. Instead, he devotes a few lines to the health problems, which sound as if no real facts are known about it."[78]

It is worth noting that activists like Oodgeroo Noonuccal, Jack Horner, Faith Bandler, and their many counterparts frequently cited Dr. Coombs's address. This was no doubt due to its strident tone but also, as Ian Langmen (another activist) reflected in a letter to Jack Horner, because "Coombs has given the best summary of the research that is progressing throughout Australia at the present time."[79] It was clear, in other words, that even by 1969, though many medical researchers were conducting surveys on Aboriginal health, very little of this data was being collated, compiled, or even compared to formulate an overall picture. In his address delivered in Sydney to the Australian College of Physicians, Dr. Coombs therefore attempted to present the closest thing yet to a "national survey" of Aboriginal health:[80]

If an Aboriginal baby is born today—

1. It has a much better than average chance of being dead within two years.
2. If it does survive it has a much better than average chance of suffering from sub-standard nutrition to a degree likely permanently to handicap it A) in its physical and mental potential; and B) in its resistance to disease.
3. It is likely in its childhood years to suffer from a wide range of disease but particularly E.N.T. and respiratory infections, from gastro-enteritis, from trachoma, and other eye infections.
4. If it reaches the teen ages it is likely to be ignorant of and lacking in sound hygiene habits, without vocational training, unemployed, maladjusted, and hostile to society.
5. If it reaches adult ages it is likely to be lethargic, irresponsible and, above all, poverty-stricken—unable to break out of the iron cycle of poverty, ignorance, malnutrition, ill health, social isolation, and antagonism. If it lives in the North it has a good chance of being maimed by leprosy and, wherever, its search for affection and companionship may well end only in the misery of V.D.
6. If it happens to be a girl it is likely to conceive a baby at an age when her white contemporary is screaming innocent adulation at some "pop" star and she will continue to bear babies every twelve or eighteen months until she reaches double figures or dies of exhaustion.
7. And so the wheel will turn.[81]

A few points are worth noting about this list. First, Coombs clearly connected Aboriginal health problems to wider issues such as housing and education, and much like medical experts at this time he also emphasized the idea of a "cycle" ("wheel") of bad health. Of special significance for urban spokespeople like Noonuccal, Coombs also drew attention to the fact that these health findings applied as much to the urban populations as to the country and rural communities: "It would be a mistake to think of these conditions being restricted to the 'outback' or far north."[82] Coombs also helped deliver this information in a way that invited his listeners to look forward with him and consider "what might be done about all this." Speaking to an audience of physicians, it is notable that Coombs closed his address with a series of rhetorical observations surely intended to compel his listeners into action and underscore their moral obligation to do so: "This is a responsibility that we all share but would you think it, Mr. Chairman, an impertinence on my part to wonder whether an especial responsibility in this matter does not lie with the medical profession?"[83] Here we can arguably see the impact of the advocacy work of medical doctors coming around full circle: The alarming research findings of doctors had compelled Coombs (a public servant) to deliver this impassioned address to the wider medical community. What's more, Coombs also sought to instill a special sense of responsibility upon the medical professionals and doctors gathered to hear his talk. The propriety of both rhetorical moves was not lost on the urban Aboriginal activists who continued to cite Coombs for the next few years.[84]

Finally, the crucial role of doctors was not simply limited to the ways in which they helped change the terms of public and political discourse about Aboriginal health; they also played a critical hands-on role once the community's free clinic was up and running in Sydney. Doctors like Fred Hollows, Ross Macleod, and David Smith not only helped set up the AMS but volunteered their services, in most cases for free, to allow the clinic to operate on next to no budget. Activist Bobbi Sykes recalled how many of the early AMS doctors even spent their own money on medical supplies and equipment to get the clinic running.[85] In terms of medical care, they provided vital services such as vaccinations, nutritional support, and emergency care. And even after hours there are stories of doctors who were "so committed" they were willing to "hang around the streets waiting for patients."[86] One doctor stood out in Sykes's memory in particular, as she recalled the work the AMS did to mitigate the effects of police brutality against Aboriginal men in the city:

One doctor in particular was quite famous to us—notorious to the white community—for actually hanging around the hotels when the police raids were on, seeing who had been thrown in the van, and at what angle, and then going to the nearest police station, and saying, "He is a patient of mine and I must see him" and, of course, they would throw him out time and time again. But there is one thing about throwing a black out and there is another thing about throwing a doctor out, and the doctor just goes to the press and gets publicity about it—and that strengthens our case.[87]

Jilpia Nappaljari Jones (Walmadjari), one of Australia's first Aboriginal nurses (who also worked at the AMS), recounted in her oral history that of all her experiences at the AMS, what she remembered most was the incredible work ethic and tireless resolve of Dr. Fred Hollows: "Most of all, I remember 'the Prof.' [Fred Hollows] and how hard he was always working to help us blacks. He dedicated his life to the health of Aboriginal people."[88]

"There Is Little Point in Fixing the Body by Destroying the Soul"

On July 20, 1971, Aboriginal activists in Sydney opened the doors to Australia's first community-run, free medical clinic for Aboriginal people. They called it the Aboriginal Medical Service. At first, the clinic operated out of a small space that was previously occupied by a coffee shop at 171 Regent Street. At this early stage activists relied solely on donations to keep the clinic afloat. Consequently, it was staffed in these days by a roster of volunteer doctors and nurses drawn from a network of sympathetic physicians and nursing sisters recruited by Dr. Fred Hollows. Activist Shirley Smith—known affectionately within the community as "Mum Shirl" on account of her central role in looking after the welfare of many of Sydney's most destitute Aboriginal people—worked as the first "field officer" for the AMS. In this role she traveled extensively across Sydney and other areas of New South Wales, meeting with patients and ascertaining their medical needs. Activist Bobbi Sykes later recalled how rudimentary this initial clinic was and how quickly the activists came to see the need for a larger space. Their premises on Regent Street, which consisted of two small rooms in a "small, long and skinny building with a toilet out the back" afforded almost no privacy to patients.[89] The tenants who lived directly above the clinic had to enter their home via the doctor's surgery, meaning that "right where the doctor was examining patients, they [the tenants] had the freedom to come and go, which they did, while the doctor was actually talking to patients and examining patients behind the screen."[90] After eighteen months of providing much needed medical care to the community from this space, the clinic moved to a new location down the block, where it was reported that they started seeing an average of 277 patients every fortnight.[91] Over the course of its first decade in operation, the AMS worked toward the provision of two major types of care: primary health care—medical, dental, and nutritional—and counseling services for drugs and alcohol, and prevention and education regarding sexual health.

Prominent Aboriginal activists who were instrumental in the creation of the AMS have recounted the origins of the clinic in a variety of settings: Gary Foley (well-known Aboriginal activist and former AMS staffer) wrote a brief history of the AMS on the occasion of its twentieth anniversary.[92] Naomi Mayers (long-serving CEO and founding member of the AMS) has shared her story in numerous publications, including an anthology about the working lives of Aboriginal Australians titled *A Story to Tell*.[93] Gordon Briscoe (prominent Aboriginal activist and founding member of the AMS) recalled his involvement in setting up the clinic in interviews, articles, and in his memoir, *Racial Folly: A Twentieth Century Aboriginal Family*.[94] And Bobbi Sykes (poet, author, Aboriginal rights activist and former "publicity officer" for the AMS) often spoke and wrote about the founding of the clinic within her official capacity as its appeals and public relations liaison.[95] Interestingly, all of their accounts portray a fairly uncomplicated series of events that led to the opening of the clinic in July 1971.

As the story goes, the life of the AMS began with a simple conversation between two prominent members of Sydney's Aboriginal community following a visit, one wet and miserable night in June 1971, to their desperately ill friend in Sydney's predominately Aboriginal suburb of Redfern. The seemingly straightforward way in which this visit prompted the idea for a community-run clinic is worth repeating in some detail since this story appears frequently in publications about the AMS.[96] In one of the more detailed retellings, activist Bobbi Sykes recalled the story for the *Reader's Digest* in 1975:

Gordon Briscoe, 32 and Shirley Smith, 49—"Mum Shirl" to every Aboriginal in Australia—were visiting a desperately ill friend. He was in a bad way, coughing up blood. "Listen, bud," Shirley demanded, "why didn't you go to hospital?"

"I queued up for four hours," the sick man told her. "Then I was told I'd have to pay $34 before I'd be treated."

Mum Shirl and Gordon looked at each other, neither surprised. Hospitals are hostile places, to an Aboriginal. Most assume that doctors, nurses and hospital administrators are racist. Some are. Poverty inhibits as well. As Mum Shirl says, "If you have pride, and nothing more, you walk away from a hospital when they start talking money. You might say you'll come back. But you don't, no matter how sick you are."

Outside the house of their dying friend, Mum Shirl and Gordon Briscoe conferred. Gordon, a person who always desperately wants to do things, asked, "Why can't we set up our own medical service?"

"Okay, let's do it," Mum Shirl said to Briscoe, a university undergraduate. "You've got education. And I'll help. Because it's going to need more than education—it's going to need a lot of hard work.[97]

According to Gary Foley (Gumbainggir), what happened next was equally swift. Briscoe and Smith called a meeting the next day, gathering some thirty Aboriginal activists, twenty-five doctors, and a handful of allies including Paul Coe, Dulcie Flower, Dr. Fred Hollows, Ross McKenna, John Russell, Chicka Dixon, and Eddie Neuman.[98] They decided then that the community would set up a shop-front medical service in Regent Street Redfern, adopting a "community-control" structure. Without any delay, on July 20, 1971, the Aboriginal Medical Service Co-Operative Ltd. was officially born. According to Sykes, it didn't take long before the clinic was attracting a sizable body of patients from within the community: "Initially, the Aboriginal Medical Service operated on an honorary 'whenever a doctor is available to work a few hours' basis, mostly in the evenings, and it was just a few weeks later, advertised only by word of mouth, that queues could be seen each night waiting for the surgery to open."[99]

Facets of this oft-repeated story suggest a kind of simplicity and common-sense approach that has clearly been important for the political identity of the clinic, as well as for its persistence in the face of numerous challenges throughout its history. Testifying to the continued salience of this common-sense and "can do" ethos, the AMS's website has put notable emphasis on the simplicity of its raison d'être and its approach to getting things done: "There was one simple reason why we got organised, and why we built our own medical service—self-determination. We knew then, as we know now, that unless we set the priorities for our community, we would never receive a service that put our priorities first."[100] Remembering and commemorating the founding of the clinic in this way—as a self-evident and uncomplicated solution—makes a great deal of sense when we consider how much voluntary support and funding the organization has had to rely on over the years. (To put it plainly, it is much easier to attract support for something that seems like a simple and obvious solution.) What's more, at every potential setback, activists and their supporters have therefore had recourse to a set of founding principles that instill a sense of possibility, hope, and purpose: "Despite funding difficulties and opposition from government on the matter of expansions, the Aboriginal Medical Service outgrew its two-room operation and now carries on a wide range of diverse activities. The Aboriginal Medical Service was started on private donations and funded itself, albeit in a limited manner, for almost the first year of its operations. This early attempt to avoid total dependence on government funds, and therefore limitations imposed by government sources, has been a major feature of the Aboriginal Medical Service ever since."[101]

A very practical set of considerations—maintaining a sense of possibility, purpose, and resiliency in the face of constant challenges—might therefore explain the somewhat understated character of stories that emphasize the clinic's overnight origins in a simple conversation between friends. However, there are important reasons to expand our understanding of the activism and the parties responsible for the creation of the clinic. In particular, it has had much broader and longer roots in Aboriginal community action and advocacy in Sydney, not just in the service of health but also other inseparable issues: antidiscrimination, lack of housing, and of legal representation in particular. To that end, any understanding of the role of health activists must begin by acknowledging the politically efficacious measures taken by community members in the 1960s as they intentionally (and sometimes unintentionally) acted to highlight, resist, or simply mitigate general Aboriginal vulnerability in the cities, and especially in the medical system. Though these people may not have seen themselves as embodying the role of "activist" at the time, and though their efforts may not have been coordinated or planned expressly as political interventions, in the aggregate, these communitywide actions and behaviors had a significant political impact on Aboriginal health reform, either by attracting unexpected attention and sympathy or by inciting more politically active community members into action on their behalf.

To identify measures taken specifically to address health issues—particularly the problem of health care access—we can first consider the way in which Aboriginal people in Sydney (and elsewhere) typically interacted with the mainstream medical system throughout the 1960s. This eventually became the subject of research by medical anthropologists in Australia during the 1970s. Jan Reid, of the Center for Medical Education at the University of New South Wales, conducted a sizable investigation into a practice of "absconding" common among Aboriginal patients admitted into both rural and urban hospitals across Australia. In a research paper, Reid described how inscrutable this practice of absconding seemed to the medical professionals who frequently encountered it: "Aboriginal patients who abscond from hospital rarely communicate to hospital staff their reasons for leaving. As medical and nursing personnel who have worked in hospitals which serve Aboriginal communities know, such departures are usually sudden and unannounced. They variously puzzle, concern, annoy, or anger those who have vested energy and resources in the patients care. At best they are viewed as ill-advised and inexplicable. At worst, they are seen as irresponsible, dangerous and negligent—sometimes as a threat to the patient's life."[102] To suggest how absconding could be mitigated, Reid conducted fieldwork with the aid of an interpreter and community guide, B. Dhamarrandji (Yirrkala). Together, they traveled across northern Australia seeking out the stated and inferred motivations of Aboriginal patients who had engaged in the practice at least once. Though Reid's research focused mostly on the Northern Territory, other sources confirm that the practice of absconding was equally common in other rural settings, as well as in the cities.[103] Reid's detailed findings offer a general picture of how and why Aboriginal patients frequently left hospital prematurely, or at least before they were advised to do so by medical personnel.

Reid's report divided the reasons for premature departures into two main categories: (1) factors related to patient responsibilities at home and to events in the community requiring the patient's presence—births or deaths, and other important events; and (2) factors related to the hospital—its procedures, staff, environment, and regulations. On the whole, Reid found that events and family obligations at home figured only marginally in explanations given by patients and their families when accounting for why they or their relations had run away from hospital. More commonly, patients and their families mentioned the perceived shortcomings of the hospital and its staff. In particular, they cited a general lack of recognition by hospital staff of the concern and responsibility (culturally) of the patient's family to provide care at times of illness; general lack of communication between hospital staff and Aboriginal patients and kin (including lack of information about medical procedures to be performed); perceived racist attitudes of medical staff toward Aboriginal patients, including toward their accounts and explanations of their own illness; a fear of medical procedures; and complaints about the general hospital environment such as restrictive visiting hours, impersonal care by medical staff, or the physically and psychologically uncomfortable settings of waiting rooms and shared wards.[104] Of all these reasons for absconding in Sydney, the Aboriginal community in Redfern experienced the worst racism at Rachel Forster Hospital on Pitt Street.[105] Mistreatment there was so common that this historical detail has featured prominently on the AMS's website in the past: "Our community would watch as white people who arrived after us, got treated before us. And then, when that was done, we would watch medical staff wander off for a coffee and a chat. Our health was not a priority. Often we just left."[106]

Compounding the problem of absconding, Aboriginal people often simply avoided the medical system altogether. As related in the story about Gordon Briscoe and Shirley Smith's sick friend, this practice of avoidance was a direct response not only to neglect and discrimination but also because general practitioners and hospitals usually insisted on cash payment in advance from Aboriginal patients. This too, was a form of overt racism since non-Aboriginal patients were not expected to do the same.[107] Institutionalized forms of racism in the mainstream medical system at this time, segregated wards, and sometimes whole blocks of hospitals—called "A wards" by patients—were still common in the 1960s.[108] Indeed, a controversy that unfolded over several "Letters to the Editor" in the *Sydney Morning Herald* in 1961 reveals that new hospitals, (such as the Public Hospital at Urbenville, Sydney) were still being planned and constructed with designated blocks for Aboriginal patients. One angry letter writer revealed the attitudes that Aboriginal patients in Sydney still commonly faced at this time: "The stock argument that this [separate 'Aboriginal block'] is necessary because some aborigines are dirty is not even relevant in this case. It is the duty of the hospital staff to keep the patients clean."[109]

The situation in Sydney was so grim that field workers from the Aboriginal Legal Service were routinely finding community members who would "literally rather die than be subjected to degrading, humiliating treatment at the hands of non-Aboriginal health workers."[110] In the late 1970s, activist Bobbi Sykes summed up the problem: "The very notion of a visit to the doctor, or even the perceived but futuristic need to visit a doctor, is a source of anxiety. Doctors, generally, because of their ignorance of the Black community, and because of their own upbringing and pre- and mis-conceptions, are so judgmental, or patronizing, or racist, that contact with them for whatever reason, is often a dreaded occasion."[111]

Rather than producing an apathetic response on the part of community members, we should recognize the actions and coping strategies of sick Aboriginal people as a political response; that is, many sick Aboriginal people actively *chose* not to subject themselves to mainstream medical services because they viewed it as an injustice and even as counterproductive to their health. Bobbi Sykes, reflecting on absconding and avoidance by Aboriginal women in particular, stated, "There is little point in fixing the body by destroying the soul."[112] This of course highlights an important point about the general relationship between the Australian medical system and its Aboriginal patients. As discussed in chapter 1, part of the federal government's goal in encouraging Aboriginal urban migration in the 1960s was to foster the process of Aboriginal assimilation into mainstream Australian culture and society. It was intended that this would be achieved in urban settings via multiple avenues, including limiting the social welfare dependency of urban Aboriginal residents by encouraging them to access social services (such as medical care) alongside other Australians. Aboriginal people were supposed to adjust and assimilate themselves into the system, both practically and culturally. The medical system thus made no accommodations whatsoever for Aboriginal cultural perspectives on illness, care, or recovery. The importance of maintaining family members close by during times of sickness, for example, was crucial within many Aboriginal communities, but Aboriginal people were expected to immediately conform to white Australian norms and expectations.[113] The purposeful rejection of this environment by Aboriginal patients through their practices of absconding and avoidance must therefore be seen as a political response and a refusal of this expectation to assimilate.

These widespread practices of absconding and avoidance were also accompanied by other common strategies for mitigating the negative and alienating environment of mainstream medical services. Namely, Reid's research revealed a widespread practice of visiting hospitals in large groups to guard against feelings of isolation and unfamiliarity.[114] The families of admitted patients would also regularly break visitation rules by staying late, arriving early, or camping out on hospital grounds in order to stay close to their relations.[115] In cases where families camped out, Reid recorded numerous testimonials of families who described the "forced isolation" of patients from relatives as "cruel," and who explained that "it is the Aboriginal way for relatives to congregate in order to watch over, and comfort the sick."[116]

As a result, Reid found many examples of encampments of various sizes that waxed and waned outside the hospital buildings according to the number of seriously ill members of the community who were admitted. This practice, Reid recorded, "has attracted the hostility of European townspeople and created a degree of discomfort and unrest among the hospital staff."[117] Moreover, the feelings of family members with respect to maintaining proximity to their sick relatives and friends were "so strong," Reid recorded, that "they are willing to camp in the most inconvenient and uncomfortable of circumstances, with little or no privacy from the stares of European visitors and staff, little or no access to toilet or washing facilities, and no shelter in the rain but that of the covered walkways between buildings."[118] While Reid's informants recognized the shortcomings of their solutions, and while many even expressed concerns that the short period of ritual singing and dancing following a death at the hospital might disturb nearby residents and other patients, most nonetheless maintained a firm conviction that "these hospitals should be different."[119] They should, one informant insisted, "cater for the needs of families of those who are seriously ill, for both they and their relatives suffer if separated at such a critical time."[120]

Upon first consideration, while these early efforts (disengagement, rejection, avoidance) might not register as a kind of activism, I argue that we should recognize these actions and coping strategies of sick Indigenous people as a political response to their situation in the cities and in the mainstream medical system. Their principled stands against mistreatment, acts of refusal and noncompliance, and their assertions of their dignity may have started as individual acts, but together, these amounted to a powerful, communitywide rejection of the mainstream medical model, its rampant racism, and the assimilationist political agenda that operated through it. And importantly, these behaviors quickly developed into nascent and gradually more sophisticated forms of organizing—from informal networks to information sharing, to eventually the enlistment of self-identified activists, who as we saw through the case of Nancy Young, worked to draw attention to the wider neglect of urban Indigenous peoples and eventually, to create their own clinics.

As a means of appealing to a largely apathetic Australian public, these more vocal Aboriginal community members worked hard throughout the 1960s and 1970s to generate public concern about the urgency of solving Aboriginal health problems. They did this in several ways. Most successfully, they seized on the newly emerging data from medical researchers described earlier to advance a discourse about Aboriginal health problems being at "crisis levels." We see early evidence of Aboriginal activists collecting this data in their direct appeals to physicians and researchers for their findings. For example, through May and September 1969, Jack Horner sent letters to various medical researchers, asking if they would "send copies of papers on Aboriginal health, which we are very interested in this year."[121] Activist Dulcie Flower (a Torres Strait Islander woman and active campaigner for the Aborigines Progressive Association and founder of the Health Committee of FCAATSI) was responsible for promoting the discourse of a "crisis" (moral and otherwise) in Aboriginal health, frequently making public statements of the following nature: "Unless this situation is rectified immediately, this state of affairs places the whole future of the Aboriginal race in jeopardy. We cannot succeed as a race of people until we are given that basic human right of enjoying good health and well being."[122]

Making the case that Aboriginal health problems required urgent attention was not hard given the overwhelmingly negative and alarming findings of medical research published in the 1950s and 1960s. Flower's remarks above highlight how, in particular, activists focused their efforts on politicizing the issue of infant mortality. The Nancy Young case and all the medical data it both reflected and generated were a critical part of this. Especially during the late 1960s and early 1970s, activists wrote articles and press releases, made public media appearances, and lobbied for international attention to be paid to the devastating reality that Aboriginal children across Australia were dying at a rate that was "the highest in the world." The intentional, political use of this medical data was explained by Flower in a report of FCAATSI's Health Committee, following their annual conference in April 1970, in which she wrote, "I am of the opinion that it is not sufficient for medical specialists to perform surveys of the Aboriginal people, table their reports, then leave it up to the various health departments to rectify the health problems of Aborigines. It appears that political action is necessary to ensure that recommendations be implemented."[123]

Flower and other outspoken activists in Sydney understood that political action was necessary if the health needs of the urban populations were to be recognized, given the overwhelmingly rural focus of the health research being done. In a statement clarifying the goals of the FCAATSI Health Committee, Flower therefore emphasized to her fellow campaigners that "at present the committee is concentrating on Sydney and NSW because of the lack of attention paid to this state and the absolute need for more research into urban Aboriginal health. We shall in the very near future extend our attention to the problems of other states and look at the question nationally."[124] One means of putting political pressure on the government was to bring international attention to the issue. Therefore, activists worked to forge connections and highlight the similarities between their own communities' struggles and those of other oppressed groups. The hope was to raise public awareness of the injustices faced by Aboriginal people in Australia to the levels garnered by civil rights violations in the United States. However, in reporting on these transnational solidarities, oftentimes the mainstream media in Australia would simply focus on the dominant society's fears about a violent form of Aboriginal activism that was seen to be growing in the cities. Where some Aboriginal activists drew parallels between their activism and the work of the Black Panthers and adopted the language and militaristic aesthetic of the American Black Power movement to make a political point, dramatic newspaper headlines (see figure 4.1) in the early 1970s tended to dwell on the threat of violence, resulting in some debate among Aboriginal activists about the best language for expressing their political goals.[125]

Transnational Solidarities, Comparisons, and Connections

When interviewed in 1972 for the ABC's *Monday Conference* television program, activists Bobbi Sykes and Paul Coe debated the reasons for using the language of Black Power in Australia. Sykes expressed reservations about the term, saying, "It is a phrase that I think is misused in this country a lot." Instead, she preferred "Black action" or "Black people in motion," since in her view those terms drew attention to the significant achievements of Aboriginal initiatives like the health service: "The legal aid, the medical service, are the classical examples of this direct black action," she stated.[126] By contrast, Coe pointed out the merits of associating their goals with other disempowered groups who also used this political language: "They want to put the black struggle where it should be, it is part of the third world movement. We are a coloured minority, whose land has been taken, who have been suppressed, and that is what's happened over the rest of the world, where Europeans/colonialists, have come into power, and this is what they've done and this is what the so-called third world movement is about."[127] However misplaced she believed the connections were in certain respects, Sykes also agreed it was probably necessary for Aboriginal Australians to actively draw these connections, if only to highlight how far behind the country was in supporting struggles for social justice: "I think the only thing that will goad Australia into doing anything is international

FIGURE 4.1 "Black Power Comes to Australia," the *Australian*, December 5, 1971: 11. The activists identified in this photo are Gary Foley (*foreground*), Billy Cragie (*right*), an anonymous field marshal (*left*), and Dennis Walker (*center*). Reproduced in Gary Foley, *A Short History of the Australian Indigenous Resistance 1950–1990*.

embarrassment."[128] The efficacy of this international embarrassment strategy became apparent in later references made throughout the 1970s by politicians, public intellectuals, and members of the general public that suggested Australia "lagged far behind the rest of the world in justice for our Indigenous people."[129] Perhaps most prominent among such public statements was prime minister Gough Whitlam's 1973 description of Australia's treatment of its Aboriginal people as "in the eyes of the world a test of the integrity and humanity of the whole people of Australia."[130]

Activists' efforts to bring Australia's mistreatment of Aboriginal people directly into the international spotlight and to situate their struggles within broader political currents of the time came to a head in 1971, the United Nation's "Year for Action to combat racism and racial discrimination."

An Indictment of This Country   175

Activists organized numerous public forums, meetings, seminars, and talks across the country about Aboriginal health inequalities and other forms of injustice. For example, on June 20, 1971, a public seminar on "Australian Action Against Racism" advertised their event as "a contribution to the United Nations' Year for Action to combat racism and racial discrimination."[131] Earlier that year, Faith Bandler also wrote letters to representatives of the Australian Council of Trade Unions, the Australian Council of Churches, the Australian Union of Students, the Australian Council of Salaried and Professional Associations, the World Council of Churches, and the Council of Public Service Organisations, calling them all to action for a "National Congress Against Racism and Racial Discrimination" that she and others from FCAATSI were organizing. In her efforts to rally the support of these organizations, Bandler made sure to assert the "obligations we all have to make the United Nations Year Against Racism and Racial Discrimination 1971, a reality."[132]

Activists didn't limit the international connections they drew to health issues alone but also invoked problems such as land dispossession, racial discrimination and violence, lack of access to housing and employment, and civil liberties. In these broader respects, activists most often compared their political, economic, legal, and social struggles to those of African Americans and Native Americans in the United States and to Black people living under apartheid in South Africa, as well as to the self-determination struggles of many decolonizing nations of the former British Empire. In a few cases activists even visited some of these other communities to build those connections. In their accounts of overseas visits, young Aboriginal activists like Chicka Dixon and Charles Perkins recalled traveling for the express purposes of gathering information that might be of use to the Aboriginal cause at home and raising awareness among these other communities of the Aboriginal struggle in Australia.

One of the best known of these diplomatic missions occurred in 1972, when Dixon led a delegation of eight other Aboriginal activists (Terry Widders, Lyn Thompson, Lilla Watson, Cheryl Buchanan, Ruby Hammond, Gerry Bostock, Ken Winder, and Phillip Long) to visit the People's Republic of China. When interviewed about the visit, activist Paul Coe told a journalist from the *Melbourne Sun* that the group intended to "seek China's support in forming an international lobby directed at shaming Australia to alter its policies towards aboriginals."[133] Several such missions also went to the United States, such as a 1970 visit by activists Bob Maza, Bruce McGuinness, Sol Bellear, Patsy Kruger, and Jack Davis, to Atlanta, Georgia, for a conference hosted by the Congress of African Peoples. Dr. Roosevelt Brown of the Congress of African Peoples had invited the activists after a visit he paid to Australia in 1969. A report in the *New York Times* quoted activist Bruce McGuinness stating the Aboriginal delegation were attending the conference because "we must make alliances with other people engaged in liberation struggles."[134] In an Australian newspaper report on the visit, McGuinness was also quoted as saying, "We will be interested in the self-help programs the US has for negroes."[135]

Learning about the self-help programs of communities in the United States was certainly as much of a priority as building useful political alliances and connections. The best example of this in the context of health care, and one that also offers an early example of connections that have since flourished between Indigenous health workers in the United States and Australia, can be seen from an article in the *Seattle Times* in September 1978.[136] Titled "Indians, Aborigines: Visitors See Parallel Problems for Two Peoples," the article reported that two "Australian Aborigines" had recently spent a few weeks in Seattle visiting "alcohol programs offered in King County, through such groups as the Seattle Indian Health Board." According to the report, Eric Conway ("an administrator of a legal service for Aborigines") and Alec Illin ("a welfare official for the Western Australia Alcohol and Drug Authority") were shocked by the extent to which circumstances facing Australian Aboriginals and Native Americans were the same. "Historic similarities" and "health problems" common among Indians and Aborigines were "uncanny," Illin told the *Times* reporter. For Conway, the parallels of "deep-seated prejudice" faced by both communities at the hands of government and medical officials were "unbelievable."[137] The men explained that the purpose of their visit was to learn from the success of alcohol treatment programs for Native Americans in Seattle. Their presence indicated that news of the city's Indigenous health activism had indeed traveled to Australia by this stage. Illin and Conway explained that they chose Seattle over other cities in the United States because "the community involvement here is amazing. It's really working." As guests of the Seattle Indian Health Board, Conway and Illin stayed at the Thunderbird Fellowship House (the SIHB's alcohol recovery center) and spent their days studying the operations of the clinic and "meeting with those served by alcohol programs here." When asked about major lessons learned from their time in Seattle, Illin emphasized that he was "most impressed by the success of treatment programs in which Indians themselves have an active administrative role."[138]

Another example of this kind can be seen from a tour Chicka Dixon made of the United States and Canada in 1975. Organized as part of a formal "study tour" sponsored by FCAATSI's "Abschol" program, Dixon and other Aboriginal students toured the United States and Canada for three months.[139] Dixon's explicit purpose in embarking on this extensive tour was to study the alcohol rehabilitation programs among African American and Native American communities.[140] He was especially attentive to how his Native hosts had been able to secure government funding, writing of his visit to the Native American Alcoholism and Drug Abuse Center in Oakland, California, that "the Director is a Mr. Erwin, who is a 24-year-old Indian— he gave me a copy of a submission for funding for their organization and also informed me that this document was confidential but due to the fact that I have similar problems with my people and was seeking guidelines he made this information available to me. I certainly am thankful for his assistance in this matter."[141]

Aboriginal activist Gary Foley recounted to me how study tours like these "occurred at a crucial moment in the ideological and philosophical development of the Black Power movement in Australia" and were of "enormous influence to both those who went to the United States and those who they were linked with back home."[142] Clearly, Aboriginal health activists used such visits not just as a form of diplomatic outreach and information gathering but also to ensure that the injustices faced by Aboriginal people in Australia were known elsewhere. These visits, and the way they shaped the articulation of Black politics in Australia, also reveal the extent to which Aboriginal health activists saw themselves and their communities as a part of broader liberation struggles.

International travel was often not financially feasible, so activists also raised international awareness about Aboriginal health disparities by writing letters to representatives of political organizations, tribal nations, and even the United Nations. In the late 1960s Dulcie Flower wrote numerous letters to overseas organizations seeking their direct support for the work of the FCAATSI Health Committee. In a private letter sent to fellow activist Daisy Marchisotti in 1968, Flower explained, "At an emergency meeting of members of the Exec. of FCAATSI, it was decided to extend our campaign to request the support of Indigenous peoples in other countries such as Africa, Indians in Canada and USA, and Papua New Guinea."[143]

If they didn't seek out connections with or appeal directly to other oppressed communities, then activists also sought to draw international attention to the crisis in Aboriginal health by emphasizing the moral implications of its continued neglect. In 1970, members of the Aborigines Advancement League strove for the greatest heights of international attention by sending a letter directly to the secretary general of the United Nations. In it, they implored members of the UN to recognize that Aboriginal people in Australia were victims of a long-standing and ongoing genocide: "This genocide started when the Europeans first invaded us almost two hundred years ago. In earlier decades their methods were open and their purposes avowed. . . . In more recent decades the techniques of the invaders have become more subtle, but we are still experiencing the same genocide because the effect of what they do, and of what they fail to do, is still to exterminate us."[144] No clearer articulation of settler colonialism's structural violence (what Patrick Wolfe has theorized as a "structure of invasion") could have been made, and the first pieces of evidence the activists offered in their letter to substantiate this genocide claim were statistics that reflected the dire state of Aboriginal health across the nation. Specifically, they cited data on Aboriginal infant mortality: "In Central Australia our infant mortality rate has been found to be 165 per thousand live births. In the Northern Territory one in every six of our children dies in its first four years of life." More broadly, the activists also explained, "Among our children and infants the disease[s] of poverty are rife: Gastroenteritis, Dysentery and Pneumonia, so that even when they survive they are debilitated, weakened, and grossly handicapped in the struggle to survive the conditions in which they live." The poor housing conditions of Aboriginal communities across the nation were also mentioned in their appeals to the international community: "The housing conditions in which we are forced to live are a major contributing factor as our diseases are these born of squalor. Whereas in rural New South Wales 67% of the non-Aborigines of Australia own the dwellings in which they live, this is true of only 9% of the Aborigines: moreover, 37% of the dwellings in which we live are only shacks, and in 51% of the dwellings there are more people than beds." Summing up their plight, activists described "the literal, physical annihilation of our people" as a "genocide" that has been due in large part "to the social framework into which the Government of Australia has thrust us."[145] In this single letter, activists gave voice to a social and historical determinants of health argument and also made the case that their health disparities must be understood as the product of systemic and structural forms of violence rooted in settler colonialism.

Activists also had a robust awareness-raising campaign at home. They utilized various forms of print media to politicize an indifferent and uninformed Australian public about the parallels between injustices at home and abroad. A common strategy was to promote specific reading material that could "give a background to the problems we [Aboriginal Australians] face today."[146] In the newsletter the AMS eventually produced and distributed for free, a list of suggested reading was regularly featured on the back page. The texts suggested over the years indicate how activists sought to educate their uninitiated readers and also reveals something of the activists' own self-understandings. Across the first twenty issues of the *Aboriginal Medical Service Newsletter*, Aboriginal-authored texts were recommended, such as *Because a White Man'll Never Do It* by Aboriginal activist and poet Kevin Gilbert and *We Have Bugger All!: The Kulaluk Story* by Aboriginal activist Cheryl Buchanan. Texts like these offered uninformed Australians a firsthand perspective on the difficulties of contemporary life as an Aboriginal person in Australia. Alternatively, Aboriginal news publications like the *Black News Service* or *Identity Magazine* were frequently suggested. These texts marketed themselves as "alternative news services," meaning they ran articles that reframed Australian news from an Aboriginal perspective. Or alternatively, Aboriginal print media often reproduced articles from other—foreign—publications, such as *Akwesasne Notes* (the political journal of the Mohawk people of Akwesasne). Including this foreign content was part of an effort to stress the similarities between Aboriginal people's experiences and those of other communities of color. In a similar vein, books by and about other marginalized peoples were also regularly recommended in the AMS newsletter's reading lists: *The Wretched of the Earth* by Franz Fanon appeared several times, as did *Bury My Heart at Wounded Knee* by Dee Brown and *The Autobiography of Malcolm X* by Malcolm X. Again, more than being just a strategic way of bringing visibility to their health issues, these connections reveal how activists saw and understood themselves and their struggles as part of wider liberation struggles.

By encouraging Australians to immerse themselves in this literature, activists also sought, at a more basic level, to make the case that Australians ought to extend the same sympathy to Aboriginal people that they seemed to have for Black South Africans, African Americans, and other communities. Targeting this kind of oversight meant that activists even directed their efforts at Australian charitable organizations like the Red Cross by highlighting the hypocrisy of the work they did for other communities before addressing the dire needs of people at home. In his private correspondence, activist Jack Horner described how in 1972, FCAATSI members and some other "young concerned Aborigines in Sydney" had planned to visit the Sydney office of the Red Cross in order to find out if they could "at least make a thorough inspection of the complex and nasty health situation of Aboriginal Australians."[147] Expressing his frustration, Horner wrote, "After all, if they can help people overseas in similar situations in Biafra and India and Bangladesh and Indonesia, they could investigate reasons for the highest infant mortality rate in the world at present being in Australia."[148]

Importantly, such comparisons and connections with other oppressed peoples were also directed at their existing support base. The aforementioned "alternative news services"—the *Black News Service: An Alternative Black News Service, Son of Lemark: The Alternative Black Community News Service, Koori-Bina: A Black Australian News Monthly, Black Liberation*—were, for the most part, consumed by Aboriginal readers. Such comparisons were thus meant to provide possible "lessons" or act as a source of inspiration for Aboriginal readers by highlighting transnational solidarities between their political struggles and those of other groups. As activist Gary Foley wrote in *Son of Lemark*, in a piece titled "Support Our Palestinian Brothers," "The problems of the Australian Aborigines are not unique and that we should examine other situations, support other oppressed groups and find if we can learn anything from their experience and vice versa."[149] Comparisons with apartheid South Africa were very common. In Queensland, where paternalistic government protection laws in the 1960s meant that the state government controlled all aspects of Aboriginal people's lives, it was often said that "the Queensland Act is almost as bad as the apartheid laws of South Africa."[150] More generally, activists such as Charles Perkins would also often invoke South Africa or the United States, where conditions of segregation dominated, in order to attract Aboriginal readers or listeners to the ideas of Black Power. In a famous speech, Perkins endorsed the use of Black Power rhetoric in Australia, stating, "Because of the scandalous race situation in this country—which, incidentally, is equal to South Africa and America in principle, if not in extent or degree—I believe that 'black power' must eventually come under consideration."[151]

Comparisons drawn with Indigenous peoples in either Canada or the United States most frequently emphasized land claims and related issues, or else they brought attention to instructive cases where Indigenous groups had succeeded in some respect. For example, a special issue of the *Black News Service* was devoted to the achievements of the American Indian Movement.[152] This was clearly aimed to foster a sense of solidarity so that Aboriginal Australians could take encouragement from the comparatively successful efforts of Indigenous people in the United States. Summing up this intended effect on Aboriginal readers, activist Gordon Briscoe would later write in a 1978 article on the subject of "Aboriginal Health and Land Rights" that "there is little comfort in the knowledge that aboriginal society in Australia is an oppressed minority. However, Aborigines can draw strength from the knowledge that in terms of black civilization outside Australia, we make up part of the majority. Equally true is that increasing pressure is mounting beyond our shores which can assist in eroding the racist attitude of white superiority."[153] Again, it was clear that Aboriginal activists saw themselves as a part of broader struggles for racial and social justice.

These activist publications achieved much more than just awareness-raising. Like the doctors who utilized their research and writing to shift the discourse around Aboriginal health away from blaming individuals for their own health problems, Aboriginal health activists also utilized the mediums of writing and publishing to aggressively attack racist assumptions about the causes of poor Aboriginal health. Some of these refutations appeared in publications aimed at the general public, such as *Black News* or *Koori-Bina*. Other forms of writing were directed specifically at government officials and offices, such as FCAATSI's 1971 Submission to the Senate Committee on Social Environment.[154] In this brief, FCAATSI's Health Committee devoted considerable attention to parsing out the relationship between poor housing conditions and the health problems rife within Sydney's Aboriginal community. They also referred back to the Nancy Young case in order to illustrate the injustice and imprudence of a social welfare and legal system that failed to recognize Aboriginal health problems as the direct result of the unhealthy social environments in which they lived: "The Nancy Young case was notable for the way that neither judge nor jury at Roma were at all inclined to take into account the effect of social conditions in Aboriginal communities upon the public health of Aboriginal children and adults."[155]

The other side of this, of course, was that activists simultaneously invited attention to prejudicial societal attitudes and institutional discrimination. In the city, activists pointed to poor housing conditions, chronic unemployment, lack of education, and social isolation. Activist Paul Coe even labeled Aboriginal malnutrition in the cities a form of "white violence."[156] In 1972, when appearing on the ABC's television program *Monday Conference*, he expressed the point sharply, stating, "For every white kid that dies from malnutrition there are six black kids. Now to me that is white violence, legalized white violence."[157] Reflecting back on this kind of advocacy that shifted the focus away from blaming Aboriginal individuals or culture, Bobbi Sykes would later celebrate the fact that, thanks to the discursive interventions of activists at the AMS, "there can no longer be doubt in anybody's mind that the social and economic conditions under which most Blacks live are an important contributory factor to the pattern of ill-health which exists."[158] There was absolutely no ambiguity in these activists' statements that the causes of Aboriginal health disparities were the result of historic and ongoing conditions of life under settler colonialism.

Once the tide of Australian indifference had started to turn by the 1970s, many individuals mentioned already—Gary Foley, Dulcie Flower, Gordon Briscoe, Shirley Smith, Bobbi Sykes, Naomi Mayers—were particularly instrumental in the early progress of the AMS. The work of these activists, the majority of whom were women, extended far beyond simply publicity and awareness-raising; they too played a hands-on role within the clinic, performing administrative and other jobs if they couldn't be of assistance to the doctors. Activists were also crucial contributors to the process of fundraising. As an embodiment of the can-do ethos so central to the origins of the clinic, these practical contributions by activists were perhaps most powerful in the message this sent to the Aboriginal community, who were, according to Shirley Smith, "skeptical" because "you get a bit brainwashed if you are black in Australia. The conditioning starts in schools; you really think, 'Why should I try? I know I can't do it.'" But, as Smith explained in her autobiography, she and others involved in the early days of the AMS were "determined to make the Aboriginal Medical Service an all-out demonstration of "yes, we can!" Thus it was essential for Aboriginals to control the medical center, with white people doing the only thing Blacks could not yet do—practice medicine."[159] In other words, through their various efforts to get the clinic off the ground, the activists themselves embodied the ideal of self-determination in action. Moreover, at a time when the civil rights movement, the Black Power movement, the Red Power movement, and the decolonizing movements of former British colonies were making waves across the world, Aboriginal health activists didn't simply see their struggles reflected in those of others; they actually saw themselves as part of a larger political narrative in which oppressed peoples all over the world were standing up for themselves, making demands for equality and self-determination. Health activists played a central role within broader Aboriginal politics at this time, since they used their concern for the health inequalities faced by Aboriginal Australians to bridge connections, both personal and conceptual, between other activist communities who were fighting against sources of inequality and discrimination. Within the wider community of Sydney, Aboriginal activists also courted the support of allies from various sectors of Australian society who would contribute to the growth of the AMS in important ways.

Allies

In the fourth issue of the *Aboriginal Medical Service Newsletter*, appeal co-ordinator Bobbi Sykes addressed the important role of the organization's non-Aboriginal allies. Somewhat cynically, she pointed out that Aboriginal concerns had to be voiced by white allies if they were to be heard and understood at all: "If these statements do not produce a sense of urgency, then I think I shall despair. We have for many years told the white public of these conditions, again it takes for a white person, in this instance, Mr. Mathews, to speak on our behalf before we are actually 'heard.'"[160] Six issues later, she reiterated these remarks, putting an even sharper point on the significance of the advocacy to be done by and within the non-Aboriginal community: "Much of the work which needs to be done then is not in the Black community, but rather in the re-education of people in the white community. THOSE WHO ARE <u>NOT</u> A PART OF THE SOLUTION <u>ARE</u> A PART OF THE PROBLEM."[161]

According to Sykes, there were some easy ways that white allies and supporters could "really put their shoulders to the work."[162] She suggested they could take measures to "help spread the word, to talk with their friends at every opportunity, to increase circulation and interest in our Newsletter and every publication concerning Blacks."[163] And she announced that "each month I shall print suggestions of methods to make this possible, book-lists for people to read, sources of relevant material for schools and homes. I shall also print suggestions for action, and will appreciate feedback from people, and any ideas which you might have."[164] The aim was to implore non-Aboriginal people to "make Black affairs a daily issue," by which it was meant they should bring the subject alive in their own homes through the introduction and discussion of relevant reading material and also by carrying this attitude into their organizations, schools, and workplaces. In other words, Bobbi Sykes and the other health activists at the AMS aimed at nothing less than a cultural sea change in the attitudes of Australians toward Aboriginal people and the problems within Aboriginal communities. More specifically, the hope was not simply to push non-Aboriginal Australians into taking on the work of advocacy, or even simply to start paying attention to Aboriginal issues, but to actually acknowledge that their own perceptions needed to change. In an exemplary expression of this idea, Aboriginal activist and Sydney University student Cheryl Buchanan implored her (mostly white) fellow student readers of *Race Relations* (a political student newsletter) to recognize that "clearly the only problem in Australia is the 'white problem.' What you, as ignorant and naïve students must do, is sort out what your values are."[165]

Activists treated their many newsletters and political publications as an efficient and effective means of speaking directly to potential white supporters. In addition to making suggestions that might educate or transform the thinking of their readers, they also filled these publications with requests and very direct suggestions about the practical measures allies could take to help out with the health movement. For example, the *Aboriginal Medical Service Newsletter* often appealed to its readers for donations, either in the form of funding or material items: "Mum Shirl now spends approximately $30 buying fruit and vegetables each week for about 50 odd families. Can you help us give the life-sustaining food that is necessary to these families and children?"[166] Such appeals for donations even applied to the funding of the newsletter itself: "Send us what you can, when you can, and we'll send you our Newsletter for as long as we can."[167] Indicating the success of such direct appeals and the willingness of their supporters to help, Bobbi Sykes noted in the next issue of the newsletter, which followed her appeal above, that "through the efforts of a truly kind woman, we have been fortunate enough to receive—on loan basis—a duplicating machine from Gestetner. This will surely end those earlier problems with regard to printing."[168] This "truly kind woman" was one of many other nameless supporters drawn from the general public who found ways and means of helping the AMS get off the ground, even if they couldn't provide donations themselves, or provide much.

If they couldn't send money, then allies held collections, bake sales, or raffles, and sent the proceeds to the AMS.[169] Numerous stories also exist of many small but consistent generosities, such as "one little old lady" who "used to come round every pension day and leave us $1," or "one man, white, dropped by each week with $50. It was a year before he told us who he was."[170] Otherwise, allies contributed their time, skills, or expertise to the clinic, as suggested by Bobbi Sykes's frequent "thank-you messages" to readers of the AMS newsletter: "We gratefully thank also those many, many, volunteers, black and white, who drop by to help, drive, type, knock in a few nails, sweep, or whatever needs to be done."[171] Long-time activist and former AMS staffer Gary Foley also recalled the essential contributions of these allies, stating that "in the early days, we really relied on others to do what we couldn't."[172]

One especially important role played by allies was in their capacity to act as witnesses to police brutality and unlawful arrests of Aboriginal people in downtown Sydney. Bob Bellear, field officer of the Aboriginal Legal Service, recounted the problem in an issue of the AMS newsletter when he described how "the paddy wagons come near closing time at the Empress Hotel, Redfern and line up two abreast. They arrest up to 30 blacks a night for drunkenness and other charges. They treat us like dirt. They won't even let a doctor in to inspect a charged man to ascertain if he is in fact drunk."[173] Appealing directly to their non-Aboriginal newsletter readers, Bobbi Sykes therefore issued an appeal "to especially you non-Aboriginal readers, to man the vigil. People prepared to act as witnesses are asked to be in the vicinity of the Empress Hotel, Regent Street, Redfern, at 9.45 any night, particularly Thursday, Friday and Saturday night. We do not want to fight the police, we just want the public to really see the conditions which are forced upon us in the dead of night."[174] Playing the role of "witness" wasn't only limited to such extreme events, but as Sykes made clear to newsletter readers, "the black community is continually harassed in this way, very 'back of the bus' type of thing, and often 'no bus.' It is important that people who want to understand what we are doing [at the AMS] realize the circumstances of our lives and the conditions under which we live. So remember, you can always speak up."[175]

Allies who made a significant contribution to the AMS didn't come only from anonymous quarters of the general public. As the Nancy Young case illustrated, individuals within the mainstream media could also be important strategic allies for the Aboriginal health movement. In their 1972 appearance on the ABC's *Monday Conference* program, Paul Coe and Bobbi Sykes reflected on the complex relationship that Aboriginal health activists had with the media. On the one hand, Coe acknowledged the effective awareness-raising outcomes of the "sensational stories" about infant mortality and police victimization.[176] But at the same time, he lamented that for the most part the press only focused on these issues instead of critically analyzing and isolating the root causes of these problems, which he described as "the destruction of our society, of our way of life and trying to offer the people no identity, no positive alternative."[177] Despite such critiques of the mainstream press as a whole, individual journalists were certainly among those the AMS counted as their important allies. For instance,

Sykes recalled the important contributions of the ABC journalist Michael Willesee when the AMS first tried to move into a bigger location.[178] As Sykes recalled, representatives of the AMS encountered great difficulties getting a building permit from the South Sydney Council that "we got so sick and tired of this that we went straight to the media. We rang up Michael Willesee and Michael sent a team down to film where we were."[179] According to Sykes, Willesee's crew managed to capture the "raw deal" that the AMS was being handed by the South Sydney Council.[180] Indicating precisely how powerful an ally the media could be, Sykes remembered that "the programme went to air one night and the next morning by special courier arrived our permit to go ahead and alter the inside of our building."[181]

Finally, while it would take some time, health activists and the AMS also eventually found both Aboriginal and non-Aboriginal allies within government. Sympathetic, outspoken, and well-positioned public servants like Dr. H. C. Coombs and Gordon Bryant were important allies in their broader advocacy for Aboriginal rights and on the subject of Aboriginal health in particular. I have already mentioned the ripple effect created by Coombs's address on "Aboriginal Health" in 1969. In addition to this, he became a close advisor to Gough Whitlam in the years before Whitlam became prime minister in 1972, and he has been credited with largely writing Whitlam's policies on Aboriginal Affairs.[182] Gordon Bryant, in addition to being a federal employee from 1957 until his appointment as the first minister for Aboriginal Affairs in 1973, was also an office-bearer in the Aborigines Advancement League and in FCAATSI during this time. For example, he played a key role in FCAATSI's early years when his electoral office—with its parliamentary phone account—became a communication hub, with members of sister organizations from other states being telephoned on meeting nights.[183] Bryant was also instrumental in organizing support for the national "Vote Yes" campaign for the 1967 referendum, and he played an important role during Nancy Young's campaign by advising Jack Horner and FCAATSI members about key strategies for approaching the Queensland state government in their appeal.[184] As Sykes pointed out in the AMS newsletter, setting aside any advocacy work these allies did within the halls of government itself, the public endorsement offered by these high-ranking officials when making public statements about Aboriginal health often did much more to gain attention and funding for Aboriginal political demands than complaints raised by the community itself.[185]

Perhaps most significantly, however, by March 1969, in the space of just three months, seven Aboriginal people were employed in various positions by the federal government: Phillip Roberts, Charles Perkins, Reg Saunders, Margaret Lawrie, Val Bryant, Patricia Conway, and Reta Merrick were dubbed by the *Aboriginal Quarterly* as members of a "Quiet Revolution."[186] Employed to occupy various roles in the Office and Council of Aboriginal Affairs, these seven appointees were selected to act as advisors to the federal government on the basis of their expertise and connections to Aboriginal communities throughout Australia. For the health activists in Sydney, Perkins, Saunders, and Lawrie were especially useful representatives to have within government given their prior working experience in grassroots political organizing, urban communities, and the health sector. It was hoped these new appointees would also be well positioned to guide and recruit additional allies within government. Speaking in 1972 about the value for the AMS of having these government allies, Bobbi Sykes reflected, "The people haven't been there for us to use in the past, and now they are there for us to use, and I think we'd be silly if we didn't take advantage of it, because you know it means money which we haven't had in the past."[187]

While the input of these various allies was undeniably crucial to the creation of the AMS and to many early successes of the Aboriginal health movement more generally, the activists themselves both courted and set the terms for allied support. As Sykes put it above, these allies could be "used by us," and as Foley explained in an interview in 1975, "the only real thing people can do is recognize that the only people who are really going to be able to solve this problem are Aboriginal people and having recognized that, determine the way in which they can support us."[188] In understanding the part played in this history by allies, it is therefore critical to recognize that activists set the agenda, even for the help they received, by asking for and accepting very specific kinds of contributions. Whatever help they may have received was therefore never an obstacle to the political goals of the clinic, which were to foster Aboriginal community control and self-determination.

· · · · · ·

For Aboriginal people in Sydney, creating their own health service was at once a practical and political solution to their inability to access health services. The AMS was therefore always more than just a health center—it represented a means for urban Aboriginal people to enact their political ideals of self-determination and sovereignty in a context (health care) that had been set up to forcibly assimilate them into the Australian mainstream.

Doctors, Aboriginal activists, community members, and individual allies within government, the media, and the public all played important roles in turning Aboriginal health from a marginal subject in Australian news and politics in the early 1960s into one of the most pressing issues confronting Australia's medical community and its national politicians by the 1970s. Health activists used the political momentum generated by current events—both at home and overseas—to shift the discourse about poor Aboriginal health and its causes from one that blamed the victim to one that recognized the social, historical, and economic determinants of health. In doing so, they called the moral culpability of the Australian government and society into question. They highlighted that the structures of inequality and exclusion that perpetuated conditions of poverty and discrimination were responsible for disproportionate health problems among Aboriginal people in both the past and present. They used medical data and statistics to argue that this structural neglect was having an especially disastrous impact on Indigenous health in cities where the Aboriginal population was largely abandoned by the state. The rural focus of most medical data at this time meant that activists also had to overcome a problem of urban invisibility. Different to the circumstances in Seattle, though, the kind of structural invisibility that Aboriginal people faced in Sydney was less bound up with institutional (government and medical) mismanagement and more a product of generalized public misconceptions that Aboriginal health was only problematic in the country. In Sydney, much like in Seattle, the urban Indigenous community thus had to fight for their community's visibility by raising awareness about the significant discrimination they faced in mainstream medical care and showing that their urban community suffered from many of the same problems as rural communities.

Aboriginal health activists in Australia pushed for many of the same solutions we saw the community in Seattle advocating for: antidiscrimination, culturally appropriate health services, and guaranteed access to and funding for medical care for Indigenous people beyond emergency services. Like Native people in Seattle, and like many other disempowered groups who were also contending against medical discrimination in the 1970s (women, Black people, LGBTQ+ people), Indigenous people in Sydney found their solution was within their own hands, and thus they established the Aboriginal Medical Service in 1971. Precisely how their ideals of self-determination and sovereignty took shape through the clinics—an idea I have been describing as "reterritorialized sovereignty"—will be explored in the following chapter with reference to both the Seattle Indian Health Board and the Aboriginal Medical Service.

5 Sovereign Bodies, Sovereign Spaces

The Seattle Indian Health Board and the Aboriginal Medical Service, 1970–2020

In 1970, Aboriginal activist and Aboriginal Medical Service (AMS) cofounder Dulcie Flower addressed a forum of health activists in Sydney and pleaded with them never to lose sight of the true meaning of "health" and by implication, the significance of their struggle to protect it: "In closing I'd like to quote Dubois who defined health as: not a state but a potentiality—the ability of an individual or social group to modify himself or itself continually not only in order to function better in the present but also to prepare for the future."[1] In 2004, just months before she died, Adeline Garcia (Haida), activist and cofounder of the Seattle Indian Health Board (SIHB), humbly recalled the impact of the work she and others had done to establish that organization and many of Seattle's other groundbreaking programs for Native Americans: "We just needed to get together and find strength to be someplace where you know somebody isn't going to be criticizing you because your skin is not the same color theirs is and you don't speak the same way. We just needed a place where we were comfortable and accepted at face value. That was important."[2]

Together, these statements encapsulate two foundational attributes of Indigenous community-controlled health services in Australia and the United States that have since given them an enduring political significance. On the one hand, Flower's comments remind us that as places that seek to protect and prioritize the health of Indigenous people, urban Indigenous-controlled health clinics are an important staging ground for the futures of these communities. On the other hand, Garcia's comments remind us that as Indigenous-controlled and Indigenous-serving places within an otherwise inhospitable and alienating environment, these clinics also serve as an "Indigenous space" in the city—a place where Indigenous people can go, not simply for medical care but for a sense of community, of belonging, or even of "home." Supporting these essential attributes, a third element also accounts for the political significance of these clinics: from the very beginning, their existence was premised on a belief that pan-Indigenous urban

communities are just as entitled as reserve or reservation-based Indige-
nous communities to the benefits of government support on the basis of
Indigenous rights. This belief, in other words, refutes that urban pan-
Indigenous communities are assimilated (and thus no longer rightly identified as Indigenous). And, importantly, it also entails an assertion that
Indigenous sovereignty (understood, in part, as the right to make claims
on the federal government) should be reconceptualized so that urban pan-
Indigenous communities are not excluded. Rather than holding to a notion
of Indigenous sovereignty that aligns with a western conception of jurisdiction over a specific territory, urban activists, via their health politics,
pushed for an enlarged view of Indigenous sovereignty that could carry
weight *in spite of* territory; they advocated for a reterritorialization of Indigenous sovereignty onto Indigenous peoples' corporeal bodies, and onto
Indigenous-run organizations that serve their communities; sovereign bodies, and sovereign spaces.

According to this model of sovereignty, the basis on which Indigenous
people can assert their sovereign rights and justly make claims against the
federal governments of the United States and Australia emanates from their
very identities as Indigenous peoples, not their residence in a particular lo-
cale. This is a model of Indigenous sovereignty that can accommodate
movement, migration, and the growth of diasporic communities, which are
realities that increasingly characterize Indigenous communities and families in the United States and Australia. Moreover, it is a model of sovereignty
that seeks to make Indigenous peoples at home wherever they choose to live.
The AMS and the SIHB, in other words, were established not simply as
responses to a health crisis but to the systemic, intentional government
neglect and disavowal of their communities—indeed the active attempt
to erase them and their ability to claim Indigenous political and cultural
identities. These clinics have thereby acted as a critical site for the expression and enactment of a form of Indigenous self-determination that has been
crucial in expanding the reach and power of the political project of Indigenous sovereignty.

· · · · · ·

The preceding chapters have shown how the pan-Indigenous urban communities in Seattle and Sydney succeeded in making the urgent health struggles
of their respective peoples visible within the United States and Australia. In
Seattle, an urban Indian health movement formed around key political goals
(visibility, space, obligation) during the 1950s to 1970s. In Sydney, key groups

(doctors, activists, allies) formed a loosely bound Aboriginal health movement during roughly the same time and prioritized similar goals. In both cities, advocacy by these groups revealed that urban Indigenous people faced various forms of structural violence within mainstream health care: exclusion, neglect and abandonment, abuse and discrimination, and a common issue of structural invisibility that activists in Seattle described as "ping-ponging." Two factors worked symbiotically to exclude them from accessing health care in all but emergency cases. On the one hand, free government health care afforded to Indigenous people as part of historic agreements and obligations applied only to Indigenous residents of reserves or reservations; people thus effectively "lost" their Indigenous rights to health care as soon as they moved into an urban area that was not their Indigenous homeland.[3] On the other hand, mainstream doctors in cities often refused—for various reasons—to treat Indigenous patients. These factors in combination meant that in the postwar period, Indigenous people who relocated to cities like Seattle and Sydney were simultaneously forced into mainstream health care on the one hand while they were actively excluded from it on the other. By the 1950s and '60s Indigenous people in cities grew increasingly wary of mainstream health services because they were inhospitable—often outright discriminatory—environments. If they weren't refused treatment from the outset, then the hostility encountered by Indigenous people once admitted into mainstream health facilities meant they were often driven away. This left many without access to health care at all.

In response to this crisis of access, activists in Seattle and Sydney were compelled by the early 1970s to take measures into their own hands. Pan-Aboriginal and pan-Indian activists set up their own free grassroots medical clinics that were run by, and which catered exclusively to, Indigenous people. The clinics were understood by these activists to be an embodiment of their sovereign rights and a place where diasporic Indigenous people in cities could experience a sense of community. Against the governments' insistence that urban relocation would result in near universal assimilation, the clinics thus stood as unambiguous proof that urban Indigenous people were not somehow becoming "less Indigenous" in the cities. By contrast, the clinics showed that while hailing from diverse nations and cultures, diasporic Indigenous people in cities nonetheless understood themselves to be a unified political and cultural group. They were distinct from the mainstream, and their community was forged in part by the experiences they faced in common within the exclusionary urban environment. Constituting some of the earliest and most visible grassroots organizations to be born from urban pan-

Indigenous identity and shared struggle, the clinics cast doubt on the legitimacy of claims that diasporic urban Indigenous communities should neither be recognized nor supported by the government. Acknowledging the significance of how the Seattle Indian Health Board and the Aboriginal Medical Service asserted a form of Indigenous identity and self-determination that neither depended on specific claims to nationhood nor required jurisdiction over a specific territory, each of the previous chapters proposed that the movements for health reform and the clinics themselves had come to represent the "reterritorialization" of Indigenous sovereignty.

The 1960s and '70s were a busy time for Indigenous political activists in both Australia and the United States. Historians have paid a great deal of attention to the significance of activist movements for territorial sovereignty or "land rights" in this time. Indeed, all the big markers of Indigenous activism from this period evince the dominance of land and territory in articulations of a newly strengthening Indigenous sovereignty movement: in the United States, the occupations of Alcatraz Island (1969), of the Bureau of Indian Affairs (BIA) offices (1972), and of Wounded Knee II (1973) loom large in the historical imaginary. In Australia, the Aboriginal Tent Embassy (est. 1972) remains perhaps the most recognizable symbol of Indigenous politics in Australia, and nothing represents more clearly the centrality of land claims to the Indigenous struggle for self-determination and sovereignty in that national context. There is little denying that land rights are, have always been, and will always be of utmost importance to the political project of Indigenous sovereignty in these two settler nations.

Yet, at the same time, the health activism studied in this book shows different projects in Indigenous politics were simultaneously forming around the concept of sovereignty. In the 1960s and 1970s Indigenous urban migrants hit up against the limitations of a territorial and juridical model of sovereignty that excluded them from continuing to receive recognition and access (to government-provided services) *as* Indigenous people. Their experiences of living in ways that cut across the territorial borders of rural and urban communities also resulted in the formation of cultural and political identities that aligned them with an Indigenous diaspora in addition to their national or tribal community. Their health struggles, and especially the structural violence (invisibility, erasure, discrimination) they encountered in mainstream urban medical settings in the 1950s, '60s, and '70s distilled new ideas about sovereignty in a particular way.

This chapter unpacks the idea of reterritorialized sovereignty by first examining the ways in which the very idea of the clinics sought to de-emphasize the necessity of a territorial and juridical model of Indigenous sovereignty, pushing instead for an ideal of practiced and embodied Indigenous sovereignty that would serve the goal of self-governance. Second, this chapter considers several ways in which attributes of the clinics counteracted specific government policies aimed at denying urban pan-Indigenous communities their rights and recognitions (or even a political voice) *as* Indigenous people simply because of where they lived. Third, I show how the quest for federal government funding represented the culmination of these efforts to assert their Indigenous rights as diasporic pan-Indigenous urban communities. Activists at each of the clinics were instrumental in influencing government legislation and policy that eventually funded urban Indigenous health. This represented a vital step in the realization of urban pan-Indigenous rights and sovereignty.

Embodied Sovereignty and Sovereign Bodies

In 1967, Pearl Warren (Makah) told a reporter of the *Seattle Post-Intelligencer* that in striving to create a place where urban Indians could receive free social services from their own people, the city's pan-Indian community did not desire "a reservation right in the middle of town." All they wanted, Warren explained, was a place "where in our most vulnerable times of feeling unwell, we could feel free and proud to be ourselves."[4] Warren's comments underscore a subtle but important difference between the politics of territorial sovereignty (or "land rights" in Australian parlance) and the model of Indigenous sovereignty that urban pan-Indigenous health activists were striving to create with their medical services. Warren expressed a special regard for the importance of Indigenous people's freedom and ability to simply *be* Indigenous at all times and in all places, but most especially when they were not in good health. Rather than seek jurisdictional control over territory, Warren asserted that health activists were simply trying to push back an assimilationist agenda that encroached into even the most vulnerable and private moments in an Indigenous person's life.

In Australia during the 1980s, celebrated Aboriginal activist Ruby Hammond wrote an op-ed for a major Australian newspaper reflecting on the close relationship between Aboriginal land rights and community-run health services. She lamented the difficulties encountered by Aboriginal activists and communities across Australia who were struggling to achieve land rights: "We are adapting every day. We have to adapt because we are living in a changing society." And yet precisely because of these challenges, she underscored the vital necessity of the work being done by Aboriginal health activists in the cities: "But the only way we will survive is if we have community-based services."[5]

Hammond's and Warren's comments call our attention to the ways we might understand the actions of Indigenous health activists in both nations as contributing to an important distinction within the broader political project of Indigenous sovereignty. In their respective efforts to serve their communities, Warren and Hammond shared a commitment to the idea that Indigenous peoples must be in charge of their own affairs— that is, be self-determining. Yet, the strategy each advocated for achieving this goal was not the acquisition of territory but rather the creation of their own community-controlled services. In their focus on self-governance, self-control, and self-reliance through these community services, Warren and Hammond both challenged the statist assumption that legal monopoly over a territory must necessarily be the only or even most effective way by which a group collectively governs itself or achieves self-determination. In fact, the innovative character of their political ambitions is evident in how Warren and Hammond each proposed a new and different social mechanism that would allow Indigenous people who had no recourse to nationhood status or to land claims as a group (the position of pan-Indigenous groups in cities) to nonetheless find ways to exist as a political community, exercise self-governance, and eventually, make claims on the federal government for financial support. Their proposal was one that also did not challenge or displace the territorial claims of the Indigenous people on whose lands they were living.[6] In Warren's words, this could be achieved not by creating a reservation in the middle of town but by creating another kind of space that would allow Native people to practice their culture freely and to feel a sense of community, especially during difficult times. In Hammond's words, this could be achieved explicitly by creating community-controlled organizations. In both instances, the intention was not just to create organizations that would allow Indigenous people to be in charge of their own medical affairs but to allow them to do this, and to receive treatment, *as* Indigenous people.

Their specific ambitions highlight a few important points that are worth emphasizing. First, their move away from a territorial model of sovereignty serves as an important reminder that many urban Indigenous people *do* have a claim to territory and nationhood status in cities. For these Indigenous people, fighting for recognition of urban communities as Indigenous communities with rights as such is about demanding that urban territory *is*

Indigenous territory.[7] This leads to a second issue: the ambitions of the health activists reinforce the fact that their claims to sovereignty were rooted in a pan-Indigenous identity rather than a national or tribal one.[8] Third, Warren and Hammond, in their respective comments, suggested the inconsequence of a specific location to the status of these "nonreservation" spaces as Indigenous, and thus they evinced the nonterritorial basis of the underlying rights they were meant to uphold.

As a practical matter, by seeking the right to be self-governing as opposed to the right to territorial sovereignty, urban Indigenous health activists made a substantive claim about the project of Indigenous sovereignty as a whole. Their efforts supported the idea that securing territory, rather than being the only expression of Indigenous sovereignty, was just one aspect of it—to be sure, an undeniably important one. But as their actions demonstrate, they believed a meaningful form of self-determination could (indeed, must) also be realized for peoples who did not seek territorial control or claims to nationhood. Hammond's insistence that "we have to adapt" also suggested that she thought it shortsighted for Indigenous people to continue as if jurisdiction over territory was the only paradigm for realizing Indigenous sovereignty. Both Warren and Hammond were in fact key proponents of the idea that control over territory *could not* be the only way in which Indigenous people pursued their sovereignty moving forward. Rather, as they and their communities sought to show with their respective health clinics, other forms of self-governance and social practices might even serve better in the long term in realizing the goal of Indigenous self-determination. To be sure, in pressing for forms of reterritorialized sovereignty, urban Indigenous health activists did not seek to displace or deny the importance of land claims (it was never an "either/or" argument); they simply intended to make room for other political endeavors and needs. Their goals were ultimately expansive; they sought to extend the reach of Indigenous sovereignty such that it could always be realized by Indigenous people in all contexts, not only when they were within the bounds of recognized Indigenous territories. This emphasized both an embodied and mobile form of Indigenous sovereignty that could literally meet Indigenous people where they were.

Understanding how postwar urbanization and the ensuing growth of an Indigenous diaspora brought on these changes in the goals of Indigenous sovereignty entails a reframing of Indigenous political activism in the 1960s and 1970s. Although at this time urban Indigenous communities led the way in political and social movements to protect sovereign homelands (Red Power, Alcatraz, Aboriginal Tent Embassy), these experiences only sharpened a collective realization among urban communities that their pan-Indigenous political and cultural life in the cities was neither represented nor protected by a territorial model of sovereignty.[9] Moreover, for many diasporic Indigenous people who lived in cities, it made little sense to think about their interests as being separate or opposed to those of reservation or reserve communities. A continuing connection with rural homelands was, for many diasporic urban people, a lived reality. Family members were not infrequently split across rural and urban locales, and it was common for the urban/rural divide to be bridged by these kinship ties. Therefore, even though territorial sovereignty may not have benefited them directly in cities, urban pan-Indigenous activists fought hard for it since territorial sovereignty benefited their families, friends, and the communities on whose lands they now resided after relocating.

Indeed, at this time, many newly urbanized Indigenous people saw themselves and reserve/reservation populations as part of the same community and as sharing in the same political struggle. Bearing this out, in the 1960s, Aboriginal urban migrants in Australia came to speak of themselves and of all Aboriginal people as "Black."[10] Much like the language of "Black Power" in Australia, the language of "Red Power" in the United States drew little distinction between how this politics and a broadened "Indian" identity applied to urban versus rural communities. In both the Indigenous Red Power and Black Power movements, a vocal anticolonialism with ties to the global decolonizing struggles of the postwar era blended with a new awareness of local constructions of race ("black" and "red"). The clinics in Seattle and Sydney therefore provided alternative plotlines to the fiction of assimilation that falsely dichotomized rural and urban Indigenous communities and erased the realities of continuing political, social, cultural, familial, and economic ties between them. Remembering back to their strategizing in the 1970s, Dr. Walt Hollow (Assiniboine-Sioux), one of the SIHB's first physicians, recalled the emphasis the early founders of the clinic placed on their treaty rights, even as urban Indians living off-reservation: "The treaty said we were to get health care. And here we could demonstrate that there were a group of Indians living in Seattle, who were not getting regular health care."[11] Drawing little distinction between the political struggles of urban and rural communities, urban health activists in particular spoke up on behalf of reserve communities, referring to them as "our brothers and sisters."[12] Such acts provided a counternarrative to the romances of assimilationist "melting pots" imagined by Australian and American national history and federal policy. Ironically though, the visibility of the territorial struggles that urban activists fought for on behalf of rural communities in the 1960s and '70s often obscured efforts to protect their own (nonterritorial) sovereignty in the cities. If the shift toward imagining forms of Indigenous sovereignty that could exist alongside but separate from territorial politics took place slowly, then community-controlled health clinics (and the political struggles that built them) were key sites in which this vision took shape.

With the clinics themselves embodying what a de/reterritorializing of Indigenous sovereignty might look like, they functioned almost as mobile mini sovereign zones or "hubs," where Indigenous people were in control of their own affairs, and where they were free to gather and associate as a community on terms they set. The "hub" is an idea drawn from the work of Renya K. Ramirez, who writes, "The hub suggests how landless Native Americans maintain a sense of connection to their tribal homelands and urban spaces through participation in cultural circuits and maintenance of social networks, as well as shared activity with other Native Americans in the city and on the reservation."[13]

According to Ramirez, "hub-making activities" common among urban Indians can include "signs and behavior" as ubiquitous as phone calling, emailing, and other virtual activities such as reading tribal newspapers on the Internet. As a cultural, social and political concept, for Ramirez the hub ultimately has the potential to "strengthen Native identity and provide a sense of belonging, as well as to increase the political power of Native peoples." She also describes "hub-making activities" as practices that "bridge tribal differences so that Native Americans can unify to struggle for social change."[14] I borrow this language of the hub, with its emphasis on urban and rural mobility and diasporic Indigenous identity and connection, as well as political and social innovation, in order to conceptualize the social, cultural, and political significance of urban Indigenous health clinics as a kind of "native hub." On this reading, understanding the clinics as "health hubs" or as I suggest, as sovereign spaces (indexing a shift away from *specific* land/territories, and which in theory could be located anywhere), registers how they expanded the project of Indigenous sovereignty considerably and provided Indigenous peoples a capacious means to exercise their sovereignty wherever they lived.

The creation of community-controlled health clinics thus reflected the reterritorialization of Indigenous sovereignty and the pursuit of self-governance on two crucial planes: at the level of Indigenous-run institutions and at the level of Indigenous people's individual corporeal bodies.

Of course, in a certain sense, this concern that individual Indigenous people exhibit agency and control over their bodies and medical affairs does not look all that different from the ordinary liberal concern that individuals have sovereign control over their own bodies. However, Indigenous health activists' concern with the bodily sovereignty of their respective community members was distinctive in several important respects. First, Indigenous bodily sovereignty required a particular social, political, and cultural context to be fully realized. The dignity and autonomy of Indigenous people in their medical affairs and their concomitant capacity to exercise bodily integrity required a set of institutions that would cater to and, at a bare minimum, not seek to erase their Indigenous identities. Activists were concerned, in other words, to make sure that their community members could enjoy individual dignity and bodily control over their medical affairs *as* Indigenous people. This is perhaps what Pearl Warren meant when she said that all the Seattle Indian community wanted was a place "where in our most vulnerable times of feeling unwell, we could feel free and proud to be ourselves."[15]

Second, while many activists no doubt shared the "liberal" aspiration that individual Indigenous persons enjoy autonomy and control over their own bodies and medical care qua individual subjects, the activists' concern with the bodily integrity and sovereignty of their communities' members manifested another set of slightly different and very distinct Indigenous normative concerns about a fundamental link that tied Indigenous peoples' sovereignty to their corporeal bodies. As Aileen Moreton-Robinson has explained in the Indigenous Australian context, "Our sovereignty is carried by the body and differs from Western constructions of sovereignty, which are predicted on the social contract model, the idea of a unified supreme authority, territorial integrity and individual rights."[16] This understanding that their sovereignty emanates from their bodies, histories, and identities as Indigenous people reflected one key sense in which health activists drew on an "embodied" understanding of sovereignty. But in another crucial sense, Indigenous peoples' very existence and their fight (over centuries) to not just be healthy but sometimes simply to live means that their sovereignty is also "embodied" through a refusal to die, or through simply existing. Structures of settler-colonial governance that attempted to decimate Indigenous communities in the United States and Australia were often manifested most acutely at the level of individual Indigenous bodies. Therefore, protecting the health and wellness of individual Indigenous persons becomes a form of resistance in this context. Understood in this way, the health of the Indigenous community and its own capacity for self-direction is predicated on ensuring the health and bodily sovereignty of its individual members. Likewise, the concern for the self-determination of individuals within that group is also advanced by the health of the community. Ruby Hammond expressed just this point when she extolled the work of the AMS in 1980, writing, "The Redfern Service, however, offers an impressive example of the advantages of such community run organisations—their total commitment to the task [of self-determination], their acceptance by the target population and their vital role in the total development of the Aboriginal community by supporting individual people and the larger community."[17]

Providing for the health of individual members in this way—via Indigenous-run organizations—was thus thought to be necessary to the self-determination of the community. The importance of creating sovereign spaces for their community members therefore indexes another important conceptual and practical shift in the project of Indigenous sovereignty as it became reterritorialized. In addition to protecting the health, safety, and freedom of Indigenous peoples' literal bodies, community-controlled organizations like the health services were another crucial staging ground from which Indigenous sovereignty could be practiced and protected, irrespective of location.[18] Indigenous-run institutions like the clinics therefore literally shifted the ground on which Indigenous sovereignty could be exercised.

Seeing the clinics in this light points to the important role that health issues played as part of the wider narrative sweep of Indigenous activism in Australian and US history. Scholars have already noted how as Indigenous communities became more diasporic in the postwar period, the need arose to protect ongoing attachments to specific territories. By contrast, we should also recognize how the concurrent efforts to protect Indigenous health in cities expanded upon the limited reach of a territorial model of Indigenous sovereignty. Rather than developing in separate and isolated ways, the history of this activism shows us that ideas about Indigenous sovereignty were multifaceted, responsive, and contested in the postwar world. Indigenous migration and mobility in Australia and the United States in the 1950s and 1960s raised all sorts of questions—for the newly relocated in particular—about the status of any rights and recognitions enjoyed by Indigenous peoples in their new settings. Did Indigenous rights travel along with the people? Was Indigenous identity lost outside of the reserve and traditional territories?

In postwar cities, where Indigenous people lost even the modicum of territorial sovereignty they had on reserves and reservations, resisting settler colonization and defending Indigenous sovereignty turned on successfully defying assimilation and asserting the continuities of their cultural and political identities regardless of where they resided. Health activists therefore often began their advocacy by doing the work of showing that Indigenous communities remained cohesive (and indeed, remained Indigenous) even if they lived in ways that cut across geographic borders and even if their cultures changed (became "pan-Indigenous") in new settings. In essence, these health activists made the all-important argument that by moving off recognized Indigenous lands, urban migrants were not forfeiting their Indigenous rights but were expanding the boundaries of Indigenous life and thus of Indigenous rights.

The SIHB and the AMS: Antidotes to Assimilation

A key premise of the termination and assimilation policies of the US and Australian federal governments in the second half of the twentieth century was that these would be emancipatory programs geared toward giving Native Americans and Indigenous Australians full civil rights, clearing the way for them to finally join the nation by removing them from their supposedly backward reserve and reservation communities and freeing them from the yoke of government welfare. In pursuing assimilationist programs, these federal governments treated Indigenous people living in the United States and Australia in ways that mirrored the immigration rhetoric of the time regarding ethnicity. Indigenous people were positioned as "new immigrants" to urban areas, requiring assistance to assimilate into the American and Australian way of life. However, few measures were taken to make sure that Indigenous people would receive the social services available to other citizens. Urban Indigenous migrants were given little guidance about how to take advantage of the services available to them, and providers (such as hospitals and doctors) were given little training in how to reach or cater to the newly urbanizing Indigenous communities.

During the 1950s and '60s, Indigenous people nonetheless found ways of making the urban environment a more hospitable place to live. In Seattle, the American Indian Women's Service League played an important role in this respect. Their social club provided an informal support network for their growing urban community, and it soon expanded to do the work of more organized forms of social service such as a food bank and clothing drive. In Sydney, the growing Aboriginal community found mutual support and a sense of belonging in the Aboriginal neighborhoods that formed in Redfern, Waterloo, and Newtown because of discriminatory housing policies that prevented Aboriginal people from accessing housing anywhere else. These neighborhoods, in turn, became the foundation for the political and cultural organizations that later formed in response to the limited options Aboriginal people had for freely socializing in the city. In particular, the Aboriginal Legal Service and the National Black Theatre Company, which formed around the same time as the AMS, were instrumental in making Sydney a safe and accommodating place for Aboriginal people and their cultures.

From the minute they opened their doors in the early 1970s, the SIHB and the AMS became instrumental in these communitywide efforts to counteract a hostile urban environment. More than just providing an alternative place for Indigenous people to seek out health care, the SIHB and AMS intentionally delivered their services and crafted their institutional identities in ways that explicitly pushed back at the assimilationist logic governing so much of Indigenous peoples' lives in cities, and which sought to either erase or deny them their identities. One important way the clinics did this was simply by fostering a pan-Indian and pan-Aboriginal cross-cultural environment within the clinics. For example, the clinics ran cultural programs such as Indigenous art fairs and art therapy programs within their premises that fostered the growth and visibility of urban pan-Indigenous culture in the cities and provided a space for community members to engage in cultural practices together. Both clinics also had open-door policies of accepting Indigenous patients regardless of tribal/national affiliation, thus reinforcing the idea that they were an inclusive, pan-Indigenous space. And since the settler-colonial history of Indigenous health has also involved the supplanting of Indigenous health care practices and the undermining of Indigenous medical knowledge, the clinics also provided facilities for a wide variety of traditional Indigenous medicine and healing practices to be used in conjunction with Western medicine, thereby showing that their communities not only possessed but held onto this knowledge even while they adopted American or Australian ways of living.[19] Once the clinics had the resources to publish their own written materials and to renovate and redesign their administrative and clinical offices, they also self-consciously incorporated artistic designs and motifs that reflected their pan-Indigenous identities. The logos of both health clinics (below) encapsulate this through their use of designs and imagery that symbolize unity.

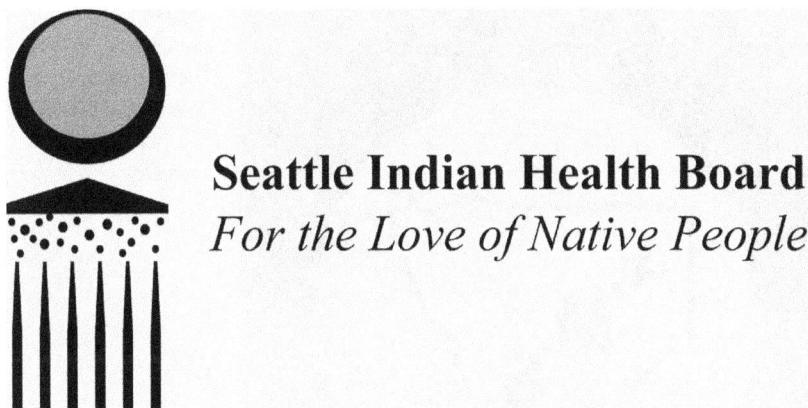

Seattle Indian Health Board

For the Love of Native People

FIGURE 5.1 Seattle Indian Health Board logo. Seattle Indian Health Board website.

Figure 5.1 shows the letterhead and logo of the SIHB. They have been described in the following way: "The Seattle Indian Health Board logo sym-
bolizes the union of the people in good health."[20] Designed by Bernie
Whitebear's brother, Lawney Reyes (Colville), the logo's symbol is drawn
from the Plains Indians symbols for healing and the medicine house.[21] The
outer circle represents continuous life, while the red inner center circle sym-
bolizes the spirit of the people. The triangle, dots, and poles represent a
stylized medicine house where health rituals and healing ceremonies are
practiced.[22] Meanwhile, the tagline "For the Love of Native People"—a later
addition coined by longtime SIHB staffer Becky Corpuz, and adapted from
a phrase that she remembered SIHB founder Adeline Garcia would often use
when describing the work of the clinic—emphasized the inclusiveness of
their clinic.[23] Together, the logo and tag line are designed to underscore that
a key aspect of the SIHB's work involves fostering the unity and inclusion
of all Native peoples in their attempts to get healthy.

As you can see in figure 5.2, the main part of the AMS Redfern's logo is
made up of the Aboriginal flag, comprising a black and red background and
yellow center circle. Designed in 1971 by Aboriginal artist Harold Thomas,
the black color of the flag represents all Aboriginal people of Australia,
while the red represents both the red earth and the red ochre used in ceremonies and symbolizing Aboriginal people's relation to the land. The yellow circle represents the sun, the provider and protector of life.[24] Overlaid
on top of the yellow circle, a white outline of the state of New South Wales
contains the letters "AMS." While Thomas originally designed the flag for
the land rights movement, it soon became a symbol representing all Aboriginal people and their many political struggles in Australia. It was first flown

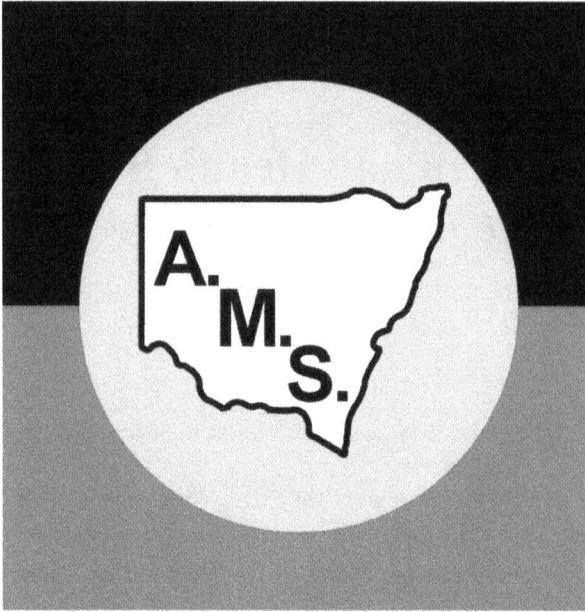

FIGURE 5.2
Aboriginal Medical
Service logo.
Aboriginal Medical
Service Redfern
website.

on National Aborigines Day in Adelaide on July 12, 1971, and was subsequently planted on the lawn of Parliament House in Canberra as part of the Aboriginal Tent Embassy from late 1972. The flag was always used as part of the AMS logo, signifying the clinic's connection to the broader Aboriginal political movement of the 1970s and underscoring its commitment to serving all Aboriginal people.

The legacy of these early endeavors to foster unity and inclusion can be seen today, not just in the continued use of these logos but also in the physical environments of the clinics—their waiting rooms are adorned with art and photographs that proudly show the cultural diversity of their communities in both the past and present. And at events they host, the SIHB and the AMS have always emphasized how the clinics function as both health and cultural institutions—like two sides of the same coin. In the 1970s, expressing this diversity at the very same time that they also showed themselves to be a unified political and cultural community meant that the SIHB and AMS asserted a distinctive pan-Indigenous identity in the cities against assimilationist government efforts to deny and discourage them from doing this.

Beyond these efforts to support a visible, diverse, and vibrant Indigenous presence in the cities, key attributes of the clinics also demonstrated how Indigenous sovereignty and self-governance could be practiced in the urban environment without recourse to territorial jurisdiction. Most obviously, the fact that the SIHB and AMS were established with an explicit mandate of being staffed and run by Indigenous personnel wherever possible was the clearest way in which they put the concept of self-determination into practice. Reflecting on precisely this point, AMS Redfern chairman Sol Bellear recalled, "We knew then, as we know now, that unless we set the priorities for our community, we would never receive a service that put our priorities first. . . . The Board of the AMS is elected by the members of our service—by our patients, by our staff, and by our community members. We do it [this way] because not only do we believe in self-determination and Aboriginal control of Aboriginal lives, but we remember all too well what life was like when we left our futures in the hands of people outside our community."[25] This approach affirmed Aboriginal control of the organization but also provided benefit to the community in the form of employment opportunities. Many positions, such as field officer, clerical, or cleaning staff did not require an extensive formal education that had been out of the reach of most Aboriginal people. Importantly, Indigenous staff had community connections, appropriate cultural knowledge, and life experience that were important assets to the clinic in its early days, and which helped make sure the AMS was an Indigenous space where Aboriginal clientele could feel comfortable.

Community control over these health services also meant, most crucially, that the medical care patients received was provided in ways that met cultural as well as health needs. For some patients this meant providing access to Indigenous medicine and healing alongside Western medicine. For many patients it meant addressing needs around family visitation or ceremony that were not accommodated in mainstream health care. For a lot of people this simply meant providing access to resources, space, and community with which to practice their Indigenous cultures. Most fundamentally, it meant providing services that reflected an Indigenous understanding of health. Representatives of the AMS have been especially clear about this over the years. To this day, their organization's understanding of health is reflected on the home page of its website: "We see health as: 'Not just the physical wellbeing of the individual but the social, emotional and cultural wellbeing of the whole community, this is a whole-of-life view and also includes the cyclical concept of life-death-life' (National Aboriginal Health Strategy 1989)."[26]

Often, what an Indigenous understanding of health also came down to was an acknowledgment of the significant impact that the context of settler colonization has had as a continuing determinant of Indigenous health. In 1978, for example, the AMS submitted a report to the Senate Standing Committee on Social Environment outlining the historical determinants of Indigenous health very explicitly: "The creation of a different life-style, the building of a completely new environment, (urban, suburban), and the eradication of many of the native creatures which provided the life-food of the indigenous people—without creating possible avenues of access to alternative food-stuffs—was, in fact, the basis of ill-health of the Black Community as we see it today."[27]

This understanding of health was also a reason for health activists to get behind the land rights movement and to stress the important health benefits of restoring Indigenous peoples' access to their lands and waterways. In the 1980s, for example, Ruby Hammond, in her work advocating for the importance of Aboriginal health in rural communities, often spoke of how "land rights is fundamental to any improvements in the health of Aboriginal people."[28]

Recognizing both social and historical determinants as key contributing factors to the health of their communities, both the SIHB and AMS have made community services like food banks and clothing drives a central feature of their services from the day they opened their doors. In recognition of how damaging a lack of access to their Indigenous cultures has also been for the health of their community members, both clinics have also made access to cultural programs a central part of the health work they do. The core role played by these community and cultural programs— and hence of social and historical determinants of health frameworks—for serving the health and well-being of their patients and communities is still evident in the work these health centers do in the twenty-first century. The beading workshop in the advertisement (featured in figure 5.3) is just one example of how the SIHB continues to enact this culturally informed approach to health care.

In these ways, the clinics have asserted the cultural distinctiveness and diversity of the communities they serve, they have taken charge of their affairs, met the cultural and health needs of their people, and rejected the assimilationist expectations imposed on their community. While such efforts testify to the successful assertion of a unique urban pan-Indigenous culture and presence in these cities, we must also recognize that these efforts simultaneously reflect the burdens of recognition for Indigenous peoples, who must often seek settler state accommodation even as they pursue sovereignty. These burdens became especially pronounced when the

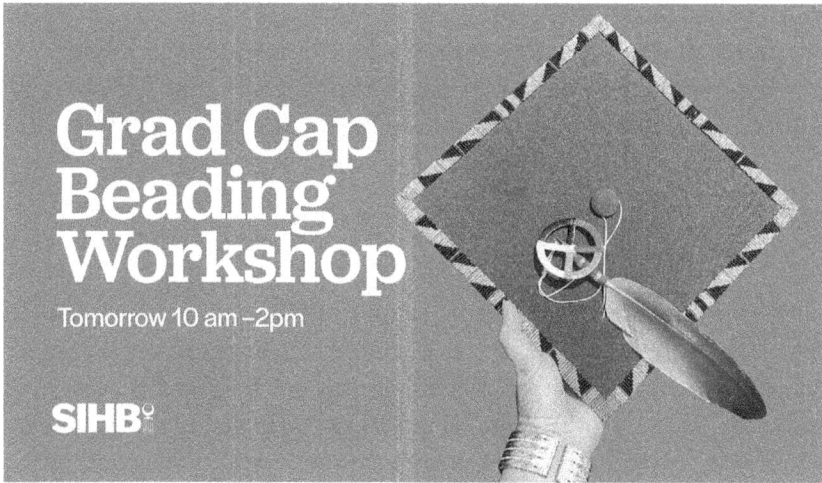

FIGURE 5.3 Example of a cultural program offered by the SIHB. This beading workshop provides an opportunity to engage in cultural practices while also resulting in greater visibility of Native culture within educational spaces. Seattle Indian Health Board, Facebook post, May 19, 2023.

clinics decided to seek government funding. In pressing the case that they should have access to government funding on the basis of their Indigenous status, it was incumbent upon the communities to "perform" their Indigeneity in much the same way that Indigenous people in the United States and Australia have also been asked to do this in the pursuit of land claims. Yet, what is remarkable about the way in which activists pursued government funds is that in addition to asserting their Indigenous right to health care on the basis of their identities, they also pressed a moral argument that the government had an obligation to do something for Indigenous communities in cities since they had promoted urban migration in the first place. Aboriginal activist Naomi Mayers (Yorta Yorta) expressed this point succinctly when she wrote, "In setting up our own [health] organization, we were saying [to the federal government], 'You were responsible for handling Aboriginal health and you have made an absolute mess of it. You have never listened, and we being Aborigines know what we want, know what causes the problems, and we know what has to be done to fix it, and we are going to make these decisions ourselves.' And we did."[29] By convincing the government to recognize their obligations to urban pan-Indigenous communities, health activists essentially succeeded in challenging an exclusively territorial model of Indigenous sovereignty. Two key federal government policies bear out the instrumental role of urban Indigenous health activists in Seattle and Sydney in extending Indigenous sovereignty to pan-Indigenous urban communities: Article V of the Indian Health Care Improvement Act (1976) in the United States, and the Whitlam government's Ten-Year Plan for Aboriginal Health (1973) in Australia.

Seeking Federal Funding: An Assertion of Urban Pan-Indigenous Rights

Initially the health clinics in both Seattle and Sydney were launched with the belief that to be self-determining, they would have to eschew reliance on any kind of government aid. Consequently, for the first few years both clinics ran on a combination of donated space, donated funding, and volunteer labor. As their client base grew however, and as the needs of the clinics expanded, both the AMS and SIHB transitioned away from this "donation" model of operations and fought for their community's right to a piece of the federal budget. This shift in approach angered the generation of activists who had been most prominent in the 1950s and early 1960s (like Pearl Warren and Mum Shirl), as they still held to the importance of remaining autonomous from government dependency of any kind. In part this was born of a concern that government funds would entail conditions and restrictions that would impinge on their ability to run their organizations as they desired. But it was also grounded in the belief that as a normative matter, the acceptance of government funding would compromise their aspiration to self-determination and autonomy. However, a younger generation of activists including Bernie Whitebear and Elizabeth Morris in Seattle, and Naomi Mayers, Gary Foley, and Chicka Dixon in Sydney, pressed both for their communities' rights to political representation within the government's Indigenous Affairs policies as well as permanent federal funding. They did not, however, conceive of the acceptance of federal funding as a moral compromise of their independence and capacity for self-determination. Where the earlier generation saw the acceptance of government largesse as a reliance on charity and beneficence that would compromise the independence of their clinics and community, the new generation of activists saw federal funding as an obligation owed to their community both on the basis of their Indigenous status and given that the dire situation urban pan-Indigenous communities were in was a government-created problem.

The younger generation of activists also saw federal funding, and the recognition that this would signal, as a means of securing their urban community a political voice *as* Indigenous peoples. In the United States, Seattle's urban Indian activists played an important part in getting the Indian Health Care Improvement Act (IHCIA) passed in 1976. Their work is little known but constitutes one of the most dramatic ways in which this community stood up for their right to a political voice *as* Native people, and for their entitlement to government-funded health care on the basis of this identity. In 1970, President Nixon had already famously asked Congress for more money to support Indian health in his message to Congress: "This administration is determined that the health status of the first Americans will be improved, and requests an additional $10 million for health programs."[30] And he had also stressed the importance of Indian participation in running these services: "These and other Indian health programs will be most effective if more Indians are involved in running them."[31] For the most part, however, Nixon's proposals were directed toward reservation communities only, and in spite of his avowed commitment to these goals, his policy initiatives were severely hampered by the fact that they tended to be too liberal for many of his Republican lieutenants to substantively endorse.[32]

With Nixon's efforts to increase the federal budget for Indian health remaining largely aspirational until the end of his presidency in 1974, US historians have widely understood that the IHCIA of 1976 was pushed through Congress by senator Henry M. Jackson, who chaired the Senate Committee on Indian Affairs in the immediate postwar years. Conventional historical wisdom holds that Jackson, formerly a stalwart of the federal government's termination-era policies, cynically changed his stripes to become an architect of the new mirror-image federal policies of tribal self-determination in the 1970s as part of a bid to clean up his race relations credentials for a run for the presidency.[33] As part of Jackson's political pivot, he introduced the IHCIA to "implement the federal responsibility for the care and education of the Indian people by improving the services and facilities of Federal Indian health programs and encouraging maximum participation of Indians in such programs."[34] Commonly referred to as "Jackson's Indian Health Care Improvement Act,"[35] the law contained five major components: increased scholarships for students in medical and health-related fields; improved funding for health services; money to upgrade or build new facilities; entitlement for eligible American Indians to receive Medicaid or Social Security services; and (most significantly for my considerations), authorization for contracts for urban Indian health clinics.

The IHCIA was the first time in US legislative history that *urban* Indians were specifically singled out for inclusion in the federal budget. In fact, the entire piece of legislation was more or less constructed around the need to get funding to the urban Indian communities. This much was made clear by journalist Mark N. Trahant in his book on Jackson's career. Trahant discusses the close relationship between Jackson's main advisor on Indian Affairs, Forrest Gerard (Blackfeet), and a Seattle pediatrician, Dr. Abe Bergman.[36] Bergman ran the outpatient clinic of the Children's Orthopedic Hospital in Seattle and also taught at the University of Washington's medical school. He was well-known for being a political activist as well as a doctor (or, as some of his colleagues complained, "a doctor as well as a political activist").[37] Between 1973 and 1975 Bergman and Gerard met several times to discuss the possibility of a general upgrade of Indian health programs. Trahant and others who have written about the IHCIA have noted that Bergman was the one who suggested the addition of an "urban mission" to the Indian Health Service.[38] But Gerard explained to Bergman that "if you went forward with a plan just to improve urban Indian health, it would fail."[39] Jackson shared Gerard's view about the difficulty of passing legislation only for urban Indians. In November 1972 he wrote to senator James Abourezk:

> Dr. Bergman suggested to me at the time of our initial discussion
> earlier in the year that I consider legislation to deal with the urban
> Indian health problem. However, he agreed with my position that it
> would be difficult to single out that category of Indian concern and not
> address attention to Indians living on Federal reservations and Indian
> communities. Following these discussions, and at my suggestion,
> Dr. Bergman traveled extensively throughout Alaska and met with
> Indian Health Officials and tribal leaders in the lower 48 states to
> discuss Indian health needs, priorities and alternative solutions. As a
> result of these efforts, Dr. Bergman, members of my personal and
> Interior Committee Staffs, met in my office and began framing a
> sweeping legislative proposal which would do much to improve the
> health status of Indian people residing on and off reservations.[40]

According to Trahant, the difficulty of passing legislation for only the urban community effectively became the impetus to devise a more comprehensive approach, which eventually became the Indian Health Care Improvement Act.[41] Bergman confirmed this to be the case many years later in a letter he wrote to the newly appointed director of the SIHB, JoAnn Kauffman (Nez Perce), in 1984: "Are you aware that the main reason the Indian Health Care Improvement Act was originally drafted was to extend IHS services to urban Indians?"[42]

What is missing from most accounts of the IHCIA is the crucial influence that Seattle's urban Indian health activists had on Bergman. In his correspondence, Bergman often spoke of how "happily, there is a lot of credit to spread around."[43] He recalled how Bernie Whitebear (Colville) of the SIHB had reached out to him in early 1973 after Bergman's work in passing significant new child-safety legislation had gained him some local media attention. Whitebear had called Bergman in order to invite him on a tour of their clinic: "He showed me around and, of course, it was a terrible place," Bergman recalled.[44] He remembered asking Whitebear what sort of help was available from the US Indian Health Service, only to be shocked that the existing funding was only for Indians living on reservations.[45] This direct exposure to the realities of how little health care was available for Indians in a city like Seattle drove Bergman to make use of his political contacts in order to press for the idea of reforming Indian health services, and specifically those for urban Indians.

The appalling lack of health services for Seattle's Native population not only motivated Bergman to bring the issue to Jackson and his staff. Once the process got underway to craft a comprehensive bill, the SIHB became the inspiration for Title V, which authorized federal funding for urban Indian health programs. Luana Reyes, Bernie Whitebear's sister and representative of the SIHB to the congressional hearings, testified before Congress on the work of the SIHB on April 3, 1974: "In 1970 the Seattle Indian Health Board began to address the complex health problems of Indian people through the promotion of culturally acceptable readily accessible health care to the Seattle area Indian community. The Seattle Indian Health Board is a community-controlled program operating on a limited evening schedule to a comprehensive primary level health delivery system with a registered patient population of over 6,000 persons. Patient records show 2,000 to 2,500 patient visits per month and the program now employs 46 people, 75% of whom are Indian or Alaskan Native."[46]

Bergman recognized these contributions in a letter to Reyes, commending her for the fact that "the SIHB was used as the model for drafting Title V. Your own testimony to the Committee in the Senate and House was influential in justifying the inclusion of that title. I am proud that such an exemplary program has been instituted in the Seattle community."[47] Forrest Gerard summed up the momentous impact of the bill: "We often speak of Indian Country, it's an old legal term. Well, the Indian Health Care Improvement Act applied Indian Country to urban Indians living in metropolitan centers."[48]

In Australia, the influence Aboriginal health activists had as part of the broader campaign to push the federal government toward accepting responsibility for Aboriginal Affairs deserves more scholarly attention. At the time the AMS was launched, the Federal Liberal/Country Party Government (under prime minister William McMahon) was still slow-moving in its acceptance of the responsibility for Aboriginal Affairs that the 1967 referendum bestowed upon them, but the political pressure applied by the AMS and their supporters helped push the government to begin fulfilling some of this responsibility, if reluctantly, in the field of health. Indeed, the first submission to the government by the AMS was made in August 1971, when they sought a total of $29,700 from the Office of Aboriginal Affairs (OAA), forerunner of the Department of Aboriginal Affairs (DAA). In response to their request for this funding, they received a mere $13,000. But this did not discourage the activists. In February 1972, they sent a second submission for $69,000 to the OAA. In response to this, the AMS received $14,000. When recalling the work it took to get even this much funding, Dr. Ross Macleod described these early efforts of the activists to secure federal funding as being akin to "getting blood from a stone."[49] Meager as this minimal financial support initially was though, Macleod also recalled how their persistence later paid off in unexpected ways. Because AMS representatives were constantly battling bureaucrats and politicians for resources, they soon became adept at negotiating, and moreover they realized the most effective means of communicating with bureaucrats was via data and by appropriating their institutional language.

In April 1973, Naomi Mayers and two of the AMS doctors, Dr. Laing and Dr. Hollows, made a formal submission to the Senate Standing Committee on Social Environment requesting that they consider funding the AMS so that it could bring its service model nationwide as a "viable, national, and successful organization." To back their submission, Mayers, Laing, and Hollows provided copious data on the health problems to be addressed and the funding required for it.[50] They were also clear to specify that such an expansion should not be accompanied by any loss of Aboriginal control. In order to make this assertion, they notably borrowed from the government's own assimilationist language, requesting that the subsidy be made available not just as a token gesture but as a substantial contribution to the emergence of the Black community as a "useful section of the Australian population."[51] The personal correspondence files of Dr. Doug Everingham (minister for health under Prime Minister Whitlam, McMahon's successor) reveal that the efforts of Mayers and other AMS representatives from this time were having a considerable impact on the health minister's discussions and plans regarding the future funding of Aboriginal health programs. For instance, in a series of letters exchanged between R. G. Walton (assistant director-general, Aboriginal Health Branch) and Everingham in 1973, numerous references were made to letters from "Ms. Mayers," indicating that she had been in frequent contact not only with the DAA but the Department of Health.[52] The exchanges between Everingham and Walton suggested that Mayers was pressuring them to contribute funds from the Health Department since support from the DAA was falling far short of the AMS's needs. In one particular set of letters, Everingham mentioned that Mayers had even pressed him for a "Treaty of Commitment" when it came to the government funding of their health clinic. On January 28, 1973, he wrote to Walton, "It is clear the issue of Aboriginal control of Health Services is bedeviled by the fact that any money allocated has to be accounted for by bureaucrats and politicians, both of whom can be vulnerable to public opinion. . . . I agree it is probable that as long as Aborigines are part of the Party–political point scoring process this will not change. It is a point very well discussed in the submission by Ms. Mayers on a 'Treaty of Commitment' in matters of their health funding."[53]

Suggesting the influence Mayers apparently had on Everingham, in a "Draft Green Paper on Aboriginal Affairs" Everingham included a subsection on a "Treaty of Commitment," writing, "Labor accepts in principle the need for a convention or treaty of commitment or covenant of settlement. It must ensure long term funding for key programs such as health, for land rights and other constitutional rights."[54] Further examples from Everingham's correspondence attest to both the persistence of AMS representatives in contacting him and the influence they were succeeding to have on his approach to Aboriginal health. On September 14, 1975, Everingham wrote to minister for Aboriginal Affairs Ian Viner, enclosing a copy of a report he had received from "Mrs. Hume, Managing Director, Aboriginal Advancement Council of W.A.," in which she detailed how "Aborigines get inadequate help, especially with health services." As Everingham explained to the minister, "This is quite consistent with other reports frequently reaching me from Aboriginal organisations and individuals, especially the Aboriginal Medical Service in Sydney, which compels me to forward these details to you."[55]

As the minister for health, Everingham reported directly to the prime minister's office and thus had considerable sway on Whitlam's health initiatives. In a series of memos exchanged between Whitlam's office,

Everingham, and Walton, it is clear that Everingham's contact with representatives from the AMS was playing a direct part in shaping his plans for a national strategy to address Aboriginal health problems. One memo in particular, dated March 1973 and addressed to Whitlam's office, expounded on the successes of Aboriginal-controlled health services. Everingham wrote of "the initiative shown by groups of Aboriginal people in establishing Aboriginal Health Services in Sydney, but now also Melbourne, Brisbane, Perth and Bairnsdale," and of how he had met with "representatives of these Services" and heard their suggestions for "the desirability of funding to develop new Services in other centres of Aboriginal population and to consider the training of Aboriginal health workers and the role of Aboriginals in training programs for health professionals."[56] According to Everingham's memo, he intended to fit this into "the national approach for the improvement of the health of Aboriginals which is being developed, with the aim of bringing about a permanent up-grading in the health status of Aboriginal people."[57] Everingham stressed that he believed "high priority" should be given by the government "to the task of raising the standard of health of Aboriginal people by the adoption of a ten year national plan to raise the standard of health of Aboriginals to the level enjoyed by their fellow Australians."[58]

In the "Briefing Notes for the Prime Minister" submitted by Everingham to Whitlam's office later that same month, and in which he drafted the prime minister's public announcement of this national plan, Everingham's language from the prior memo reappeared verbatim: "As a first step my colleague the minister for Health approved a national plan with the following objective 'to raise the standard of health of the Aborigines of Australia to the level enjoyed by their fellow Australians.' This campaign is being planned and coordinated in stages and aims to achieve its goal at the end of ten years."[59] Therefore, when Gough Whitlam announced his Ten Year Plan for Aboriginal Health, this was not simply the first time that a comprehensive national program and commitment to funding for Aboriginal health had been pursued in Australia; it was also a significant achievement for the community of Aboriginal activists at the AMS, who had lobbied Everingham directly and sought to influence his policy decisions. As Whitlam explained in his speech announcing the plan, "The active participation of the Aborigines themselves has been sought and every encouragement is being given for them to be involved in all aspects of the plan."[60] As the persistence and requests of Mayers and others from the AMS made clear, this outcome was a direct result of the pressure they had applied on Everingham's office.

On the crucial issue of funding for Aboriginal-controlled health clinics, the AMS activists had also made sure to continually engage Everingham's and Walton's offices directly on the matter of maintaining their clinic's autonomy in spite of the government's financial support. This issue came up in a number of different ways, as for instance, when Naomi Mayers wrote to Walton to express her outrage over the government's insistence on being involved in its staffing issues. Perhaps due to their cordial relationship, Everingham rather than Walton replied to this letter, writing, "While I can understand that you see the need for prior approval of staff as a straightjacket, perhaps a reasonable requirement would be prompt (e.g., within 30 days) notification of staff changes <u>after</u> the event. If the Department will not accept this, I believe you are entitled to an explanation."[61] This exchange, and the candor of Mayers's tone in her letter to Walton ("This condition is a straitjacket [sic] we cannot wear. IS THAT UNDERSTOOD?") exemplified the persistence with which AMS activists insisted that their funding should not be attached to any strings that would take the control of their organization out of the community's hands.[62] This underscores the extent to which AMS activists viewed the provision of government funding not as something they should have to bargain for but as something they were owed—a significant symbolic recognition of their Indigenous rights and status and of obligations owed to them on that basis.

Acquiring funding for their clinics was both a symbolic and practical victory of inordinate proportions for the communities in Seattle and Sydney but also for Indigenous peoples more widely across these settler nations. This would henceforth shape the future of urban Indigenous health care. The activists were cautious in the 1970s about accepting this government funding, even as they celebrated getting it, and the reasons for their guarded attitudes have, in the years since they secured these funds, been substantiated. Arguably, nowhere is the structural violence within Indigenous health care clearer in the twenty-first century than in matters of funding.

The Endurance of Structural Violence

In February 2006, the George W. Bush administration proposed eliminating the urban Indian health program established as Title V of the Indian Health Care Improvement Act, arguing that urban Indian health organization clients could instead use federally supported community health centers that serve the general public in the United States. No funding increase for community health centers was included to offset the additional expense of new

Indian patients or to provide community health center staff members with relevant cultural competency training. The lack of advance consultation with urban Indian health professionals led to a national outcry among urban Indians. Prominent American Indian and Alaska Native organizations testified before Congress against the cuts and reminded Congress that the federal government's responsibility does not end at the reservation border.

In April 2016, Australian Aboriginal health activists Dr. Jackie Huggins and Mick Gooda of the "Close the Gap Campaign" called on the Australian government to make Aboriginal and Torres Strait Islander health a priority in the federal budget. Responding to the threat of serious budget cuts to Indigenous health, including federal support for Aboriginal community-controlled health services, Dr. Huggins warned that any reduction in Indigenous health funding in the federal budget would have serious implications for Aboriginal and Torres Strait Islander peoples. Despite the achievements of Aboriginal community-controlled health services in raising the status of Indigenous health, Huggins warned that Aboriginal people continue to face a life expectancy at least ten years less than non-Indigenous Australians. Rather than rewind the clock on their political achievements, she stressed it was time for the government to respond with strong political will and redouble efforts to "close the gap."

These recent events are a stark reminder that the Indigenous health activism examined in this book has an ongoing history. Much as I have argued in relation to the activism of the 1950s, '60s, and '70s, urban Indigenous health activists in Australia and the United States today still face the need to defend their rights and status *as Indigenous peoples* in their efforts to protect their health services from federal budget cuts and continued neglect. Their eligibility for continued government support *as Indigenous peoples* remains at stake, emphasizing that health care continues to be an especially fraught context in which Indigenous people assert their rights and work to push back against structural forms of Indigenous elimination.

Especially in the United States, recent history has demonstrated the endurance of this structural violence. Nowhere do we see this more clearly than in the structure of the Indian Health Service (IHS) budget. According to the US census, approximately 76 percent of self-identifying Native Americans live in urban areas today, yet on average only 1 percent of the IHS budget has been allocated to urban Indian health care. Data shows that many of the recurring health problems faced by Native Americans in general are more acute for those living in urban areas. According to IHS, Native youth residing in cities "are at greater risk for serious mental health and substance abuse problems, suicide, increased gang activity, teen pregnancy, abuse, and neglect."[63] These persistent health problems are often compounded by urban Indians' inadequate access to health care services. The Kaiser Family Foundation has found that "the share of IHS funding going toward urban programs over time has not reflected the overall demographic shift of American Indians away from reservations."[64] Therefore, the insufficiency of the 1 percent budget allocation has been repeatedly underscored by Native American health advocates. As Dr. Bonnie Duran explained in the *American Journal of Public Health* in 2005, "More than 60 percent of members of US tribes reside outside their home reservations at least part of the year, but only 1 percent of the IHS budget is earmarked for urban Indian health care." Not only is federal government funding of urban Indian health care inadequate to cover the needs of this population, but due to the ways in which services are restricted through compacting agreements and geographic restrictions, in the case of urban communities, these services often simply aren't available to them.[65]

Therefore, in the United States, while the existence of Title V has been hugely significant, the failure of federal funding allocations for urban communities to catch up with and meet the needs of the vastly expanding urban population is a serious problem.[66] The reluctance of the government to change its funding structures in order to allocate a larger portion to urban Indians or to bring the funding of the IHS as a whole up to a level that would meet the needs of Native communities (both reservation and urban), as well as the active and repeated attempts by successive administrations to actually scale back the funding for urban Indian health, must be recognized for how this continues an assimilationist policy agenda and is thus continuous with an original reluctance to fund urban health programs at all.

The COVID-19 pandemic also brought the consequences of the chronic underfunding of Indigenous health to light in staggering ways. Early in 2020, an article in the *Lancet* reported that in Australia, "government policy and funding (or a lack thereof), are political determinants that directly impact the ability of Aboriginal Community Controlled Health Organizations (ACCHOs) to provide services that are accessible and attentive to the needs of their communities, which in turn shapes health outcomes. Given the short-term government funding modalities placed upon ACCHOs, and their restricted health infrastructure, and workforce capacity it is imperative that additional government resources to support the control of COVID-19 be made rapidly and easily accessible to deal with increasing cases."[67] Within the same article, a comparison was drawn to the state of Native American health care funding in the United States: "Comparatively, in the U.S., health, socioeconomic, and cultural inequities among Native Americans have contributed to their overrepresentation among COVID-19 cases. Similar concerns have been expressed by Native American leaders, emphasising the limited capacity of the U.S. Indian Health Service to respond to the pandemic due to a chronic lack of government funding, and restricted health infrastructure."[68]

These continuing realities of funding shortfalls and a resistance to recognizing, let alone acting, on the urgency of continuing medical neglect and need, especially in urban Indigenous communities, shows how structural inequalities are on the one hand produced by these persistently inadequate and underfunded health services, but on the other hand, in the case of urban Indigenous health care in particular, colonial agendas of the past are also maintained by a system that in effect (through underfunding) denies federal health services to urban Indigenous communities in the present. When we understand the historically persistent nature of these funding shortfalls, and in the case of urban pan-Indigenous communities, the assimilative reasons for the original and ongoing barriers to accessing government-provided health care placed on them, it seems the case of Indigenous health care must be recognized for what it is: the persistence of colonial, racialized, and spatial modes of governance through health policy.

Despite the immense challenge that COVID-19 did pose to underfunded Indigenous health services in both the United States and Australia, what the pandemic also showed was the historical legacy and success of Indigenous self-determination within health care, and the resiliency of the alternative structures of care established through their health clinics (something I explore more in this book's epilogue). At a time when news headlines were dominated, for the most part, by revelations about how fragile our health care systems are, a steady trickle of stories reported on the surprising triumphs of Indigenous communities, many of whom successfully fought off the worst of COVID-19 despite being at disproportionate risk and disadvantage: "Indigenous Communities Demonstrate Innovation and Strength Despite Unequal Losses During COVID-19"; "Native Americans in Minnesota Keep COVID-19 at Bay"; "Indigenous Leadership Points the Way Out of the COVID Crisis"; "American Indians Have the Highest Covid Vaccination Rate in the US"; "How Native Americans Launched Successful Coronavirus Vaccination Drives: 'A Story of Resilience'"; "In the Early Days of Covid-19, Indigenous Leaders Used Their Voice and Averted a Catastrophe"; "Why Australia's Real Covid-19 Success Belongs to the First Nations."[69] These headlines make sense when we understand the history of Indigenous health activism in these nations.

· · · · · ·

This book has advanced a series of central claims. A key question my research surfaces is how urban pan-Indigenous community formation hastened a reframing and reconceptualizing of the project of Indigenous sovereignty. In both Australia and the United States, a good deal of this political reimagining about sovereignty occurred in the context of struggles over access to health care in the 1950s, '60s, and '70s. This in turn has suggested the unique significance of urban Indigenous health care as a site for explaining how Indigenous-state relations dramatically shifted between the 1950s and 1970s, and likewise how the relationship between place and Indigenous sovereignty became more fluid, if not reterritorialized, in this time.

The comparative nature of this book has underscored the systemic and structural dimensions of the historical and ongoing experiences of structural violence in health care experienced by Indigenous people under conditions of settler colonialism. Even though activists in Seattle and Sydney may not necessarily have influenced one another, I have shown that their struggles were grounded in a common reaction against, and refusal of, the spatial logics of settler-colonial governance and the persistence of structures of elimination within health care settings. By identifying a set of shared ideals (self-determination, Indigenous control) that grounded these clinics, we see that their parallel histories also connect them to broader movements within health reform usually not associated with Indigenous communities or actors. While it remains beyond the scope of this book to fully explore the ways in which these connections were made and acted on by Indigenous activists, it is nonetheless clear that the efforts of urban Indigenous health activists in the United States and Australia reflected transnational aspirations at the time for accessible, culturally appropriate, needs-based health care with a focus on prevention and social justice. For example, we can fruitfully connect the histories of the Indigenous clinics to the People's Free Medical Clinics set up by the Black Panthers in the 1970s and the women's health clinics established around the same time. Indeed, in a short autobiographical article published in the 1990s, Naomi Mayers reflected on precisely these sorts of connections and solidarities fostered by activists at the AMS. She wrote, "The women's health movement copied the Aboriginal community–controlled services. We also get requests for information from overseas countries, for example Ghana and

Uganda, on how to go about setting up a community-controlled health service."[70] That these other social groups did not invoke the language of sovereignty only underscores the special way in which Indigenous political actors connected their health struggles to a history of settler colonialism and its persistent efforts to deny them their identities and rights as Indigenous peoples.

Another significant argument underscored by the comparative history in this book is that we should reframe our understanding of Indigenous politics in the postwar period, elevating the significance of health as a galvanizing political issue and recognizing the existence of quieter forms of activism that did not attract the same attention as protest movements for territorial sovereignty. Against the backdrop of postwar urbanization, this book has also given attention to less obvious struggles that mobilized diasporic urban Indigenous communities in their early days of formation. What this has revealed is that in both the United States and Australia, health was often a significant factor in people leaving reserves and reservations. I have asserted that this should also shift our historiographies on Indigenous mobility and migration in the twentieth century.

Significant legacies of the health activism I have examined here also warrant emphasis. First, the successes of the clinics in Seattle and Sydney have contributed to the proliferation of community-controlled health services as *the* health care model for Indigenous primary care in both the United States and Australia. In the United States today, forty-one community-controlled urban Indian health clinics exist nationwide.[71] In Australia, there are currently over 140 Aboriginal community-controlled health organizations (ACCHOs) across the country, serving both rural and urban populations.[72] It is widely recognized that these services have been essential not only in terms of improving Indigenous access to health care but also as significant providers of Indigenous employment and centers of Indigenous health research. The greater access to health services that these clinics provide, while not enough to completely counteract the deep-rooted historical determinants of health that still negatively impact Indigenous people, can be credited with important advances in Indigenous health outcomes. Hence on a purely practical level, the activism examined in this book has been profoundly important in shaping Indigenous health services and outcomes for the better in both the United States and Australia since the 1970s.[73]

At the level of Indigenous political discourse and activism, these clinics have also had an important shaping influence. Health struggles in particular distilled a crucial fact: settler colonialism has not only happened to land;

it has also happened to people. If Indigenous sovereignty is meant to be the answer to settler colonization, what urban Indigenous people's experiences with health care access brought to the surface was an understanding that sovereignty must therefore also speak to the struggles of people whose experiences of colonization are not limited to exclusion or detachment from land. Instead, as health disparities make explicit, forms of colonial injustice are often experienced first at the level of people's corporeal bodies. This focus on the colonization of Indigenous people's literal human bodies is an underlying tenet running through much Indigenous political activism today, and it begs further investigation to flesh out the possible ways in which postwar urban Indigenous health activism might have played a role in contributing to the development of this current direction within Indigenous politics.

Another legacy of this health activism is that it reminds us that Indigenous sovereignty is a political framework that has constantly shifted in meaning and manner of deployment. Through these changes, the insistent and persistent self-definition of Indigenous peoples through a discourse of sovereignty (like the "reterritorialized" forms of sovereignty considered here) can be understood as a response to continuing settler colonialism. Persistently claiming their sovereignty and including multiple sociocultural and political issues under this rubric has been a strategy in and of itself, not merely to deflect the reinvention of settler-colonial practices of elimination but to reassert a politically empowered self-identity that exists within, beside, and against settler colonization. In this way, Indigenous health activists in both the United States and Australia have embodied a politics of existence as resistance.

Epilogue

Refusing Settler Colonial Harm in Health Care

• •

On December 14, 2020, almost a year into the COVID-19 pandemic, the Seattle Indian Health Board's chief research officer, Abigail Echo-Hawk (Pawnee), shared the following public post on her Facebook page: "It's done. After 6 months of starting and stopping as trauma ebbed and flowed, it's done. Sewing body bags is harder than I thought. Never thought I'd write those words but also never expected a box of body bags instead of the PPE we asked for at our urban Indian clinic. Yes, this is one of the body bags they sent us, and yes I turned it into a ribbon dress."[1] Turning a body bag into something beautiful and symbolic of Indigenous peoples' survival was not easy for Echo-Hawk, but she explained it was something she had to do: "I'm making something that takes the shit they do to us, and reconstructs it into strength and beauty. . . . We will not let them harm our babies, our next generations. The words are ones I repeat in my head everyday, I am the tangible manifestation of my ancestors resiliency."[2]

"They" and "them" did not need to be named for Echo-Hawk's followers on social media to understand that she was referring to the same structures and systems within US society that have historically harmed and attempted to eradicate Native peoples for centuries. In this single extraordinary act of refusing settler-colonial harm, Echo-Hawk encapsulated so many generations of Indigenous struggle and resistance. The dress, according to Echo-Hawk, took shape "as a stream of ancestral consciousness."[3] What this became in physical form features vibrant colors and intricate embellishments with mirrors, red handprints, and writing: "I stitched the ribbons with the color of prayer, red. The sleeves are interwoven with toe tags that come with body bags, and ribbons. The string that would be tied to the toe of a body is now fringe. The stitching is jagged in places mimicking autopsy stitching. The pieces of historical trauma. The mirrors honor my heart sister Shawna, a fierce Northern Cheyenne mother and auntie, mirrors deflect and reflect back to those who dare try to cause us harm."[4]

In one of many interviews that Echo-Hawk did since creating the dress, she explained the meaning of the personal mantra, "I am the tangible manifestation of my ancestors' resiliency," that appears repeatedly in her handwriting and is sewn alongside the body bag's zipper: "I come from a tribe in Oklahoma that in the 1830s was estimated at being a population of 38,000." By the census of 1910, the tribe numbered less than 700. "I'm literally the descendant of genocide survivors," said Echo-Hawk. "And it is because of their resiliency, and their fight to survive that I can thrive."[5] "Each ribbon is prayer," Echo-Hawk also explained. "Each stitch is prayer." And thus, she described that as she lovingly crafted the dress, she had to let go of her anger. When making a prayer—which the dress, in so many ways is—"you can't come from a place of bitterness," she explained. "It's my responsibility to instead be in a place of peace and a place of loving our people. And for me, that means advocacy, and continuing to push for justice."[6]

This place of "loving our people" describes the very same spirit with which Indigenous activists created their health clinics in the 1970s. Adeline Garcia, one of the Seattle Indian Health Board's (SIHB) founders, would often say that the work they did was "for the love of Native people." This has since become the clinic's slogan, and this ethos of community care is apparent in all the work they do. Indeed, despite the early setback with their request for COVID-19 personal protection equipment, the SIHB went on to prove itself a model for how to respond to a pandemic. How they did this was a combination of several things, but at its heart was the community-based approach that founded the clinic in the first place. Esther Lucero (Diné), the CEO of SIHB, explained that when it came to vaccine distribution, this meant prioritizing not just health care workers and elders but those providing services that were essential to the community: "We reached out to Chief Seattle Club and we vaccinated their staff. We reached out to Mother Nation, which is an organization that is a shelter for women experiencing domestic violence, the United Indians of All Tribes because they serve families and pregnant women and they also operate a daycare. We vaccinated their staff and then also the Urban Native Education Alliance because they serve our youth and families."[7] Meanwhile, they also vaccinated marginalized community members like those experiencing homelessness, along with culture keepers and traditional healers. Early on, they were able to vaccinate all patients over the age of fifty, and they prioritized working with Seattle Public Schools to vaccinate their Special Education department. SIHB was able to execute this community-based approach thanks to a long history of caring for their community in these ways.

After the body bags incident, and reminiscent of the health activism in Seattle during the 1960s and '70s, the SIHB also leveraged to their advantage the media exposure that this incident brought. Besides getting the supplies they had originally asked for from government entities, this allowed them to attract donations from the local community. And because of their ability to pivot to the challenges that arose due to the pandemic, unlike many government-funded institutions, SIHB also managed to avoid layoffs or furloughs of any of its employees. They also made sure unhoused elders had access to food, hygiene stations, and a warm place to go. They also established a pop-up testing site at Chief Seattle Club so that unhoused relatives could walk right up. "We have been defined as a model program as to how to address a pandemic from a community-based approach," Lucero said.[8] These successes didn't only reflect traditions of community care, self-reliance, and self-determination; they also demonstrated the community's expansive understanding of health and the fact that they conduct themselves in line with Indigenous cultural values. Patients of SIHB are called "relatives," explained SIHB chief operating officer Ryan Gilbert.[9] And in all their efforts to motivate community members into preventative action, whether it was handwashing, mask-wearing, or getting vaccinated, SIHB workers could rely on their traditions of community care to do the work of advocacy for them. As reflected in the public health campaigns of both clinics during the pandemic, cultural traditions and values were central in their organizations' efforts to fight COVID-19 in Seattle and in Sydney alike. With public health messaging that reflected values like, "Protect our Future Generations," "Be a Good Relative," "Be a Good Ancestor," and "Keep Our Mob Safe," it is clear that for both Aboriginal Australian and Native American communities, cultural values were central in the protection of their peoples' health and a motivator for good public health behavior.

These public health campaigns also showed how crucial the sovereignty and self-determination of Indigenous communities and their health clinics were to their success in dealing with the pandemic. By centering the concept of nationhood in their "#VacciNATION" campaign, for example, the SIHB's public health messaging was a nod toward the significance of Indigenous political sovereignty in their health struggles. We also saw this reflected more broadly across the United States by the choice of many Indigenous health clinics and communities to prioritize the vaccination of elders and language and culture keepers. This meant that communities could prioritize the protection of their Indigenous identities and their sovereignty in ways that the state or government might not. In both the United States and Australia, many Indigenous communities exercised self-determination by articulating and enforcing rules on who could enter their communities, often implementing far stricter measures than those enacted by local municipalities, such as closures and checkpoints.[10] Self-determination in their health care also meant that communities produced their own educational material in their own languages. The Northern Land Council in Australia, for example, produced YouTube videos about COVID-19 in seventeen different Indigenous languages.[11] Crucially, sovereignty in the management of their health care has also meant that Indigenous leaders have advocated for the collection of Indigenous-specific COVID-19 data, with clear data sovereignty agreements related to access, control, ownership, and possession of the data. This advocacy around data collection in health care has arguably become one of the most urgent issues brought to light by the pandemic. Studies are starting to reveal that one of the biggest ongoing problems faced by Indigenous communities in the context of health care today is a basic but chronic problem of invisibility in health data.[12] In the twenty-first century, Indigenous invisibility within mainstream health care has evolved from simply the problem of exclusion from routine care that was rampant in the 1950s, '60s, and '70s and now encompasses the much more complex issue of systemic erasure of Indigenous people from health data, and the exclusion from funding (and ultimately care) that this can produce.

Abigail Echo-Hawk has been one of the most outspoken advocates on the importance of data sovereignty for Indigenous people in the face of a deepening problem of data erasure and invisibility. In one interview, she explained, "As data advocates, we have been saying for many years that American Indians and Alaska Natives are some of the most racially misclassified within hospital records."[13] She said a big issue right now is the fact that lots of people are being misclassified by hospital staff as white or Latinx, or something else. She experienced this firsthand when her son was hospitalized in Seattle. The condition itself was stressful enough, but so was Echo-Hawk's discovery of the racial designation hospital workers had given her son: "I had to go to the administrator and I had to argue with her that my son was not white, he was in fact American Indian or Alaska Native," explained Echo-Hawk. And moreover, she noted, "My experience isn't unique."[14] Studies in places like Washington and Oregon have shown that many patients there were racially misclassified in hospital discharge records—often miscoded as white, or with missing race information. During the pandemic, Echo-Hawk made it one of her priorities to expose how this was even more likely to happen to COVID-19 patients, who may not be in a condition to clarify their identity, and when relatives may not have been allowed to accompany them to the hospital. "The implication of that is, we effectively disappear within the data," she explained.[15] Putting a sharp point on it, Echo-Hawk has sometimes described this as a "data genocide."[16] Her understanding of what this means reflects the deep structures of violence that Indigenous people continue to face within health care: "I believe that eliminating us in the data through racial misclassification and non-collection of the data is an ongoing act of institutional racism that is resulting in the continuing genocide of American Indians and Alaska Natives. It effectively eliminates us. And as a direct result of that, then the resources that our community needs aren't being directed to us because the government is making data-driven decisions."[17]

Like the dress she sewed from body bags, Echo-Hawk's vital research and advocacy with respect to decolonizing Indigenous health data (which she does alongside others at the Urban Indian Health Institute—one of twelve tribal epidemiology centers across the United States) is a refusal of the settler-colonial violence that continues to pervade health care. Speaking of the dress, Echo-Hawk wrote, "I'll never accept their body bags for our people, all I will accept is a world where we are thriving, ever continuing. That is our past, present and our future."[18] In the United States and Australia, Indigenous health activists continue, as they always have, to imagine and create better futures for the health of their people. And they do it with love.

Notes

Introduction

1. Erik Ortiz, "Native American Health Center Asked for COVID-19 Supplies. It Got Body Bags Instead," *NBC News*, May 5, 2020, www.nbcnews.com/news/us-news/native-american-health-center-asked-covid-19-supplies-they-got-n1200246.

2. Adakai, et al. "Health Disparities."

3. Crosby, "Virgin Soil Epidemics," 289–99.

4. Diamond, *Guns, Germs, and Steel.*

5. Jones, *Rationalizing Epidemics*; Kelton, *Epidemics and Enslavement*; Cameron, Kelton, and Swedlund, *Beyond Germs*; Kelton, *Cherokee Medicine*; Reséndez, *Other Slavery.*

6. For example, as Jeffrey Ostler notes, the spread of smallpox, which may have started as a virgin-soil issue in the early 1600s, was also due to warfare, such as when tribes from the Great Lakes and Ohio Valley were recruited to fight for the French against the British and subsequently spread the disease to their people upon their arrival home. While immunity may have been a factor in this case, the war was the pivotal one. Similarly, Hernando de Soto's arrival in the Southeast spread disease, but it was the trade of Native slaves that was largely responsible for massive death tolls, as Indigenous peoples were already weakened from war and its concomitant consequences, including malnutrition, exposure, and lack of care. These same conditions made Native peoples more susceptible to other diseases, including cholera, typhus, malaria, dysentery, tuberculosis, and more. See Jeffrey Ostler, "Disease Has Never Been" *The Atlantic*, April 29, 2020.

7. Dunbar-Ortiz, *An Indigenous Peoples' History*, 40.

8. Ostler, "Disease Has Never Been."

9. Jen Deerinwater, "Historic Injustices Against Native People Put Them at Greater Risk of COVID-19," *Truthout*, April 3, 2020, https://truthout.org/articles/historic-injustices-against-native-people-put-them-at-greater-risk-of-covid-19/; Nick Estes, "The Empire of All Maladies: Colonial Contagions and Indigenous Resistance," *Baffler* 52, July 2020.

10. Ostler, "Disease Has Never Been."

11. John, "Violence of Abandonment."

12. Wolfe, *Settler Colonialism.*

13. Wolfe, "Patrick Wolfe on Settler Colonialism," 347.

14. Reading, "Structural Determinants," 5.

15. Reading, "Structural Determinants," 5.

16. Greenwood, de Leeuw, and Lindsay, *Determinants of Indigenous Peoples' Health.*

17. McCallum and Perry, *Structures of Indifference*, 62–63.

18. Kelm, *Colonizing Bodies*.

19. Razack, *Race, Space and the Law*; McCallum, "This Last Frontier"; Stevenson, *Life Beside Itself*; Razack, *Dying from Improvement*; Lux, *Separate Beds*; Geddes, *Medicine Unbundled*; Greenwood, de Leeuw, and Lindsay, *Determinants of Indigenous Peoples' Health*; McCallum and Perry, *Structures of Indifference*.

20. Reading, "Structural Determinants," 12.

21. Dhillon, *Prairie Rising*; Doenmez, "Carrying Water"; Coulthard, *Red Skin, White Masks*; Hobart and Kneese, "Radical Care: Survival Strategies"; Kowal, *Trapped in the Gap*; Kristjansson, "Refusing Child-Stealing States"; Lea, *Bureaucrats and Bleeding Hearts*; Million, *Therapeutic Nations*; Watson, *Raw Law*; Moreton-Robinson, *White Possessive*.

22. Povinelli, *Economies of Abandonment*.

23. Kauanui, "Structure, Not an Event."

24. Simpson, *Mohawk Interruptus*, 7–8.

25. Whitebear, "Taking Back Fort Lawton," 3.

26. Whitebear, "Taking Back Fort Lawton," 3.

27. American Indian Women's Service League Inc., *Indian Center News* 3, no. 1 (February 1963): 4.

28. Under the social media tag #justiceforjoyce, an especially harrowing example emerged from Canada in September 2020, calling into serious public scrutiny the way that Indigenous people are treated in its health care system. In her last moments, while tied to a hospital bed, Joyce Echaquan, a thirty-seven-year-old First Nations (Atikamekw) woman who had been hospitalized for stomach pains, pleaded for someone to help her. In crisis, she started recording live on Facebook, screaming for help and saying she was being overmedicated. Near the end of the seven-minute video, hospital staff can be heard talking in her room. Two women are recorded calling Echaquan stupid, questioning her life choices, saying she's only good for sex and that she would be better off dead. "And who do you think is paying for this?" one of them is heard saying. Echaquan, a mother of seven, died soon after. In the wake of Joyce Echaquan's death, similar stories emerged from across Canada. In October 2020, Georges-Hervé Awashish died in another Quebec hospital in Chicoutimi, where only four days earlier he had complained to his family that he overheard nurses making racist and discriminatory remarks about him. In October 2021, Marylynn Matchewan, a forty-four-year-old Native woman from the Algonquins of Barriere Lake, reported that she was treated poorly by staff after being admitted to Montreal's Sacre-Coeur hospital. Ms. Matchewan told the *Globe and Mail* that she was left to sit on a chair with her own filled bedpan and that no one responded to her calls for help: "I sat there in my pan for two hours," she said. In recent history, perhaps the most widely known case of medical neglect leading to an Indigenous person's death was the tragic passing of Brian Sinclair, a non-Status Anishinaabe resident of Winnipeg, who was left untreated in a major downtown hospital for over thirty-four hours. He ultimately died, in plain sight, from an easily treatable infection. As McCallum and Perry have discussed in their book about his death, Sinclair was effectively, indeed literally, "ignored to death." See McCallum

228 Notes to Introduction

and Perry, *Structures of Indifference*. For news reportage on these other cases, see Jesse Feith, "Indigenous Woman Records Slurs by Hospital Staff Before Her Death," *Montreal Gazette*, September 30, 2020; Jesse Feith, "Indigenous Man Dies in Chicoutimi Hospital After Complaints of Racist Remarks," *Montreal Gazette*, October 15, 2020; Kristy Kirkup, "Algonquin Woman Raises Concerns About Hospital Treatment After Car Crash," *Globe and Mail*, October 15, 2021.

29. Mayers, "Growing to Meet," 146.

30. See Panaretto, et al., "Aboriginal Community-Controlled Health Services"; Urban Indian Health Commission and Robert Wood Johnson Foundation, *Invisible Tribes*; Anderson, *Koorie Health in Koorie Hands*.

31. Numbers cited by the IHS are from the US census, which reported in 2010 that 78 percent of American Indians and Alaska Natives reside in urban areas. See Indian Health Service, *Strategic Plan 2017–2021*. In its most recent reporting, the IHS relies on the 2020 census, which reported that 87 percent of the US American Indian/Alaska Native population live in urban areas. See Indian Health Service, "About Urban Indian Organizations." In Australia, Indigenous health organizations rely on numbers from the Australian Bureau of Statistics, which reported in 2021 that "the majority of Aboriginal and Torres Strait Islander people lived in cities and non-remote areas (84.7% or 688,262 people). This includes: 41.1% in Major Cities of Australia (334,259 people); 25.1% in Inner Regional Australia (203,876 people); 18.5% in Outer Regional Australia (150,118 people)." See Australian Bureau of Statistics, "Census of Population and Housing." In both cases, it should be noted that census data is imperfect, and in the case of Indigenous peoples, relies on self-reporting. For particular concerns over the accuracy of the 2020 US census data, see Mike Schneider and Morgan Lee, "Tribal Nations Face Less Accurate, More Limited 2020 Census Data Because of Privacy Methods," *Associated Press*, September 9, 2023; Carly Graf, "Census Undercount Threatens Federal Food, Health Programs on Reservations," *High Country News*, May 12, 2022; National Council of Urban Indian Health, "Urban American Indian Undercount."

32. As an example of how the language of sovereignty is engaged in these ways, in 2015, academics, curators, and artists gathered at the University of South Carolina for a panel discussion on the topic of "Power in Native Art: American Indian Artistic and Aesthetic Sovereignty." In publicity for the event, they described the animating questions and problems to be addressed by the event as follows: "The ability of artists to express themselves through their works is often taken for granted today. Many Indigenous artists, however, confront challenges in both the creation and display of their works. This panel will focus on issues of power in American Indian art: who has the power to control artistic expression, how Indigenous artists use their power to address issues that face American Indians, and the power of indigenizing the curation process. The panel will feature national and regional academic leaders in discourses concerning Indigenous artistic sovereignty." (See Missick Museum, "Power in Native Art" Facebook event page. For the event's program see, Missick Museum, "Power in Native Art.")

33. Barker, "For Whom Sovereignty Matters," 19–21.

34. Moreton-Robinson, *Sovereign Subjects*, 2.

35. This language of "fringe dwellers" lasted well into the twentieth century as well. See for example, Australian Department of Territories, *Fringe Dwellers*.

36. Thrush, *Native Seattle*, 54–59.

37. I have not reproduced the painting here on account of its crude and offensive imagery, but the painting can be viewed here: Earle, *Natives of N. S. Wales*, Trove website.

38. This has been an enduring way of framing and disparaging Aboriginality. For example, in 2002, Sydney photographer Patricia Baillie spent time with the Aboriginal community in Redfern and documented their experiences of displacement within the neighborhood. In an article written about her time spent photographing the community, Baillie reflected on how the residents were constantly being monitored and moved by the local council on account of their custom of congregating and socializing outdoors: a kind of moral policing of Aboriginal presence on the streets today that we might regard as continuous with the colonial practice of the past. She wrote, "The community at The Block is no more. I have watched it being gradually destroyed. The quiet groups, sitting drinking, often by a campfire, were moved from one place to another. Originally, they were near the train station; people coming and going from the country would pass and be greeted. When the Community center was built, this group were forced to move but still came on Tuesday and Wednesday and had the free meal. Afterwards they would sit peacefully under a big spreading mulberry tree, and chat. Then the mulberry tree was cut down." See Baillie, "Pictures from The Block."

39. For example, in an article from the *Sun* in January 1961, Australian minister for the territories Paul Hasluck expressed this very concern, saying, "The problem of assimilating a nomadic people into a civilization foreign to them is an age old one. Too often it leaves them stranded half-way between both worlds and at just that point—in humpies on towns' edges—where they lose their self-respect and the respect of others for them." *Sun*, January 27, 1961.

40. Huhndorf, *Going Native*; Deloria, *Indians in Unexpected Places*; O'Brien, *Firsting and Lasting*.

41. O'Brien, *Firsting and Lasting*, 107.

42. Deloria, *Indians in Unexpected Places*, 3–5.

43. Furlan, *Indigenous Cities*, 3.

44. Miller, *Indians on the Move*, 8.

45. Cahill, Blansett, and Needham, *Indian Cities*, 5.

46. Cahill, Blansett, and Needham, *Indian Cities*, 5.

47. LaGrand, *Indian Metropolis*; Thrush, *Native Seattle*; Karskens, *Colony*.

48. Hahn, *Nation Under Our Feet*; Kelley, "Black Poor"; Scott, *Weapons of the Weak*; Gerring, "Perils of Particularism"; Leff, "Revisioning US Political History"; Ortner, "Resistance and the Problem"; Fowler, "Politics"; and Berezin, "Politics and Culture."

49. Hahn, *Nation Under Our Feet*, 3.

50. Hahn, *Nation Under Our Feet*, 3.

51. Hahn, *Nation Under Our Feet*, 3.

52. Zoller, "Health Activism," 343.

53. Zoller, "Health Activism," 355.

54. Nelson, *Body and Soul.*

55. Nelson, *Body and Soul.*

56. Nelson, *Body and Soul,* xii.

57. Cornell, *Return of the Native,* 152.

58. For example, reformative goals "forgo fundamental change in the structure of Indian-White relations in favor of a redistribution of services, resources, or rewards within that structure, as for example, through the appointment of Indians to positions of authority in the Indian Bureau . . . or the maximization of economic returns to Indians from natural resource development." On the other hand, "transformative goals," according to Cornell, "envision not simply a redistribution of rewards within the prevailing structure of Indian-White relations, but also a fundamental reordering of those relations, as for example, through the re-opening of treaty negotiations between the United States and Indian nations or ending the plenary power of Congress in Indian affairs." Cornell, *Return of the Native,* 152–53.

59. Cornell, *Return of the Native,* 153.

60. Seeking federal funds was, somewhat ironically, grounded in the "segregative" aspiration to establish funds for separate Indian medical services that reflected and catered to their special status as Indians.

61. Indian Affairs Task Force, *People Speak,* 116.

62. Indian Affairs Task Force, *People Speak,* 116.

63. Smith, *Decolonizing Methodologies.*

64. McCallum and Perry, *Structures of Indifference,* 19.

65. McCallum and Perry, *Structures of Indifference,* 19.

Chapter 1

1. Norman, author interview.

2. Norman, author interview.

3. Norman, author interview.

4. The Thunderbird Treatment Center is a subsidiary organization of the SIHB. It was established in 1974 in response to the high rates of alcoholism among Seattle's urban Native community. When it first opened, it was called the Thunderbird Fellowship House, and it consisted of a fifteen-bed residential alcoholism treatment program. In 1976, Thunderbird Fellowship House relocated to a larger facility, increasing its size to forty-six residential treatment beds. Today, it describes itself more broadly as a "chemical dependency service," and it includes both inpatient residential and outpatient care for adults and teens. In addition to offering individual chemical dependency assessments, inpatient and outpatient services, treatment support, and medical support, the SIHB emphasizes that its approach to chemical dependency can incorporate traditional Indian medicine practices as part of patient health care plans for detoxification. On its website, the SIHB explains that these practices can include the use of the SIHB's on-site sweat lodge, talking circles, and consultation with their traditional Indian medicine liaison. See Seattle Indian Health Board, "Thunderbird Treatment Center." This mixture of

traditional and nontraditional approaches has been typical of all services offered by the SIHB since it started.

5. For instance, he has spent many years as a volunteer for the Statewide Poverty Action Network and the Chief Seattle Club—a shelter and community center for indigent Native people in Seattle.

6. Norman, author interview, part 7.

7. Tucker, author interview, part 2.

8. Tucker, author interview.

9. Tucker, author interview.

10. Tucker, author interview.

11. Tucker, author interview, part 5.

12. Tucker, author interview.

13. Tucker, author interview.

14. This is a claim that requires further investigation. I make the assertion here that women were overrepresented among medical migrants on the basis of compelling evidence suggested by early sociological and anthropological research conducted by researchers in both countries. For instance, Pamela Beasley's study on Aboriginal households in Sydney and J. Norelle Lickiss's study on Aboriginal children in Sydney indicated that women were predominantly the drivers of their family's relocation, and that many placed a high value on medical care. See Beasley, "Aboriginal Household in Sydney"; Lickiss, "Aboriginal People of Sydney." Though only a small sample, evidence from my interviewees in Seattle and Sydney also seem to reflect this trend. What can be gleaned from government files, such as the relocation files of the Bureau of Indian Affairs, also suggests that women were overrepresented among medical migrants, but more research must be done. It is beyond the scope of this project to fully account for this fact, thus in asserting this claim here I also acknowledge that this is a line of research that should be pursued in further depth in the future.

15. I want to thank Brianna Theobald for making this insightful observation in her engagement with my work.

16. For more on this early precursor as well as the later relocation policy, see Fixico, *Urban Indian Experience*, 8–25.

17. Historians usually designate the "termination era" in federal Indian policies as the mid-1940s to mid-1960s. The termination policy, articulated in House Concurrent Resolution 108 (HCR 108) in 1953, intended to dismantle tribal sovereignty and abrogate all obligations to Native Americans as promised in the 374 treaties signed with the United States. Shortly after adopting HCR 108, Congress passed Public Law 280, an act that authorized select states to assume criminal and civil jurisdiction over reservations without tribal consent. Both maneuvers sent troubling signals: Proponents of termination envisioned nothing less than liquidating the tribal land base and abandoning the obligations and responsibilities that the United States had accepted when it entered into treaties and agreements with tribes. Riding on the crest of a war fought in the name of democracy and freedom, proponents of termination evoked images of emancipation, integration, equality, and full citizenship to bolster public support. The idea of terminating tribes was thus a man-

ifestation of the assimilationist racial egalitarian ideals that informed postwar race relations more generally. (Indeed, the same set of ideals and very similar policies prevailed in Australia too, as I will discuss later.) As part of the push toward termination, the Bureau of Indian Affairs instituted a formalized relocation program starting in 1952. For more on termination and relocation, see Fixico, *Termination and Relocation*.

18. At the time of Australian federation in 1901, Aboriginal people were excluded from the rights of Australian citizenship, including the right to vote, the right to be counted in the census, and the right to be counted as part of an electorate. In addition, they were not subject to commonwealth laws and benefits in relation to wages and social security benefits such as maternity allowances and old age pensions. Control over all matters—including health—relating to Aboriginal people remained in the hands of state governments (except in the case of the Northern Territory, which was under the commonwealth government). The result was that specific conditions and regulations varied from state to state, although the overall position and status of Aboriginal people remained relatively similar across the country. Between 1900 and the 1960s there was some progress in the campaign for Aboriginal citizenship rights, but the gains were usually subject to strict conditions. In 1949 the commonwealth granted voting rights to Aboriginal ex-servicemen and ex-servicewomen. It is often stated that the 1967 referendum granted citizenship and the right to vote to Aboriginal people for the first time. This is not strictly true. In 1962, the Commonwealth Electoral Act was amended so that all Aboriginal and Torres Strait Islander people could vote. Unlike the situation for other Australians, voting was not compulsory. The 1967 referendum is significant in that two specific changes were made to the Australian Constitution: Section 21: "The Parliament shall, subject to this Constitution have power to make laws for the peace, order and good government of the Commonwealth with respect to: . . . (xxvi) the people of any race, other than the aboriginal people in any state, for whom it is necessary to make special laws"; and Section 127: "In reckoning the numbers of people of the Commonwealth, or of a State or other part of the Commonwealth, aboriginal natives should not be counted." The result of changing these two sections of the Constitution was to give the commonwealth power to make laws for Aboriginal people (which until this time resided with the states) and to make it possible to include Aboriginal people in the census, which in effect made them count as Australian citizens for the first time. (Under Section 127, this was not possible.) For more on the referendum, see Attwood and Markus, *1967 Referendum*. For more on the history of Aboriginal inclusion in the Australian nation see McGregor, *Indifferent Inclusion*.

19. Fixico, *Termination and Relocation*, 128–31.

20. Erna Gunther, "Estimated Indian Population in the State of Washington, as of June 1957," unpublished manuscript, Acc. No. 614-70-20, Erna Gunther Papers, Box 9, File 4, University of Washington Archives, Seattle, WA; "History of the Seattle Indian Health Board," 6.

21. For more on population estimates, see "History of the Seattle Indian Health Board."

22. Johnny, author interview, part 1.

23. The Seattle Indian Health Board later estimated that between 1950 and 1965 approximately 3,500 Indians were "officially" relocated to Seattle by the BIA, meaning that a high number of Indians who moved to Seattle in the postwar years did so unassisted. See Seattle Indian Health Board, "Position Paper on the BIA."

24. Attwood and Markus, *1967 Referendum*, vi–viii.

25. Broadly speaking, there were three types of spaces formally set aside by the government specifically for Aboriginal people to live on: (1) Aboriginal reserves were parcels of land set aside for Aboriginal people to live on; these were not managed by the government or its officials. From 1883 onward, Aboriginal people who were living on unmanaged reserves received rations and blankets from the Aborigines Protection Board—later the Aborigines Welfare Board—but remained responsible for their own housing; (2) Aboriginal missions were created by churches or religious individuals to house Aboriginal people and train them in Christian ideals and to also prepare them for work. Most of the missions were developed on land granted by the government for this purpose. Around ten missions were established in New South Wales between 1824 and 1923, although missionaries also visited some managed stations. Many Aboriginal people have adopted the term "mission" or "mish" to refer to reserve settlements and fringe camps generally; and (3) Aboriginal "stations" or "managed reserves" were established by the Aborigines Protection Board from 1883 onward and were managed by officials appointed by that board. Education (in the form of preparation for the workforce), rations housing, and rudimentary medical (first aid) care tended to be provided on these reserves, and station managers tightly controlled who could, and could not, live there. Many people were forcibly moved onto and off stations. Managed stations in New South Wales included Purfleet, Karuah, and Murrin Bridge near Lake Cargellico. In addition, many other Aboriginal people did not live on Aboriginal missions, reserves, or stations, but in towns or in fringe camps on private property or on the outskirts of towns, on beaches, and riverbanks. There are many such places across the country that remain important to Aboriginal people. For more on Aboriginal reserves, stations, and missions, see Doukakis, *Aboriginal People, Parliament.*

26. For firsthand accounts of this movement back and forth between rural and urban areas, see Tatz and McConnochie, *Black Viewpoints.*

27. Rowley, *Outcasts in White Australia*, 364.

28. Wait, "Migration of People," 7.

29. F. Wells, "Taste of a Bitter Utopia," *Sydney Morning Herald*, February 28, 1966.

30. Beasley, "Aboriginal Household in Sydney," 138.

31. Lovejoy, "Costing the Aboriginal Housing Problem," 81.

32. Beasley, "Aboriginal Household in Sydney," 148.

33. Beasley, "Aboriginal Household in Sydney." As we will see in chapters to follow, in circumstances of poverty, it was also women who would marshal resources to make sure everyone was fed, not only in terms of their own families but in the larger Aboriginal community in the city. Indeed, the prominent role of women in the early organizing and social support work that eventually developed into more sophisticated forms of community organizing around health issues is a

feature of the political activism I describe in later chapters, in relation to both Seattle and Sydney.

34. For example, immediately after World War II, the Australian federal government expressed interest in enfranchising all Aboriginal people who met a prescribed standard of literacy, numeracy, and good character. Yet since Aboriginal Affairs were a state responsibility, determination of who met these standards was made in cooperation with state authorities. Consequently, the federal government, in enacting its *Commonwealth Electoral Act 1949*, took the path of least resistance, extending the commonwealth franchise to all Aboriginal people entitled to vote at the state level. See McGregor, *Indifferent Inclusion*, 68.

35. The one exception to this was the community of Aboriginal people living at the government-run La Perouse reserve, just on Sydney's outer metropolitan limits.

36. Chicka Dixon cited in Tatz and McConnochie, *Black Viewpoints*, 33.

37. For detailed discussion, see chapter 4.

38. Weibel-Orlando, *Indian Country, L.A.*, 22.

39. Danziger, *Survival and Regeneration*, 22.

40. Gale, *Urban Aborigines*, 27.

41. Gale and Wundersitz, *Adelaide Aborigines*, 106.

42. Fixico, *Termination and Relocation*, 191.

43. Gale, *Urban Aborigines*, 13.

44. LaGrand, *Indian Metropolis*, 7.

45. See, for example, Waddell and Watson, *American Indian in Urban Society*.

46. For newer work that challenges and brings nuance to this older view within the historiography, see Miller, *Indians on the Move*. Miller usefully classifies this older historiography to which I refer here as a "first wave of scholarship on urban American Indians." See Miller, *Indians on the Move*, 8. I would place Miller's work in a nascent "third wave" alongside that of scholars like Brianna Theobald, Sasha Maria Suarez, Holly Miowak Guise, and others, who are showcasing—in quite specific but also representative ways—how Native histories (and especially Native women's histories) in the contexts of twentieth-century cities and migration can offer examples of a profound diversity in "urbanization" stories, a carefully exercised agency among many Native migrants, and oftentimes a legacy of lasting impact and success for sustaining their communities. A recent edited collection also exemplifies this latest wave of scholarship: Cahill, Blansett, and Needham, *Indian Cities*. This "third wave" follows a "second wave" of scholarship from the 1990s to early 2010s, when historians like Ned Blackhawk, Coll Thrush, James LaGrand, and others asserted the need for histories that pushed beyond the one-dimensional discourses of urban Indian poverty and dislocation. I should note that while the "third wave" of scholarship is filling some significant gaps in the historiography of urban Indian migration, mobility, and community formation, it still neglects a sustained analysis of health issues.

47. See McGregor, *Indifferent Inclusion*; Morgan, *Unsettled Places*.

48. National Council of Indian Opportunity, "Transcripts of a NCIO Public Forum before the Committee on Urban Indians in Minneapolis-St. Paul, March 18–19, 1969," Records of the National Council on Indian Opportunity, 1968–1974, RG0220, Box 116.

49. Corpuz, author interview, part 3; Johnny, author interview, part 2; Butterfield, interview by Teresa Brownwolf-Powers.

50. To be sure, a newer generation of historians is taking a fresh look at relocation histories, adding important nuance, new interpretations, and some much-needed complication to the older historiography in this area. In these newer histories we are seeing a greater attentiveness to Native agency within migration and relocation experiences. Two important new histories that update our understanding of the BIA's relocation program and the history of Native American urbanization in the twentieth century are Miller's *Indians on the Move* and Brianna Theobald's *Reproduction on the Reservation*. Theobald's work, in particular, supports many of the assertions I make in this chapter about the central role Native women played in these histories of migration and relocation. While more tightly focused on experiences that specifically highlight Native women's reproductive histories, Theobald's work draws on an invaluable archive of additional stories and experiences centered on Native women's migration into cities with a focus on their health. Importantly, she also discusses these histories with an attention to "self-relocatees." See Theobald, *Reproduction on the Reservation*, especially chapter 4.

51. Again, Theobald's work is an invaluable resource for understanding some of the health pressures on reservation communities, particularly as they impacted Native women.

52. DeJong, *If You Knew the Conditions*, 2.

53. Commissioner of Indian Affairs, *Annual Report, Report of Field Matron*, 135.

54. Commissioner of Indian Affairs, *Annual Report, Report of Field Matron*, 135.

55. At this time, the Office of Indian Affairs was under the auspices of the War Department (1824–49), hence the dispensation of medical care was made available to small numbers of Native people living near military posts. These services were provided by army medical staff and due to poor resourcing were usually minimal. Where services were provided, the delivery system was inefficient, with vaccines often arriving late or not at all. Doctors remained in short supply. Indian agents thus frequently wrote members of Congress and officials in the War Department seeking additional funds and increased medical personnel and supplies, but usually to no avail. See, for example, De Jong, *If You Knew the Conditions*, 2.

56. Evans, Saunders, and Cronin, *Exclusion, Exploitation, and Extermination*, 100.

57. This should be read with double meaning in terms of protecting the settlers from them and also protecting the Indigenous peoples themselves.

58. The first treaty to specifically address the health of American Indians was the 1832 treaty with the Winnebago (Ho Chunk) Nation, made at Tock Island, Illinois. Article 5 of the treaty committed the United States to provide "for the service and attendance of a physician at Prairie du Chien, and of one at Fort Winnebago." (See "Treaty with the Winnebago, September 15, 1832," 7 Stat. 370, art. 5.) In 1854–55, the United States consummated fourteen treaties containing medical provisions with tribes in the Pacific Northwest. In 1867–68, seven of the Peace Commission treaties, signed with the tribal nations on the Great Plains and in the Southwest, contained medical provisions. Medical facilities and physicians were increasingly important to tribes by the middle of the nineteenth century. In the 1854 Chasta,

Scoton, and Umpqua treaty talks, for example, treaty commissioner Joel Palmer reported to commissioner of Indian Affairs George Manypenny that while retaining certain parcels of land was important to the Northwest Coastal Indians in consideration of the treaties, the federal pledge to establish schools and a hospital among them "contributed very much to overcome their objections." In the 1855 Nisqually and Puyallup treaty, Washington territorial governor Isaac Stevens informed the Indians, "The paper . . . gives you mechanics and a Doctor to teach you and cure you. Is that not fatherly?" See *Ratified Treaties 1854–1855*, RG 75, T-494, National Archives and Research Administration, Roll 5. Where medical provisions were not specifically listed, most treaties asserted federal protection of tribes in exchange for land or a pledge by tribes to not engage in political intercourse with other foreign states. This has generally been interpreted to mean that the United States would provide the means to preserve the health of the Indians. This fiduciary responsibility is supported by federal court rulings and legislation and is the basis of the federal Indian trust responsibility.

59. DeJong, *If You Knew the Conditions*, 156.

60. White et al., *Tuberculosis Among the North American Indians*, 92–93.

61. White et al., *Tuberculosis Among the North American Indians*, 92–93.

62. Cleland, "Disease amongst the Australian Aborigines," 158.

63. Bennett, *Australian Aboriginal*, 127.

64. DeJong, *If You Knew the Conditions*, 45.

65. Meriam, *Problem of Indian Administration*, 189.

66. Meriam, *Problem of Indian Administration*, 189.

67. The fight against trachoma was largely fought by "providing separate towels in the boarding schools, displaying posters in Indian communities, and in a small amount of rather ineffective segregating of cases in schools." Meriam, *Problem of Indian Administration*, 189.

68. Meriam, *Problem of Indian Administration*, 208–16.

69. Meriam, *Problem of Indian Administration*, 7.

70. Meriam, *Problem of Indian Administration*, 31, 312.

71. Meriam, *Problem of Indian Administration*, 99–100.

72. US Department of Health, Education, and Welfare, *Health Services for American Indians*, 165.

73. Cited in Foard, "Health of the American Indians," 1405.

74. Foard, "Health of the American Indians," 1404–5.

75. US Bureau of Indian Affairs, *Annual Report 1954*, 35.

76. US Department of Health, Education, and Welfare, *Health Services for American Indians*, 165.

77. US Bureau of Indian Affairs, *Annual Report 1941*, 434.

78. Theodore D. Hegg, "Health Survey of the Muckleshoot Indians—University of Washington, 1967," RG112, King County Health Department, Public Health Director's Files, Ser 9, Box 13, King County Archives Seattle, WA.

79. Townsend, "Observation on Indian Health," 31, 42.

80. Townsend, "Observation on Indian Health," 31, 42.

81. Parron, *Alaska's Health*, vi–29.

82. Foard, "Health of the American Indians," 1404.

83. Parron, *Alaska's Health: A Survey*.

84. Garcia, author interview, part 3.

85. Norman, author interview, part 1.

86. Chisholm, author interview, part 3.

87. Biskup, *Not Slaves, Not Citizens*, 111–12.

88. Cited in Evans, Saunders, and Cronin, *Exclusion, Exploitation, and Extermination*, 97.

89. Beck, *Enigma of Aboriginal Health*.

90. Beck, *Enigma of Aboriginal Health*, 11–12.

91. Beck, *Enigma of Aboriginal Health*, 11–12.

92. Rowley, *Outcasts in White Australia*.

93. Saggers and Gray, *Aboriginal Health and Society*, 124; Biskup, *Not Slaves, Not Citizens*, 116.

94. Cited in Biskup, *Not Slaves, Not Citizens*, 224.

95. Cited in Biskup, *Not Slaves, Not Citizens*, 247.

96. Wagner, "Aboriginal Infant Mortality," *Lamp*, September 1981, 9–10.

97. Moodie, *Aboriginal Health*, 26–27.

98. Moodie, *Aboriginal Health*, 30–33.

99. Wagner, "Aboriginal Infant Mortality," 14.

100. Wagner, "Aboriginal Infant Mortality," 9–10.

101. Duguid, *No Dying Race*, 24.

102. Berndt and Berndt, *End of an Era*, 72.

103. Berndt and Berndt, *End of an Era*, 72.

104. Berndt and Berndt, *End of an Era*, 71–72.

105. Berndt and Berndt, *End of an Era*, 71–72, 76–77.

106. Stevens, *Aborigines in the Northern Territory*, 101.

107. Ingram, author interview, part 2.

108. Ingram, author interview.

109. Chisholm, author interview, part 7.

110. Ingram, author interview, part 4.

111. Chisholm, author interview, part 3.

112. Gale, *Urban Aborigines*, 88.

113. Gale, *Urban Aborigines*, 88.

114. Gale, *Urban Aborigines*, 257.

115. In the course of interviewing prominent Aboriginal activist Gary Foley, he had strong words to say about the role of *Dawn* and *New Dawn* in setting a lot of people up for disappointment. Foley, author interview, part 8.

116. C. W. Ringley, "Narrative Summation of Relocation Operations of Fiscal Year 1959, Western Washington Agency," RG75, Bureau of Indian Affairs Western Washington Agency Employment Assistance Case Files 1958–71, Box 0186, National Archives, Seattle, WA.

117. Ringley, "Narrative Summation."

118. Ringley, "Narrative Summation."

119. Ringley, "Narrative Summation."

120. Aborigines Welfare Board NSW, *Dawn*, February 1952, 1.

121. Aborigines Welfare Board NSW, *Dawn*, February 1952, 1.

122. Aborigines Welfare Board NSW, *Dawn*, February 1953, 6.

123. Aborigines Welfare Board NSW, *Dawn*, February 1952, 19.

124. Bureau of Indian Affairs Western Washington Agency, *New Horizons*, September 1959, 2.

125. Bureau of Indian Affairs Western Washington Agency, *New Horizons*, February 1960, 5.

126. Bureau of Indian Affairs Western Washington Agency, *New Horizons*, September 1959, 6.

127. Bureau of Indian Affairs Western Washington Agency, *New Horizons*, September 1959, 6.

128. Bureau of Indian Affairs Western Washington Agency, *New Horizons*, September 1959, 6.

129. Peter Williams, Letter to the Editor, in Aborigines Welfare Board NSW, *Dawn*, February 1962, 3.

130. Fred H. Claymore, "March 1959 Narrative Report of the Western Washington BIA Relocation Office," RG75, BIA Western Washington Agency Employment Case Files 1958–71, Box 0186, National Archives, Seattle, WA.

131. Claymore, "March 1959 Narrative Report."

132. Claymore, "March 1959 Narrative Report."

133. BIA Western Washington Agency, *New Horizons*, March 1959.

134. BIA Western Washington Agency, *New Horizons*, March 1959.

135. BIA Western Washington Agency, *New Horizons*, September 1957.

136. Aborigines Welfare Board NSW, *Dawn*, April 1953, 1.

137. Aborigines Welfare Board NSW, "Home Hints," *Dawn*, August 1952, 13.

138. Aborigines Welfare Board NSW, "In the Garden," *Dawn*, May 1952, 21.

139. Aborigines Welfare Board NSW, "Home Hints," *Dawn*, May 1952, 21.

140. Saxby, "We Must Have Pride: A New Living Standard," *Dawn*, May 1953, 1.

141. BIA Western Washington Agency Branch of Relocation Services, newsletter (*New Horizons*), September 1957, RG75, Western Washington Agency Employment Assistance Case Files 1958-71, Box 0186, National Archives, Seattle, WA.

142. BIA Western Washington Agency Branch of Relocation Services, newsletter (*New Horizons*), September 1957, RG75, Western Washington Agency Employment Assistance Case Files 1958-71, Box 0186, National Archives, Seattle, WA.

143. Jimmy Cook, "Happy Indian," *Seattle PI*, April 1959, RG75, Western Washington Agency Employment Assistance Case Files 1958-71, Box 0186, National Archives, Seattle, WA.

144. Note that at this time, universal health care was not yet available in Australia. This only came about in 1975. Nonetheless, as I discuss further in the next chapter, prior to 1975 Australian citizens had access to forms of medical insurance and subsidized care. When the AWB sought to push Aboriginal people toward accepting the benefits of "full citizenship," what they therefore sought to encourage among Aboriginal people was simply use of mainstream health services in the same manner as regular citizens.

145. Aborigines Welfare Board NSW, *Dawn*, July 1953, 8.

146. Aborigines Welfare Board NSW, "Our Real Citizens: More Exempted Aborigines," *Dawn*, July 1953, 8.

147. For a full discussion of the history of these institutions see, Lomawaima, *They Called It Prairie Light*; Child, *Boarding School Seasons*; Jacobs, *White Mother to a Dark Race*.

148. Aborigines Welfare Board NSW, *Dawn*, July 1952, 1.

149. BIA Western Washington Agency, New Horizons, RG75, BIA Western Washington Agency General Correspondence 1952–68, Box 0026, National Archives, Seattle, WA.

150. Again, at the time, this citizenship in both cases did not entail rights to health care, but from the perspective of both national governments, by accepting the cultural norms of "full citizenship," this was supposed to make it possible for Indigenous people to receive medical treatment at mainstream health facilities just like regular Australian and American citizens.

151. Ramirez, *Native Hubs*; Carpio, *Indigenous Albuquerque*.

152. Carpio, *Indigenous Albuquerque*.

Chapter 2

1. For more on the life of this joke and its continuing relevance to Native communities throughout the United States, see Richie and Heape, *Don't Get Sick After June*.

2. Foley, author interview, part 10.

3. National Council of Indian Opportunity, "Transcripts of a NCIO Public Forum before the Committee on Urban Indians in Dallas TX, February 13–14, 1969," RG0220, Records of the National Council on Indian Opportunity, 1968–74, Box 116, US National Archives II, College Park, MD.

4. "Hospitals Accused of Race Discrimination," *Sydney Morning Herald*, February 1967.

5. "Hospitals Accused of Race Discrimination."

6. These intragroup tensions have grown in the twenty-first century, leading to cases of conflict and competition between reservation and urban communities over federal funding for Indian health care. While it is beyond the scope of this project to discuss these tensions at length, this warrants further attention.

7. Nash, "Remarks by Commissioner of Indian Affairs Philleo Nash at Conference of Superintendents in Denver, Colorado, October 16, 1961," RG75 Western Washington BIA Records, General Correspondence, 1952–68, Box 11 and 19, National Archives, Seattle, WA.

8. Nash, "Remarks by Commissioner."

9. Nash, "Remarks by Commissioner."

10. To be sure, it is important to underscore that when considering this dynamic in the Australian case, the issue at stake was less about the explicit loss of comprehensive health care on reserves (because given the lack of federal oversight over Aboriginal Affairs in Australia before 1967, this did not exist in the same way that

the IHS existed to provide health care to Native Americans). What was at stake, however, was the loss of Aboriginal "wardship" status in the cities. This was again a complex issue. Because, although losing wardship status was advantageous in terms of freeing Aboriginal people from government surveillance and control, it also meant that Aboriginal people lost what small modicum of recognition and obligations they had been granted on reserves in virtue of their status as Indigenous peoples.

11. Nash, "Remarks by Commissioner."

12. Nash, "Remarks by Commissioner."

13. Nash, "Remarks by Commissioner."

14. Shaw to Scheele, July 22, 1955, Acc 1885, William Lewis Paul Papers, Box 1, University of Washington Special Collections, Seattle, WA.

15. Shaw to Scheele.

16. The Meriam Report (1928), whose official title was *The Problem of Indian Administration*, was commissioned by the Institute for Government Research (IGR, better known later as the Brookings Institution) and funded by the Rockefeller Foundation. The IGR appointed Lewis Meriam as the technical director of the survey team, to compile information and report on the conditions of American Indians across the country. Meriam submitted the 847-page report to the secretary of the interior, Hubert Work, on February 21, 1928. The report combined narrative with statistics to criticize the Department of Interior's implementation of the Dawes Act and overall conditions on reservations and in boarding schools. The Meriam Report was the first general study of conditions impacting Native people since the 1850s, when the ethnologist and former US Indian agent Henry R. Schoolcraft had completed a six-volume work for the US Congress. The Meriam Report provided much of the data used to reform American Indian policy through new legislation: the Indian Reorganization Act of 1934. It strongly influenced succeeding policies in land allotment, education, and health care. The report found generally that the US federal government was failing at its goals of protecting Native Americans, their land, and their resources, both personal and cultural. In its section on health care services provided by the government to Native Americans, the report states, "The hospitals, sanatoria, and sanatorium schools maintained by the [Indian Health] Service, despite a few exceptions, must generally be characterized as lacking in personnel, equipment, management, and design." The government, although it had numerous on- and off-reservation health care institutions, did not provide sufficient care for Indian patients. The report noted, "The most important single item affecting health is probably the food supply." A further setback facing health care on Indian reservations was a general lack of knowledge of the Native languages by health care providers. See Meriam, *Problem of Indian Administration*.

17. For example, in 1947, after the closure of the Tulalip Indian Hospital in 1944, the Indians of the Tulalip Tribe sent a formal demand to their Indian agent, demanding, "Now, therefore, be it unanimously resolved by the Tulalip Tribes meeting in regular annual session at the Tulalip Agency this 5th day of April, 1947, a quorum present, that the need for financial assistance for medical and hospital care for the Indians of the Tulalip Tribes continues to be a vital problem and it is requested

that this need be presented to the Commissioner of Indian Affairs and our State Representatives in United States Congress and that they be requested to make available the necessary funds to meet this situation" (Parks to Gross, "Resolution, 5th April, 1947," RG75, BIA Portland General Subject Files, 1934–52, Box 1509, National Archives, Seattle, WA).

18. DeJong, *Plagues, Politics, and Policy*. For instance, a 1954 article in the *American Journal of Public Health* summed up the arguments, citing that obvious advantages of the transfer included obtaining new facilities, equipment, and technology; unshared control of funds by medical officers who understood better than the Indian service bureaucrats what a public health program needed; easier access to specialized services and the broad competencies of the Public Health Service; and staffing benefits. See "The Indians' Health and Public Health."

19. Senate Committee on Indian Affairs, *Aspects of Indian Policy*, 4, 16.

20. Fixico, *Termination and Relocation*, 49. The Hoover Commission recommended a new Department of Natural Resources be created for all remaining Indian programs.

21. For example, members of the American Medical Association had long favored withdrawal of assistance unless they were given full control of the Indian medical service. See Braasch, Branton, and Chesley, "Survey of Medical Care," 221.

22. The Johnson-O'Malley Act was a law of the US Congress passed on April 16, 1934, to subsidize education, medical attention, and other services provided by states to Native Americans, especially those not living on reservations. The act was part of the Indian New Deal of the 1930s to help offset costs of tax-exempt Indians making use of public schools, hospitals, and other services.

23. Authority already existed in a 1938 law that provided for the collection of fees from those non-Indians able to pay. (See US Congress, *Providing for Medical Services, House Report no. 641*, 2–3). Chapman argued such a law would help recruit physicians because they would provide care to a "greater variety of patients" and would be able to increase their pay through private practice on the side (while still being contractually bound to provide care for Indians). An initial bill passed the House on June 20, 1949, but the Senate failed to act. See Commissioner of Indian Affairs, *Commission on the Organization*, 66. The Hoover Commission suggested Public Health Service physicians be detailed to the Indian Service for a minimum of three and preferably four or five years so they would better understand the needs of the Indian community they served.

24. US Department of the Interior, *Annual Report*, 1952, 395. Myer argued final decisions regarding the closure of any health facility would not be made without tribal consultation. The Ft. Berthold Tribal Council, State Health Council, the state hospital, medical and pharmaceutical associations, and the State Commission on Indian Affairs all supported the plan.

25. Interior Secretary Chapman supported this but called for several modifications, including various measures to protect Indian priority at such facilities. For example, any hospital that had been transferred was supposed to preserve Indian access and priority over non-Indians. At Indian health facilities, non-Native patients were only to be admitted when insufficient hospital beds or health facilities

were available for them locally. Moreover, non-Native access at Indian health facilities was permissible only if Native people were not utilizing such services. Congress ultimately deferred to Chapman's concerns when it enacted Public Law 291 in 1952. It also granted the secretary statutory authority to transfer any Indian hospital to state or local agencies. The secretary was also empowered to enter contracts for health facilities with any federal, state, or territorial government (or relevant political subdivision) if this would better serve the health needs of Indians. See US Congress, *Providing for Medical Services, House Report no. 797*. The revised bill (HR 4815) allowed physicians to contract for services but without becoming federal employees, prioritized Indian access to services, and provided procedures for the disposition of funds from non-Indian patients. See US Congress, *Providing for Medical Services, Senate Report no. 1095*.

26. Fixico, *Termination and Relocation*, 46.

27. In the realm of health, this was a proposition first made apparent in the divestiture of some Indian health responsibilities to state and local governments that was already underway in the late 1940s, which I discuss below.

28. US Congress, "Concurrent Resolutions: Indians."

29. See US Congress, *An Act to Transfer*.

30. US Department of the Interior, *Annual Report*, 1955, 231.

31. US Department of Health, Education, and Welfare, *Annual Report*, 1955, 122.

32. US Department of Health, Education, and Welfare, *Indian Health Highlights*.

33. US Department of Health, Education, and Welfare, *Indian Health Highlights*.

34. Department of Health, Education, and Welfare, Public Health Service, Division of Indian Health. "Tacoma Indian TB Hospital, Hospital Directive HD-Clin.-6," December 12, 1956, RG90 Records of the Public Health Service: Indian Health Service, Tacoma Indian Hospital Reports 1929–59. Box 18, National Archives, Seattle, WA.

35. For more on the early history of health services provided to Aboriginal people, see Franklin and White, "History and Politics," 1–37.

36. Franklin and White, "History and Politics," 27.

37. Cited in McGregor, *Indifferent Inclusion*, 247.

38. An Aboriginal station (also referred to colloquially as a reserve, mission, or settlement) was a community occupying reserve lands that was managed by resident government officers (usually a "teacher-manager" and his wife). They usually contained a school and a clinic and served as a depot for the allocation of blankets, rations, and other supplies to Aboriginal people. In the Northern Territory, Queensland, New South Wales, and South Australia, stations had comprehensive programs dealing with housing, employment, education, and health. Staff of between six and twelve people implemented the programs. In 1969, New South Wales had forty-five reserves in total. Until 1965, sixteen of these were managed by a resident staff and were known most commonly as stations. Vocational training and employment were not common on NSW reserves, but education and welfare services, including health, were offered. Reserves, unlike reservations in the United States, were not owned by or considered to be under the jurisdiction of Aboriginal people. All Aboriginal reserves are owned by the governments

concerned, and their continued existence is not guaranteed in any special way. Generally, reserves were established and terminated by the states without reference to Parliament or anyone else. The exception to this was South Australia, where reserves could be reduced in size only by an act of Parliament. In the past, some states took measures to contain Aboriginal residents on reserves, and so absconders in Western Australia and Queensland, for example, were returned to settlements by force. By the late 1960s, though, Aboriginal people were not forced to stay on reserves. Indeed, they were encouraged to treat them as a springboard for movement into cities, as part of an effort to assimilate them. See Aboriginal Affairs, *Answering Your Questions About Aborigines*, 4th Edition, 1969, A1851, E. G. Whitlam Personal Papers, Box 6819, National Archives of Australia, Sydney.

39. Franklin and White, "History and Politics," 27–28.

40. As I explain in chapter 4, this often led to the complete oversight of urban populations in favor of the more populous and visible rural communities.

41. For more on the Australian government's pursuit of assimilation under Hasluck, see McGregor, *Indifferent Inclusion*, especially chapter 5.

42. Macintyre, *Poor Relation*, 22–25.

43. Macintyre, *Poor Relation*, 23.

44. Macintyre, *Poor Relation*, 23–24.

45. In terms of Australian immigration policy at the time, this was also reflected in the White Australia Policy, which favored the immigration of those deemed more able to assimilate, like Europeans.

46. Jones, author interview, part 7.

47. These issues are discussed in detail in chapter 4.

48. Harris, in National Council of Indian Opportunity, "NCIO Public Forum on Indian Opportunity, Dallas-Forth Worth TX, February 13, 1969," ARC6120300, RG0220, Records of the National Council on Indian Opportunity, 1969–1974, Box 116, National Archives II, College Park, MD, 24–25.

49. Harris, "NCIO Public Forum," 24.

50. Harris, "NCIO Public Forum," 24.

51. Harris, "NCIO Public Forum," 24.

52. Tahmahkera, "NCIO Public Forum," 24.

53. Tahmahkera, "NCIO Public Forum," 29.

54. Tahmahkera, "NCIO Public Forum," 29.

55. Harris, "NCIO Public Forum," 29.

56. Tahmahkera, "NCIO Public Forum," 29.

57. Harris, "NCIO Public Forum," 29.

58. Tafoya, "NCIO Public Forum," 29.

59. Palmer, "NCIO Public Forum," 30.

60. Edwards, "NCIO Public Forum," 47.

61. Edwards, "NCIO Public Forum," 47.

62. Edwards, "NCIO Public Forum," 47.

63. Edwards, "NCIO Public Forum," 47.

64. Harris, "NCIO Public Forum," 47.

65. Harris, "NCIO Public Forum," 47.

66. Harris, "NCIO Public Forum." The irony, of course, is that as American citizens, Native people could not claim a "right" to health care. In effect then, what Harris's comments actually sought to encourage among American Indians was a demand for equal treatment. By pushing the forum attendees to invoke their status as American citizens, she therefore meant to encourage them to stand up for their civil rights in the face of discrimination.

67. Washington State Indian Conference 1956, "Minutes of Meeting," Acc No. 614–001, Erna Gunther Papers, Box 9, University of Washington Special Collections, Seattle, WA.

68. "Minutes of Meeting."

69. "Minutes of Meeting."

70. "Minutes of Meeting."

71. "Minutes of Meeting."

72. "Minutes of Meeting."

73. "Minutes of Meeting."

74. Hollow, author interview, part 11.

75. Again, recall that this was not citizenship in a legal sense so much as a cultural or social one (see chapter 1).

76. Aboriginal Affairs, *Answering Your Questions*.

77. Aboriginal Affairs, *Answering Your Questions*.

78. Aborigines Welfare Board NSW, *Dawn*, April 1956.

79. Aborigines Welfare Board NSW, *Dawn*, April 1956.

80. The ability to pay for one's medical care was frequently held up by the government as a sign of successful assimilation, not only in Australia but in the United States too. For example, in pushing back against this assimilationist logic, spokesperson for the Alaska Native Brotherhood William Lewis Paul found it necessary to point out in a letter to Dr. Hynson, the medical director of the Public Health Service in Washington State, that "you state that in order that the Indians may learn to assume an increasingly greater responsibility for their own welfare, they should assume personal responsibility for such [medical] cost as is expected of others. But you must note that there has been a serious depletion of our fisheries, which is our principal if not entire source of income, and for this the government is to blame. You will have to assume that an Indian cannot pay unless there be good evidence to the contrary." See Paul to Hynson, June 27, 1956, Paul Papers, Acc 1885, Box 1.

81. Aborigines Welfare Board NSW, *Dawn*, December 1953.

82. Mitchell, "Aborigines in the Greater Sydney Area," 10.

83. Mitchell, "Aborigines in the Greater Sydney Area," 10.

84. Monash University, *Proceedings of a National Seminar on Health Services for Aborigines, Monash University 14–17 May 1972*, MS314–20, Box 2, Australian Institute for Aboriginal and Torres Strait Islander Studies Archives, Canberra.

85. Anon., "Health Services: Availability and Adequacy of Existing Services," Monash University, *Proceedings of a National Seminar*.

86. Anon., "Health Services for Aborigines in South Australia," Monash University, *Proceedings of a National Seminar*.

87. Anon., "Health Services for Aborigines."

88. Anon., "Health Services for Aborigines."

89. Anon., "Health Services for Aborigines in Western Australia," Monash University, *Proceedings of a National Seminar.*

90. Aborigines Welfare Board NSW, *Dawn*, February 1953.

91. Aborigines Welfare Board NSW, *Dawn*, July 1953.

92. Aborigines Welfare Board NSW, *Dawn*, July 1953. The June 1952 issue also contained tips on "how to keep fit" and suggested its reader could construct a homemade punching bag to develop boxing skills.

93. David. P. Bowler (medical superintendent Townsville Hospital), "Some Problems Facing an Administrator in Improving Health Services for Aborigines," Monash University, *Proceedings of a National Seminar.*

94. Bowler, "Some Problems Facing an Administrator."

95. Lickiss, "Aboriginal People of Sydney."

96. Lickiss, "Aboriginal People of Sydney," 6.

97. Lickiss, "Aboriginal People of Sydney," iii.

98. Lickiss, "Aboriginal People of Sydney," iii.

99. Lickiss, "Aboriginal People of Sydney," ix.

100. Bowler, "Some Problems Facing an Administrator."

101. D. J. Wilson, "Training Health Workers for Future Programmes," Monash University, *Proceedings of a National Seminar.*

102. Gordon Briscoe, "Voluntary Health Services in the Metropolitan Area," Monash University, *Proceedings of a National Seminar.*

103. Briscoe, "Voluntary Health Services."

104. Briscoe, "Voluntary Health Services."

105. Briscoe, "Voluntary Health Services."

106. Dr. R. E. Coolican, "Role of the General Practitioner in the Health Team," Monash University, *Proceedings of a National Seminar.*

107. Coolican, "Role of the General Practitioner."

108. Sister Pat McPherson, "Role of the Public Health Nurse," Monash University, *Proceedings of a National Seminar.*

109. Briscoe, "Voluntary Health Services."

110. I refer here to Part V of the 1976 Indian Health Care Improvement Act, which I discuss in detail in later chapters.

111. In using this language of the "hub," I draw from the work of anthropologist Renya K. Ramirez, who writes in her book *Native Hubs* that "the hub suggests how landless Native Americans maintain a sense of connection to their tribal homelands and urban spaces through participation in cultural circuits and maintenance of social networks, as well as shared activity with other Native Americans in the city and on the reservation. Urban Indians create hubs through signs and behavior, such as phone calling, emailing, memory sharing, storytelling, ritual music, style, Native banners, and other symbols. Some of these hubs are, therefore, not based in space but include virtual activities, such as reading tribal newspapers on the Internet and emailing. Moreover, the hub as a cultural, social, and political concept ultimately has the potential to strengthen Native identity and provide a sense of belonging, as well as to increase the political power of Native peoples." She also

describes "hub-making activities" as practices that "bridge tribal differences so that Native Americans can unify to struggle for social change." See Ramirez, *Native Hubs*, 3–8. I borrow this language of the hub, with its emphasis on urban and rural mobility, and diasporic Indigenous identity and connection, as well as political and social innovation, in order to conceptualize the social, cultural, and political significance of urban Indigenous health clinics as a kind of "native hub."

Chapter 3

1. The NCIO was established by Executive Order 11399 of March 6, 1968. The mission of the council was to encourage and coordinate the introduction of federal programs to benefit the American Indian population, appraise the impact and progress of such programs, and to suggest ways to improve the programs to meet the needs and desires of the Indian population. The council was terminated on November 26, 1974, under the provisions of section 2 of the act.

2. In July 1970, Nixon issued a "Special Message to Congress" in which he laid out his Indian policy: "This, then, must be the goal of any . . . national policy toward the Indian people: to strengthen the Indian's sense of autonomy without threatening his sense of community." (See Nixon, "Special Message to the Congress," 564–67.) Accordingly, Nixon proposed a number of legislative measures to bolster tribal self-rule, cultural survival, and economic development. Most notably, these included the restoration of the sacred lands of Blue Lake to Taos Pueblo (a substantive act of justice as well as a symbolic gesture of good faith), measures for placing greater control of education in the hands of Indian communities, and legislation defining procedures by which tribes might assume administrative control of federal programs without extinguishing the trust relationship. In words and substance, the Nixon administration essentially developed a blueprint for self-determination policy. Yet, however progressive, Nixon's Indian policy initiatives were unfortunately hampered by the fact that they tended to be too liberal for many of his Republican lieutenants to substantively endorse. See Fixico, *Bureau of Indian Affairs*, 152.

3. Bill Jeffries, "Transcripts of the National Council of Indian Opportunity Public Forum in Spokane WA, November 4, 1970," RG220, Records of the National Council on Indian Opportunity, 1968–74, Box 116, Folder 2, 201, US National Archives II, College Park, MD.

4. Jeffries, "Transcripts of the National Council," 201.

5. Jeffries, "Transcripts of the National Council," 201.

6. Jeffries, "Transcripts of the National Council," 201.

7. Jeffries, "Transcripts of the National Council," 201.

8. Jeffries, "Transcripts of the National Council," 201.

9. Jeffries, "Transcripts of the National Council," 201.

10. Bob Jim, in "Transcripts of the National Council," 201.

11. Earl Old Person, in "Transcripts of the National Council," 202.

12. Jim, "Transcripts of the National Council," 201.

13. Jim, "Transcripts of the National Council," 201.

14. Jeffries, "Transcripts of the National Council," 201.

15. See Donna Nylander, "Letter to the Editor," *Ellensburg Daily Record*, November 23, 1970; "Donations for Kidney Machine Give Ernie New Lease on Life," *Bulletin*, Bend, OR, December 17, 1970; A Report of the Martial Arts World, *Black Belt Times*; "600 Bricks Shattered for Charity," *Black Belt Magazine*, Los Angeles, July 1971, 13; Roy Blount Jr., "The Magic Number is Sixkiller: Washington Quarterback Sonny Sixkiller Is a Cherokee, but His Passing Arm, Not His Heritage Has Made Him a Hero," *Sports Illustrated*, October 4, 1971; Lawrence Altman, "Artificial Kidney Use Poses Awesome Questions," *New York Times*, October 24, 1971.

16. Fox and Swazey, *Courage to Fail*, 345. The Passage of Public Law 92-603 amended the Social Security Act, making end-stage renal failure patients the first victims of catastrophic illness singled out for special coverage of their treatment costs by the federal government.

17. See Garcia, author interview; Corpuz, author interview; Krouse and Howard, *Keeping the Campfires Going*.

18. For example, see Shoemaker, *Negotiators of Change*; Krouse and Howard, *Keeping the Campfires Going*; Barr, *Peace Came*; Mihesuah, *Indigenous American Women*; Erdrich and Tohe, *Sister Nation*; Sleeper-Smith, *Indian Women and French Men*; Perdue, *Cherokee Women*.

19. Krouse and Howard, *Keeping the Campfires Going*.

20. Krouse and Howard, *Keeping the Campfires Going*.

21. Nickel, *Assembling Unity*; Suarez, "Indigenizing Minneapolis."

22. Theobald, *Reproduction on the Reservation*; DeLisle, *Placental Politics*.

23. Sunnie R. Clahchischiligi, "Women Have Long Been the Leaders in Navajo Culture. Now They're Steering the Fight Against Covid," *Guardian*, November 20, 2020.

24. Butterfield, interview by Brownwolf-Powers.

25. Butterfield, interview by Brownwolf-Powers.

26. Butterfield, interview by Brownwolf-Powers.

27. Butterfield, interview by Brownwolf-Powers.

28. American Indian Women's Service League, "Indian Center: 1960–1964," unpublished paper, Papers of the American Indian Women's Service League, Teresa Brownwolf-Powers Archive, Seattle, WA.

29. Butterfield, interview by Brownwolf-Powers. Many of my interviewees also recalled this practice. For example, see Ralph Forquera, author interview, part 4; Johnny, author interview, part 2.

30. Butterfield, interview by Brownwolf-Powers.

31. Butterfield, interview by Brownwolf-Powers.

32. Butterfield, interview by Brownwolf-Powers. My interviewees also discussed the importance of this service to these men. See Forquera, author interview, part 4; Johnny, author interview, part 2.

33. Warren cited in Andrews, *Women's Place*, 187–88.

34. Samuel Miller, "Exit Report—December 8, 1958," BIA Branch of Relocation Services Special Study on Returnees, RG75, Bureau of Indian Affairs Western Washington Agency Records, Employment Assistance Case Files, 1958–71, Box 0186, National Archives, Seattle, WA.

35. Gerald R. Edwards, "Exit Report—May 2, 1962," BIA Branch of Relocation Services Special Study on Returnees, RG75, Bureau of Indian Affairs Western Washington Agency Records, Employment Assistance Case Files, 1958–71, Box 0186, National Archives, Seattle, WA.

36. Joan M. Finkbonner, "Exit Report—May 2, 1962," BIA Branch of Relocation Services Special Study on Returnees, RG75, Bureau of Indian Affairs Western Washington Agency Records, Employment Assistance Case Files, 1958–71, Box 0186, National Archives, Seattle, WA.

37. Claymore to Ringley, July 3, 1957, RG75, Bureau of Indian Affairs Western Washington Agency Records, General Correspondence, 1952–68, Box 0026, Folder "Admin," National Archives, Seattle, WA.

38. Claymore to Ringley.

39. Claymore to Ringley.

40. Claymore to Ringley.

41. McIntyre to Pryse, January 2, 1952, RG75, Bureau of Indian Affairs Portland Area Office Area Director General Subject Files 1951–57, Box 3, National Archives, Seattle, WA.

42. Jeffries, "Transcripts of the National Council," 201.

43. Hollow, author interview, part 4.

44. Lawrence, "Indian Health Service."

45. Lawrence, "Indian Health Service," 412.

46. Shelby Gilie, "Indians Charge Medical Care Inadequate," *Seattle Times*, May 1, 1971.

47. Gilie, "Indians Charge."

48. Gilie, "Indians Charge."

49. Gilie, "Indians Charge."

50. American Indian Women's Service League, *Indian Center News*, July 1969.

51. Garcia, interview by Brownwolf-Powers.

52. Garcia, interview by Brownwolf-Powers. In later years, this sort of community knowledge about "friendly doctors" would be most useful as a tool of health activism as well. When the community later went about setting up their Indian health clinic and needed to call on the voluntary service of medical doctors, this community knowledge about which doctors were likely to be sympathetic to their cause was indispensable.

53. Gilie, "Indians Charge."

54. National Council of Indian Opportunity, "Transcripts of a NCIO Public Forum Before the Committee on Urban Indians in Dallas TX, February 13–14, 1969," RG0220, Records of the National Council on Indian Opportunity, 1968–74, Box 116, US National Archives II, College Park, MD.

55. Don Hannula, "City Life Proves Difficult for Many," *Seattle Times*, July 6, 1968.

56. Nathan J. Smith, "The Nutritional Status of a Group of Urban Indian Families Living in Seattle," unpublished paper, December 1969, Acc No 1988-005, Frederick Haley Papers, Box 13, University of Washington Special Collections, Seattle, WA.

57. Blount, "Magic Number Is Sixkiller."

58. American Indian Women's Service League, *Indian Center News* 9, no. 3 (December 1970): 8.

59. Jeffries, "Transcripts of the National Council," 201.

60. Altman, "Artificial Kidney Use."

61. Hollow, author interview, part 4. Crowfeather's case was repeatedly mentioned in interviews as well as casual conversations I held with community members in Seattle in 2013.

62. Garcia, interview by Brownwolf-Powers.

63. See Forquera, author interview, part 2; Hollow, author interview, part 2.

64. See Butterfield, interview by Brownwolf-Powers; Garcia, interview by Brownwolf-Powers; Bentz, interview by Brownwolf-Powers.

65. Butterfield, interview by Brownwolf-Powers.

66. American Indian Women's Service League, *Indian Center News* 1, no. 1 (February 19, 1960): 1.

67. American Indian Women's Service League, *Indian Center News* 1, no. 1 (February 19, 1960): 1.

68. American Indian Women's Service League, *Indian Center News*, 1960–69.

69. American Indian Women's Service League, *Indian Center News* 3, no. 17 (November 13, 1962): 1.

70. Seattle Indian Health Board, "History 1970–1975."

71. Garcia, interview by Brownwolf-Powers; Butterfield, interview by Brownwolf-Powers; Olsen, author interview; Hollow, author interview; Forquera, author interview.

72. American Indian Women's Service League, *Indian Center News* 1, no. 1 (February 19, 1960): 1.

73. American Indian Women's Service League, *Indian Center News* 3, no. 1 (February 19, 1963): 4.

74. American Indian Women's Service League, *Indian Center News* 3, no. 17 (November 11, 1963): 5.

75. Seattle Indian Health Board, "History 1970–1975," 42.

76. Forquera, author interview, part 5.

77. Forquera, author interview.

78. Seattle Indian Health Board, "Proposal Brief: Kinatechitapi Indian Clinic," March 15, 1971, 5287-02, Mayor Wes Uhlman Papers, Subject Files, Box 73, Seattle Municipal Archives, Seattle, WA.

79. Hilda Bryant, "Loneliness Is the White Man's City," *Seattle Post-Intelligencer*, 1970.

80. American Indian Women's Service League, *Indian Center News* 8, no. 7 (March 1970): 6.

81. Seattle Indian Health Board, "Report, 1976," 5287-02, Uhlman Papers, Subject Files, Box 73, Folder 8.

82. Wood to Bentz, August 20, 1971, 5287-02, Uhlman Papers, Subject Files, Box 73, Folder 6.

83. Fox and Swazey, *Courage to Fail*, 291.

84. It is helpful to think about this work done by the AIWSL in the context of what ethnic studies scholars have written about ethnic identity formation as a collective political project, as always being engaged both with internal group dynamics and relationships to the outside. See, for example, Conzen et al., "Invention of Ethnicity"; also, Brubaker, *Ethnicity Without Groups*.

85. Anderson, *Imagined Communities*.

86. The salmon bake is still an ongoing event in Seattle.

87. Old Person, in "Transcripts of the National Council," 201.

88. Hannula, "City Life Proves Difficult."

89. The full quotation in which Bernie Whitebear explained this phenomenon of being "ping-ponged" is worth repeating here: "Indians had little experience in preventative health care, seeking assistance only in emergency or life-threatening circumstances. This situation was the result of our people being ping-ponged from one hospital to the next under the mistaken assumption that the Federal government was responsible for the welfare of all Indians. In reality . . . the Bureau of Indian Affairs (BIA) and the Indian Health Services (IHS), had developed a policy that in effect meant that 'once you left the reservation, you were no longer Indian.'" See Whitebear, "Taking Back Fort Lawton," 3.

90. Urban Indian Task Force, *"People Speak: Will You Listen?"* 116.

91. Jeffries, "Transcripts of the National Council."

92. Pearl Warren, "Seattle's Indian Center," *Everett Herald*, October 28, 1967.

93. Bryant, "Loneliness Is."

94. Bryant, "Loneliness Is."

95. American Indian Women's Service League, "Indian Center: 1960–1964," 2–3.

96. American Indian Women's Service League, "Indian Center: 1960–1964," 2–3.

97. Warren, cited in Bryant, "Loneliness Is."

98. Warren, cited in Bryant, "Loneliness Is."

99. Butterfield, interview by Brownwolf-Powers.

100. Pearl Warren, *Indian Center News*, February 19, 1965: 2.

101. American Indian Women's Service League, "Indian Center: 1960–1964," 1.

102. Warren, *Indian Center News*, February 19, 1965: 2.

103. See, for example, LaGrand, *Indian Metropolis*, 138; Arndt, "Indigenous Agendas," 36; Weibel-Orlando, *Indian Country, L.A.*, 88.

104. Sixkiller to Wheeler, June 20, 1969, RG 0220, Records of the National Council on Indian Opportunity, 1968–74, Box 8, National Archives II, College Park, MD.

105. American Indian Women's Service League, "Indian Center: 1960–1964," 1.

106. Butterfield, interview by Brownwolf-Powers.

107. It is important to note too, that these ambitions were also inclusive of Seattle's host tribe and ongoing traditional stewards, the Duwamish, who in the absence of federal recognition, also lacked access to government-funded health care.

108. Garcia, interview by Brownwolf-Powers.

109. National American Indian Council, "Report on American Indian Poverty, 1970," Acc No 1988-005, Haley Papers, Box 11.

110. Robert L. Bennett, cited in Hilda Bryant, "The Red Man in America," *Seattle Post-Intelligencer*, February–March, 1970, 10.

111. Bernie Whitebear, cited in "Mayor, Indians Discuss Lawton Use," *Seattle Times*, February 17, 1971.

112. Seattle Indian Health Board, *Free Clinic for Seattle's Indians*, Pamphlet, RG 0220, Records of the National Council on Indian Opportunity, 1968–74, Box 8, National Archives II, College Park, MD.

113. Pearl Warren, "Our President's Message," *Northwest Indian News*, February 19, 1960.

114. Seattle Indian Health Board, "History 1970–1975," 6.

115. Seattle Indian Health Board, "History 1970–1975," 6.

116. Seattle Indian Health Board, "History 1970–1975," 31.

117. American Indian Women's Service League, *Indian Center News*, February 1970.

118. At first, these volunteer doctors where mostly white, but as more Native people became trained in medicine, the SIHB eventually set up a relationship with the University of Washington School of Medicine to allow its graduates to complete a residency at the SIHB. Dr. Walt Hollow, whom I interviewed in Seattle, was the first Native person to graduate from the University of Washington School of Medicine and to complete a residency at the SIHB. Gillian Marsden, Sharyne Shiu-Thornton, and Ralph Forquera, "The History of the Seattle Indian Health Board 1970–1975: The Early Years." Unpublished paper, April 2007, p. 11.

119. Marsden, Shiu-Thornton, and Forquera, "The History of the Seattle Indian Health Board," 11; Hollow, author interview, part 2.

120. Marsden, Shiu-Thornton, and Forquera, "The History of the Seattle Indian Health Board," 10.

121. Bryant, "Loneliness Is."

122. Marsden, Shiu-Thornton, and Forquera, "The History of the Seattle Indian Health Board," 8.

123. In November 1969, approximately 200 Native American activists who were part of the American Indian movement seized the abandoned federal penitentiary on Alcatraz Island in San Francisco Bay. For nineteen months, these activists occupied the island to draw attention to conditions on the nation's Indian reservations. Alcatraz, the activists said, symbolized conditions on reservations: "It has no running water; it has inadequate sanitation facilities; there is no industry, and so unemployment is very great; there are no health care facilities; the soil is rocky and unproductive." In a final symbolic act, the occupiers offered to buy Alcatraz from the federal government for "$24 in glass beads and red cloth." This very successful case of American Indian activism had inspired Bernie Whitebear and others in Seattle to stage a similar protest at Fort Lawton. For more on the influential role the Alcatraz occupation had on Seattle's activist community, see Reyes, *Bernie Whitebear*.

124. Richard Simmons, "Indians Invade Ft. Lawton," *Seattle Post-Intelligencer*, March 9, 1970.

125. "Army Disrupts Indian Claim on Ft. Lawton," *Seattle Post-Intelligencer*, March 9, 1970.

126. Hilda Bryant, "City, Indians in Accord on Lawton Center," *Seattle Post-Intelligencer*, November 15, 1971: A20.

127. Marsden, Shiu-Thornton, and Forquera, "The History of the Seattle Indian Health Board," 9.

128. Marsden, Shiu-Thornton, and Forquera, 9.

129. See Wes Uhlman, Announcement of Fort Lawton Agreement—November 14, 1971, 5287-02, Uhlman Papers, Subject Files, Box 73.

130. Marsden, Shiu-Thornton, and Forquera, "The History of the Seattle Indian Health Board," 10.

131. Marsden, Shiu-Thornton, and Forquera, "The History of the Seattle Indian Health Board," 10.

132. Hollow, author interview, part 3.

133. Hollow, author interview.

134. Hollow, author interview.

135. Hollow, author interview.

136. For instance, a treaty signed at Fort Laramie in 1868 promised that "the United States hereby agrees to furnish annually to the Indians the physician, teachers, carpenter, miller, engineer, farmer, and blacksmiths, as herein contemplated, and that such appropriations shall be made from time to time, on the estimate of the Secretary of the Interior, as will be sufficient to employ such persons."—Article XIII, Treaty of Fort Laramie (1868), www.archives.gov/milestone-documents/fort-laramie-treaty.

137. See, e.g., Treaty with the Makah, 12 Stat. 939, art. 11 (Jan. 31, 1855) ("And the United States further agrees to employ a physician to reside at the said central agency, or as such other school should one be established, who shall furnish medicine and advice to the sick, and shall vaccinate them; the expenses of said school, shops, persons employed, and medical attendance to be defrayed by the United States and not deducted from the annuities."); Treaty with the Klamath, 16 Stat. 707, art. 5 (Oct. 14, 1864) ("The United States further engages to furnish and pay for the service and subsistence . . . for the term of twenty years of one physician."); Treaty with the Kiowa and Comanche, 15 Stat. 581, art. 14 (Oct. 21, 1867) ("The United States hereby agrees to furnish annually to the Indians the physician . . . and that such appropriations shall be made from time to time, on the estimates of the Secretary of the Interior, as will be sufficient to employ such [person].")

138. See also US Department of Health and Human Services, Indian Health Service, *Indian Health Service Gold Book*, 8.

139. The 1921 Snyder Act in which Congress funded Native American health care is not to be confused with the more famous 1924 Snyder Act (also sponsored in the US Congress by representative Homer P. Snyder of New York), which "granted" birthright citizenship to all American Indians.

140. See US Department of Health and Human Services, Indian Health Service, *Fact Sheet* (Jan. 2015), citing the US Constitution, the Snyder Act of 1921, the Transfer Act of 1954, Indian Sanitation Facilities and Services Act of 1959, the Indian Self-Determination and Education Assistance Act (enacted in 1975), Indian Health Care Improvement Act of 1976, the Indian Alcohol and Substance Abuse Prevention and

Treatment Act of 1986, and the Indian Child Protection and Family Violence Prevention Act of 1990 as "not an all-inclusive list" of legal bases for federal services to American Indians and Alaska Natives; Shelton, *Legal And Historical Roots.*

141. IHS, *Fact Sheet* (2015).

142. Treaty of Medicine Creek, 1854, art. 10, https://goia.wa.gov/tribal-government /treaty-medicine-creek-1854.

143. Hannula, "City Life Proves Difficult."

144. Hannula, "City Life Proves Difficult."

145. Reyes to Morris, undated letter, Papers of the American Indian Women's Service League, Teresa Brownwolf-Powers Archive, Seattle, WA.

146. Bernie Whitebear, "National Health Service Corps," *Northwest Indian News,* April 1972.

147. Whitebear, "National Health Service Corps."

148. These problems will be discussed in detail in chapter 5.

149. Hilda Bryant, "Indians and Blacks: Historical Similarities With a Difference," *Seattle Post-Intelligencer,* 1970.

150. Loyd, *Health Rights,* 5.

151. Nelson, *Body and Soul,* 81.

152. Forquera, author interview, part 5.

153. Authorizes appropriation for purposes of this title of $5 million in fiscal year 1978, $10 million in fiscal year 1979, and $15 million in fiscal year 1980.

154. Forest Gerard, cited in Trahant, *Last Great Battle,* 89.

Chapter 4

1. Whitlam, "Statement by Leader."

2. Whitlam, "Statement by Leader."

3. Mountford, *Records of the American–Australian,* 32.

4. Pamela Beasley, "The Aboriginal Household in Sydney," Pamela Beasley Papers, MLMSS 8885, Box 7, State Library of New South Wales, Sydney. (Parts of this study were later published in 1970. See Beasley, "Aboriginal Household in Sydney," in *Attitudes and Social Conditions,* 133–89.)

5. Bobbi Sykes, *AMS Newsletter* 1, no. 1 (March 1973).

6. Little more than a storefront office at the time it was started, the AMS was the nation's first Aboriginal community-controlled health clinic. Today, more than 140 such organizations exist across both urban and rural Australia, and they have been credited with achieving such vast improvements in Aboriginal health as increased life expectancy, lowered risk of child mortality, and the proliferation of Aboriginal health workers across all sectors of the medical field. According to the website of the National Aboriginal Community Controlled Health Organisation (NACCHO), which formed in 1975 and remains the peak body representing all 160 community clinics today, these health services are the "living embodiment of the aspirations of Aboriginal communities and their struggle for self-determination." (See National Aboriginal Community Controlled Health Organisation, "About Us.") It should be noted that while the movement of community-controlled health services is

undoubtedly a success in terms of both health and political interventions, Aboriginal health in Australia still falls far below the national norm. For an up-to-date and detailed account of the health status of Indigenous Australians today, see Australian Indigenous Health Info Net, "Overview of Australian Indigenous Health."

7. These appalling conditions would become a focal point of the public debate sparked by her conviction.

8. Marchisotti to Horner, August 15, 1969, FCAATSI Records, MLMS2999, Box 4, State Library of New South Wales, Sydney.

9. Nancy Young, transcript of "Interview with Nancy Young at Brisbane Gaol by C. Smith and D. Marchisotti. August 18, 1969," unpublished source, MLMS2999, FCAATSI Records, Box 4.

10. "Manslaughter Appeal: Uni Takes Up Case," *Sydney Morning Herald*, April 29, 1969.

11. Young, transcript.

12. A specialist later determined that Evelyn Young had been suffering from a vitamin deficiency, and so the treatment for gastroenteritis was subsequently claimed to have been incorrect. See Felix Arden, "Testimony of Felix Arden in the Court of Criminal Appeal, Queensland: The Queen V Nancy Kate Florence Young," 1969, MLMS2999, FCAATSI Records, Box 4.

13. Young, transcript.

14. Young, transcript.

15. "Govt. to Examine Scurvy Report," *Sydney Morning Herald*, May 2, 1969.

16. "Scurvy Factor in Baby Deaths," *Sydney Morning Herald*, July 3, 1969.

17. For example: "Gastro Death—Gaol for the Mother," *Melbourne Sun*, April 25, 1969.

18. "Scurvy Factor in Baby Deaths," *Sydney Morning Herald*, July 3, 1969.

19. Kalokerinos, "Some Aspects."

20. "Scurvy Factor in Baby Deaths," *Sydney Morning Herald*, July 3, 1969.

21. Jack Horner, "Federal Council for Advancement of Aborigines and Torres Strait Islanders—Press Statement Re: Ms. Nancy Young, July 19, 1969," MLMSS2999, FCAATSI Records, Box 4.

22. Leabeater to FCAATSI, April 28, 1969. FCAATSI Records, MLMSS2999, Box 4.

23. Foster to the Secretary of the Sydney University Law Society, April 30, 1969, MLMSS2999, FCAATSI Records, Box 4.

24. Erica Parker to the Editor, *Sydney Morning Herald*, April 30, 1969.

25. "Manslaughter Appeal." *Sydney Morning Herald*, April 29, 1969.

26. Jack Horner took the lead in this letter-writing campaign. For example, see Jack Horner to the Premier of Queensland, the Hon. J. Bjelke-Petersen, May 9, 1969; Jack Horner to George Spall, Queensland Council for Aborigines and Torres Strait Islanders, August 1, 1969; Jack Horner to Mr. Stephen Comino, Solicitor, Stephen Comino & Cominos, August 22, 1969; Jack Horner to Mrs. Win Brehson, August 26, 1969; Jack Horner to Mr. Laurie Bryan, August 26, 1969; Jack Horner to Mrs. D. Marchisotti, Publicity Officer FCAATSI, August 29, 1969; Jack Horner to Stephen Comino & Cominos, Solicitors, August 29, 1969; Jack Horner to Mr. Gordon Bryant, Member of Parliament, September 8, 1969; Jack Horner to Dr. A. Kalokerinos,

September 8, 1969; Jack Horner to Mrs. Daisy Marchisotti, September 11, 1969; Jack Horner to Comino and Cominos, September 11, 1969; Jack Horner to John Carrick, September 17, 1969 (MLMSS2999, FCAATSI Records, Box 4).

27. Australian Broadcasting Commission, "Out of Sight."

28. ABC, "Out of Sight."

29. ABC, "Out of Sight."

30. Macleod, author interview, part 5. The significance of this television program within the history of Australian investigative reporting is also underscored by the fact that a fully accessible HD stream of the program holds a prominent place on the ABC's website.

31. Horner, "Federal Council for Advancement of Aborigines and Torres Strait Islanders—Press Statement Re: Ms. Nancy Young," 19 July 1969. (New South Wales State Library, FCAATSI Records MLMSS2999, Box 4).

32. It is commonly misunderstood that this change also conferred citizenship rights, such as the vote, to Aboriginal people, but this was not the case. The Australian Constitution, unlike the American one, makes no reference to citizenship. It is simply not that kind of constitution. It is instead a compact designed by rulers to meet the needs of government and capital, and so it is concerned instead with the parliament and its powers, the executive and the judiciary, the states, and finance and trade. Legislative changes made prior to the referendum in 1967 had already seen many Aboriginal people gain or regain the formal rights of Australian citizens. For more on this, see Attwood and Markus, *1967 Referendum.*

33. As Australian historians Bain Attwood and Andrew Markus have pointed out, the amendment to section 51 (xxvi) did not in fact compel greater federal involvement in Aboriginal Affairs as it could have. Furthermore, no provision of the Constitution prior to 1967 barred the commonwealth from enacting "general laws" affecting Aboriginal people: federal legislation of a general nature (such as welfare provision) applied to Aboriginal people in their status as Australian citizens. Moreover, the commonwealth could have further enlarged its sphere of influence in this area by using another part of the Constitution (section 96), by which the federal government provides specific purpose or ties grants to the states. In short, the importance attached to the referendum presents something of a puzzle in Australian national history. According to Attwood and Markus, the significance of the referendum is to be found less in the actual words of the Constitution and more in the stories or narratives that were told about these, and the changes demanded by those who campaigned the longest and hardest for the referendum. In their eyes, the referendum was of the utmost importance, and in the end their account of the proposed changes as a matter of rights for Aborigines and of a greater commonwealth role in Aboriginal Affairs persuaded most Australians and has been the version of events passed down in popular national memory. See Attwood and Markus, *1967 Referendum.*

34. Evidence of this popularized memorialization can be seen, for example, in current teacher resources and high school curricula used in Australian high school classrooms. An instructional resource for teachers in Victoria, for example, reads, "The 1967 Referendum is extremely significant to Aboriginal Australians. It represented the end of official discrimination and the promise of full and equal citizen-

ship. The overwhelming 'Yes' vote also signaled that white Australians were ready to embrace social and political reform and expected the Federal government to do take the lead." See Victorian Curriculum and Assessment Authority, "1967 Referendum."

35. Attwood and Markus, *1967 Referendum*; McGregor, *Indifferent Inclusion*.

36. McGregor, *Indifferent Inclusion*, 141.

37. Barry Christophers, untitled document, MS 7992, Barry Christophers Papers, Box 2, Folder "Mrs. Young," National Library of Australia, Canberra.

38. We cannot discount the significance of the cold war context in understanding the attention garnered by these health issues. If there were ever a time Australia's national politicians felt the eyes of the world upon them, this was it. It was imperative for the geopolitical considerations of cold war alliances and potential hot spots in Asia, that Australia be seen to live up to the ideological promises of the free world. In this new heightened atmosphere, having a population with the highest infant mortality rate in the world was a source of national embarrassment. Indeed, Soviet propaganda frequently centered on the mistreatment of Native Americans by the United States (see Kyrova, "Native Americans, Socialist Propaganda").

39. In addition to heading up the letter-writing campaign that secured support for Nancy Young's appeal from lawyers, politicians, doctors, and other activist organizations, FCAATSI's Jack Horner also engaged in various public speaking events to spread the word about Nancy Young's innocence and the injustice of her conviction. For example, on April 29, 1969, Horner addressed a meeting convened by the New South Wales Law School Law Society, with a paper titled "The Social Background to the Nancy Young Case." See Jack Horner, "The Social Background to the Nancy Young Case," April 29, 1969, MLMSS 2999, FCAATSI Records, Box 4.

40. Mayers, "Growing to Meet the Work's Demands," 146.

41. Crotty, "Anemia and Nutritional Disease," and Lee, "Enteritis on Palm Island," were typical of this research.

42. Moodie, *Aboriginal Health*, viii–ix.

43. Moodie, *Aboriginal Health*, viii–ix.

44. Bandler to Madgwick, October 30, 1972, MLMSS 2999, FCAATSI Records, Box 1: Folder 6.

45. Barry Christophers, "Medical Plea for Aborigines," *Sydney Morning Herald*, May 10, 1957.

46. Christophers, "Medical Plea for Aborigines."

47. Christophers, "Medical Plea for Aborigines."

48. "Child Health Scandal," *Sunday Telegraph*, February 22, 1970.

49. Dr. L. Lazarus, "Letter to the Editor: Malnutrition and Aborigines," *Sydney Morning Herald*, March 2, 1972: 6.

50. Dr. L. Lazarus, "Letter to the Editor: Critical," *Australian*, March 7, 1972: 8; Dr. L. Lazarus. "Letter to the Editor," *Canberra Times*, March 14, 1972: 9.

51. For another example of a letter sent to newspaper editors by medical doctors, see Dr. Bernard Walsh (Royal South Sydney Hospital), "Treatment of Natives Shocking," *Sydney Morning Herald*, July 17, 1959.

52. Princess Anne was seen to be an approachable and suitable figurehead to get behind their cause since she "publicly stated a certain interest in Aboriginal

children, and she did this as the President of the Save the Children Fund." See Armstrong to Bryant, April 8, 1970, MLMSS 2999, FCAATSI Records, Box 1.

53. Armstrong to Bryant.

54. Armstrong to Bryant.

55. Aborigines Welfare Board NSW, *Report of the Aborigines Welfare Board New South Wales, for the Year Ended June 20, 1960*, MLMSS 2999, FCAATSI Records, Box 4.

56. Aborigines Welfare Board NSW, *Report of the Aborigines.*

57. Aborigines Welfare Board NSW, *Report of the Aborigines.*

58. Colin Allison, "Aborigines Live '20 to 30' in Mt. Druitt Homes," *Sydney Morning Herald*, September 9, 1970. See also Keith Finlay, "Just Give Our Kids a Go," *Australian Women's Weekly*, October 12, 1971.

59. Colin Allison, "Sydney's Forgotten Blacks: Welfare Staff Use Own Money to Help Needy," *Sydney Morning Herald*, September 18, 1972.

60. Allison, "Sydney's Forgotten Blacks."

61. Dr. B. Nurcombe, "Natives Brain Damage Linked to Diets," *Australian*, July 11, 1970, Pearl Gibbs Papers, MLMS 6922, Box 2, State Library of New South Wales, Sydney.

62. Macleod, author interview, part 2.

63. Mrs. D. Marchisotti, "Letter to the Editor," *FCAATSI News*, no. 5 (January 1971): 2.

64. Kalokerinos to Christophers, October 26, 1969, Christophers Papers, MS 7992, Box 2, Folder "Mrs. Young."

65. Barry Christophers, "Untitled Document," 1969, Christophers Papers, MS 7992, Box 2, Folder "Mrs. Young."

66. Christophers, "Untitled Document." While the language did not exist at the time, in the twenty-first century we can readily recognize what Christophers refers to here as the social determinants of health.

67. Lickiss, "Aboriginal Children in Sydney," 202; Lickiss, "Aboriginal People of Sydney," iii.

68. Lickiss, "Aboriginal People of Sydney," vi.

69. Graham Williams, "Deprived—from Cradle to Grave," *Sydney Morning Herald*, July 1, 1969.

70. Williams, "Deprived."

71. Williams, "Deprived."

72. Pamela Beasley, *Report of the Sydney Aboriginal Population—June 1966*, MLMSS 8885, Beasley Papers, Box 7.

73. Pamela Beasley, "City Aborigines and Overcrowding," June 1967, MLMSS 8885, Beasley Papers, Box 7.

74. Eugene D. Stockton, "Domestic Situation of Aborigines in Sydney," unpublished paper, 1971, MLMSS 8885, Beasley Papers, Box 7.

75. University of Adelaide, *Urban Aborigine.*

76. Oodgeroo Noonuccal (formerly Kath Walker), interviewed on "Urban Aborigine," *Radio University*, 18–19.

77. Noonuccal, interviewed on "Urban Aborigine."

78. Noonuccal, interviewed on "Urban Aborigine."

79. Langman to FCAATSI, November 19, 1969, MLMSS 5866, Hannah Middleton Papers, Box 7, New South Wales State Library, Sydney.

80. H. C. Coombs, "Aboriginal Health—Paper delivered to Australasian College of Physicians—Sydney, June 5, 1969," MLMSS 5866, Middleton Papers, Box 7. Among the studies Coombs consulted were a report on infant health in the Northern Territory by professors Maxwell and Elliot of Adelaide University during 1965–66; a survey conducted by Dr. J. J. Elphinstone in 1957 and 1958 of the dietary habits of Aboriginal communities in Western Australia (both rural and urban); and the 1967–68 research of Dr. Edna Gault, Dr. Krapinaki, and Dr. Stoller, who investigated the mental health of Aboriginal adolescents in Victoria. As Coombs himself stated at the beginning of his address, though the information gathered from such surveys and comparisons was "far from complete" and had not been "brought together by competent authorities in a systematic way," he had tried, as far as possible, "to present the available data as objectively as I can, refraining from comment or attempts to lay blame."

81. Coombs, "Aboriginal Health."

82. Coombs, "Aboriginal Health."

83. Coombs, "Aboriginal Health."

84. For example, in 1970, Aboriginal activist Alice James composed a press release titled "Continued Genocide by Apathetic Australians" in which she detailed "the health problems such as our people are forced to tolerate because of the lack of interest and an unwillingness on the part of supposedly responsible governments." She explicitly referred to the address made by Coombs and quoted his seven-point conclusion in order to assert that "governments cannot plead ignorance." Dr. Coombs, chairman of the Commonwealth Office of Aboriginal Affairs, in an address stated quite clearly, "If an Aboriginal baby is born today—it has much better than average chance of being dead within two years." See Alice James, "Continued Genocide by Apathetic Australians," Press Release November 5, 1970, MLMSS 6222, Vivienne Abraham Papers, Box 13, New South Wales State Library, Sydney.

85. Roberta (Bobbi) Sykes, "Lecture to Monash University Black Australian Studies Course, 1974: Aboriginal Medical Service, Redfern," *Aboriginal Issues: Health* 1, no. 1 (June 1976): 7.

86. Sykes, "Lecture to Monash University."

87. Sykes, "Lecture to Monash University."

88. Jones, author interview, part 10.

89. Sykes, "Lecture to Monash University," 7.

90. Sykes, "Lecture to Monash University," 7.

91. Aboriginal Medical Service, "Aboriginal Medical Service Cooperative Ltd: Seven-Year Progress Report, 1971–1978," unpublished report, MS1417, Miscellaneous Pamphlets, Australian Institute of Aboriginal and Torres Strait Islander Studies (AIATSIS): Canberra ACT.

92. Foley, *First Twenty Years*.

93. Gallagher, *Story to Tell*.

94. Briscoe, *Racial Folly*.

95. Bobbi Sykes, "The Aboriginal Medical Service," *New Doctor*, no. 8 (April 1978), MLMSS5866, Middleton Papers, Box 7; Bobbi Sykes and Stephen Johnson, "Listen, Bud. Why Didn't You Go to Hospital?" *Readers Digest*, October 1975: 3.

96. For other retellings of this story, see Gary Foley, "Aboriginal Health in Our Hands," *Black National Times*, May 19–24, 1975: 8–9; Foley, *First Twenty Years*.

97. Sykes and Johnson, "Listen, Bud," 3.

98. Foley, *First Twenty Years*.

99. Sykes, "Aboriginal Medical Service."

100. Aboriginal Medical Service, Redfern, "History."

101. Aboriginal Medical Service, Redfern, "History."

102. J. Reid and B. Dhamarrandji, "Curing, Not Caring: Why Aboriginal Patients 'Abscond.'" *New Doctor*, no. 8 (April 1978): 27.

103. These other sources include interviews with doctors and nurses who worked in Sydney hospitals during the 1960s, the testimony of activists, and news stories from the time, as well as correspondence between activists and Aboriginal hospital patients seeking out the support of political organizations like FCAATSI. For other references to the practice of absconding, see Aboriginal Medical Service, Redfern, "History"; Testimony by Father Ted Kennedy, "Hospitals Accused of Race Discrimination," *Sydney Morning Herald*, May 5, 1979; Macleod, author interview; Jones, author interview; Green to Horner, November 15, 1964, MLMSS 2999, FCAATSI Records, Box 11.

104. Reid and Dhamarrandji, "Curing, Not Caring," 31.

105. Foley, "Aboriginal Health," 8–9.

106. Aboriginal Medical Service, Redfern, "History." It is important to note that Rachel Forster wasn't the only hospital in Sydney to treat Aboriginal patients this way; it was simply the worst offender given its geographical proximity to Redfern.

107. Foley, "Aboriginal Health," 8–9.

108. Green to Horner.

109. David McPherson, "N.S.W. Hospital Uses Colour Bar," *Sydney Morning Herald*, January 2, 1961.

110. Foley, *First Twenty Years*, 5.

111. Sykes, "White Doctors & Black Women," 35.

112. Sykes, "White Doctors & Black Women."

113. Reid and Dhamarrandji, "Curing, Not Caring," 29.

114. Reid and Dhamarrandji, "Curing, Not Caring," 31.

115. Reid and Dhamarrandji, "Curing, Not Caring."

116. Reid and Dhamarrandji, "Curing, Not Caring."

117. Reid and Dhamarrandji, "Curing, Not Caring."

118. Reid and Dhamarrandji, "Curing, Not Caring."

119. Reid and Dhamarrandji, "Curing, Not Caring."

120. Reid and Dhamarrandji, "Curing, Not Caring."

121. Horner to Coppard, May 26, 1969, MLMSS 2999, FCAATSI Records, Box 1; Horner to Dr. Thompson, June 5, 1969, MLMSS 2999, FCAATSI Records, Box 1; Horner to Dr. Arnold, June 5, 1969, MLMSS 2999, FCAATSI Records, Box 1; Horner

to Grenville, July 10, 1969, MLMSS 2999, FCAATSI Records, Box 1; Horner to Maxwell, August 18, 1969, MLMSS 2999, FCAATSI Records, Box 1.

122. Dulcie Flower, "FCAATSI Health Committee Report 1969," MLMSS 2999, FCAATSI Records, Box 5.

123. Flower, "FCAATSI Health Committee Report 1969."

124. Flower, "FCAATSI Health Committee Report 1969."

125. For example, Gary Foley, who is pictured in the bottom-center of Figure 4.1, was a key figure in this effort to connect the Black Power movements of the United States and Australia. (See Foley, author interview.)

126. Bobbi Sykes on *Monday Conference*, Australian Broadcasting Channel, Transcript: 10:00 P.M. Monday, March 20, 1972, MLM 2999, FCAATSI Records, Box 1, Folder 2.

127. Paul Coe on *Monday Conference*.

128. Sykes on *Monday Conference*.

129. Newsletter of the Ad-Hoc Women's Committee for Justice for Aborigines, MLMSS 6222, Abraham Papers, Box 13. See also numerous newspaper articles that picked up on this language of comparison: "Aboriginal Health Among the Worst," *Sydney Morning Herald*, November 29, 1973; Williams, "Deprived."

130. Whitlam, "Aboriginals and Society."

131. New South Wales Australian Council of Churches and the Trade Union Education & Research Centre, Pamphlet: *Australian Action Against Racism—June 20, 1971*, MLMSS6222, Abraham Papers, Box 13.

132. Bandler to Hawke (Australian Council of Trade Unions), April 8, 1971, MLMSS 2999, FCAATSI Records, Box 1.

133. "Aboriginal Mission Leaves for China," *Melbourne Sun*, October 23, 1972.

134. Bruce McGuinness, "Aborigines Must Make Alliance," *New York Times*, September 6, 1970.

135. Bruce McGuinness, "Aborigines to Study in USA," *Northcote Leader*, September 2, 1970.

136. Jack Broom, "Indians, Aborigines: Visitors See Parallel Problems for Two peoples," *Seattle Times*, September 25, 1978.

137. Broom, "Indians, Aborigines."

138. Broom, "Indians, Aborigines."

139. Abschol was initially set up, as its name suggests, to support university scholarships for Aboriginal students. It was a committee of the National Union of Australian University Students. When the committee realized that the lack of applications was due to lack of suitably qualified students, it began considering other ways of encouraging Aboriginal tertiary education. Through the 1960s, Abschol affiliated with the Federal Council for the Advancement of Aborigines and Torres Strait Islanders (FCAATSI). It later broadened its concerns, becoming a political pressure group concerned particularly with the issue of land rights. For instance, working parties of Abschol helped erect buildings for the Gurindji at Wattie Creek. During winter 1968, a twenty-four-hour national vigil was organized by Abschol for all capital cities to draw attention to the federal government's failure to negotiate on the issue of land rights. In 1972, Abschol was also a strong supporter of the

Aboriginal Tent Embassy. Despite these broader commitments, Abschol did not lose sight of its original goal and assisted several Aboriginal students in their journeys through university during the 1970s.

140. Chicka Dixon, "Report by Mr. Chicka Dixon—Aboriginal Overseas Study Award Holder of His Study Tour to USA and Canada, May–August 1975": 12, unpublished manuscript, MS 6000, Shirley Andrews Papers, Box 6, National Library of Australia, Canberra.

141. Dixon, "Report by Mr. Chicka Dixon," 6.

142. Foley, author interview, part 8. See also Foley, "1970 Black Power Conference in Atlanta, Georgia," The Koori History Website Project, last accessed March 16, 2024, www.kooriweb.org/foley/images/history/1970s/ustrip/usdx.html.

143. Flower to Marchisotti, August 13, 1968, MLMSS 2999, FCAATSI Records, Box 2.

144. Aborigines Advancement League, Letter to the Secretary General of the United Nations, October 15, 1970, MLMSS 6222, Abraham Papers, Box 13.

145. Aborigines Advancement League, Letter.

146. Aboriginal Medical Service, *AMS Newsletter*, no. 10 (January 1974).

147. Horner to Klugman, May 17, 1972, MLMSS 2999, FCAATSI Records, Box 1.

148. Horner to Klugman.

149. Gary Foley, "Support Our Palestinian Brothers," *Son of Lemark: The Alternative Black Community News Service*, no. 2., MLMSS 6222, Abraham Papers, Box 13.

150. Black Resource Centre, "Legal Racism in Queensland," *Black Liberation*, no. 2 (November 1975), MLMSS 6222, Abraham Papers, Box 13.

151. Charles Perkins, "Black Power in Australia?" Public Speech, University of New England, 1968, MLMSS 2229, FCAATSI Records, Box 4.

152. *Black News Service* 2, no. 5 (August 1976).

153. Gordon Briscoe, "Aboriginal Health and Land Rights," *New Doctor*, no. 8 (April 1978).

154. FCAATSI, "Submission to the Senate Committee on Social Environment," 1971, MLMSS 2999, FCAATSI Records, Box 4.

155. FCAATSI, "Submission to the Senate Committee."

156. Coe on *Monday Conference*.

157. Coe on *Monday Conference*.

158. Bobbi Sykes, "The Aboriginal Medical Service," *New Doctor*, no. 8 (April 1978).

159. Smith and Sykes, *Mum Shirl*, 111.

160. Smith and Sykes, *Mum Shirl*, 1; Bobbi Sykes, *Aboriginal Medical Service Newsletter*, no. 4 (June 1973): 1.

161. Sykes, *Aboriginal Medical Service Newsletter*, no. 4 (June 1973): 2.

162. Sykes, *Aboriginal Medical Service Newsletter*, no. 4 (June 1973): 2.

163. Sykes, *Aboriginal Medical Service Newsletter*, no. 4 (June 1973): 2.

164. Sykes, *Aboriginal Medical Service Newsletter*, no. 4 (June 1973): 2.

165. Cheryl Buchanan, *Race Relations News Letter*, no. 7 (March 1974): 1, MLMSS8885, Beasley Papers, Box 4, Folder 9.

166. Sykes, *Aboriginal Medical Service Newsletter*, no. 5 (August 1973): 3.

167. Sykes, *Aboriginal Medical Service Newsletter*, no. 4 (June 1973): 2.

168. Sykes, *Aboriginal Medical Service Newsletter*, no. 5 (August 1973): 3.

169. Sykes, *Aboriginal Medical Service Newsletter*, no. 2 (August 1973): 1.

170. Sykes and Johnson, "Listen, Bud," 5.

171. Sykes, *Aboriginal Medical Service Newsletter*, no. 1 (November 1973).

172. Foley, author interview.

173. Bob Bellear, *Aboriginal Medical Service Newsletter*, no. 5 (August 1973).

174. Sykes, in *Aboriginal Medical Service Newsletter*, no. 5 (August 1973).

175. Sykes, *Aboriginal Medical Service Newsletter*, no. 3 (August 1973): 2.

176. Coe on *Monday Conference*.

177. Coe on *Monday Conference*.

178. Bobbi Sykes, "Aboriginal Medical Service, Redfern," Unpublished Lecture to Monash University Black Australian Studies Course, 1974, MLMSS 6222, Abraham Papers, Box 8.

179. Sykes, "Aboriginal Medical Service, Redfern."

180. Sykes, "Aboriginal Medical Service, Redfern."

181. Sykes, "Aboriginal Medical Service, Redfern."

182. Rowse, *Obliged to be Difficult*, 112.

183. National Museum of Australia, "Gordon Bryant."

184. Bryant to Horner, September 8, 1969, MLMSS 2999, FCAATSI Records, Box 4.

185. Sykes, *Aboriginal Medical Service Newsletter*, no. 4 (June 1973): 1.

186. "A Quiet Revolution," *Aboriginal Quarterly* (March 1969): 14–15.

187. Sykes on *Monday Conference*.

188. Foley, "Aboriginal Health," 8–9.

Chapter 5

1. Dulcie Flower, "Health Committee Report, 1969–1970," MLMSS 2999, FCAATSI Records, Box 5, State Library of New South Wales, Sydney.

2. Adeline Garcia, quoted in KUOW Interview Transcript.

3. In Australia it is important to note this works slightly differently because of the absence of treaties and also in the sense that before 1967, the federal government did not have responsibility for Aboriginal Affairs; this was in the hands of the states. Thus when Aboriginal people moved off reserves, missions, and stations, they did not lose any officially designated rights as Indigenous persons. The status they lost (or which the government claimed they had "given up") by moving to the city was that of their wardship. But the outcome was much the same for Aboriginal people in cities as it was for urban Indians; the government denied any obligation to provide them services on the basis of their Indigenous identity. As I have said elsewhere, this effectively worked to enshrine the spatial logics of colonial governance in health policy since it worked to confine Indigeneity to specific locales (i.e., the reserve/reservation).

4. Hilda Bryant, "Loneliness Is the White Man's City," *Seattle Post-Intelligencer*, 1970, 50.

5. Ruby Hammond, "Land Rights: Key to Aboriginal Health," *Sydney Morning Herald*, 1982. (Precise date unknown, but newspaper clipping can be found in MLMSS 5886, Hannah Middleton Papers, Box 7, New South Wales State Library, Sydney).

6. In Seattle, this is Duwamish territory; in Sydney this is the ancestral homeland of the Gadigal people of the Eora Nation.

7. The actions of the health activists did not challenge these claims. As the previous chapter showed, in Seattle and Sydney, health activists were equally committed to advocacy for territorial sovereignty. In Seattle, we saw an expression of this kind of urban Indigenous politics in the Fort Lawton takeover.

8. In some cases (especially in Seattle, where treaties signed by Pacific Northwest tribes guaranteed the provision of medical supplies and doctors), people did conceive of their Indigenous rights to health care in cities as an explicit continuation of their tribal rights. For people in this situation, they did often press their claims to government-supported health care in cities on the basis of specific tribal/national identity. In general however, most people in the United States and Australia seemed to think of their political demands for urban Indigenous health care in terms of a complex combination of identities—both tribally specific and pan-Indigenous—which is why I have stressed the pan-Indigenous element above. This is a set of distinctions that begs much further consideration beyond the scope of the current project.

9. Or at least, politically achievable territorial sovereignty.

10. Jones and Hill-Burnett, "Political Context of Ethnogenesis"; McGregor, *Indifferent Inclusion*.

11. Hollow, author interview.

12. *Black News Service*, 1977, 3.

13. Ramirez, *Native Hubs*, 3.

14. Ramirez, *Native Hubs*, 3–8.

15. Bryant, "Loneliness Is."

16. Moreton-Robinson, *Sovereign Subjects*, 2.

17. Hammond, "Land Rights: Key."

18. To relate this to an example from contemporary Indigenous politics, when we think of the significance of movements to guard against cultural appropriation within Indigenous politics today, or the significance of discussions around visual sovereignty among Indigenous people in the United States today, one might suggest a political lineage back to these early forms of organizing around health care access because of the ways in which this emphasized thinking about the different sites on which/from which Indigenous sovereignty could be enacted (i.e., the body).

19. For example, a list of the "Traditional Indian Medicine" offered today by the SIHB's Thunderbird Treatment Center can be seen here: Seattle Indian Health Board, "Thunderbird Treatment Center."

20. Seattle Indian Health Board, "Vision, Missions, Values."

21. Seattle Indian Health Board, "History 1970–1975," 50.

22. Seattle Indian Health Board, "History 1970–1975," 50.

23. Corpuz, author interview, part 4.

24. Harold Thomas, *Land Rights News*, July 1995, 3.

25. Sol Bellear, "AMS: Here for Our Community, Here to Stay!" *Redfern Voice*, May 2014.

26. Aboriginal Medical Service Redfern, "About Us."

27. Aboriginal Medical Service Submission, 97A48/69; AMS Submission to the House of Representatives Standing Committee on Aboriginal Affairs, 466–68, 490; Aboriginal Medical Service, *Seven Year*, 1.

28. Hammond, "Land Rights: Key."

29. Mayers, "Growing to Meet."

30. Nixon, "Special Message to the Congress."

31. Nixon, "Special Message to the Congress."

32. Fixico, *Bureau of Indian Affairs*, 152.

33. Trahant, *Last Great Battle*, 8–11.

34. US Federal Government, PL 94-437 Indian Health Care Improvement Act.

35. Trahant, *Last Great Battle*, 81.

36. Trahant, *Last Great Battle*, 85.

37. Redman, *Dance of Legislation*, 17.

38. Redman, *Dance of Legislation*, 82; Trahant, *Last Great Battle*, 86.

39. Gerard, cited in Trahant, *Last Great Battle*, 88.

40. Jackson to Abourezk, November 29, 1973, Acc 4177–4, Abe Bergman Papers, Box 1, University of Washington Special Collections, Seattle, WA.

41. Trahant, *Last Great Battle*, 86–87.

42. Bergman to Kauffman, March 30, 1984, Acc 4177–4, Bergman Papers, Box 1.

43. Bergman to DuVal, November 1, 1976, Acc 4177–4, Bergman Papers, Box 1.

44. Trahant, *Last Great Battle*, 86.

45. Trahant, *Last Great Battle*, 86.

46. Luana Reyes, "Statement to Senate Committee on Interior and Insular Affairs—April 3, 1974," Acc 4177-002, Bergman Papers, Box 1.

47. Bergman to Reyes, December 19, 1977, Acc 4177-002, Bergman Papers, Box 1.

48. Trahant, *Last Great Battle*, 89.

49. Macleod, author interview, part 5.

50. Aboriginal Medical Service, "Submission to Senate Standing Committee on Social Environment—April 17, 1973, Canberra," Misc. Pamphlets, New South Wales State Library, Sydney.

51. Aboriginal Medical Service, "Submission to Senate."

52. For example, see in MS 7346, Doug Everingham Papers, National Library of Australia, Canberra, Box 21: Walton to Everingham, January 16, 1973; Walton to Everingham, January 19, 1973; Everingham to Walton, January 19, 1973; Everingham to Walton, January 28, 1973; Walton to Everingham, February 3, 1973; Everingham to Walton, February 20, 1973; Everingham to Walton, March 3, 1973.

53. Everingham to Walton, January 28, 1973, MS 7346, Everingham Papers, Box 21.

54. Doug Everingham, "Draft Green Paper on Aboriginal Affairs—by Doug Everingham," MS 7346, Everingham Papers, Box 21.

55. Everingham to Viner, September 14, 1975, MS 7346, Everingham Papers, Box 21.

56. Doug Everingham, "Memorandum," March 1973, MS 7346, Everingham Papers, Box 21.

57. Everingham, "Memorandum."

58. Everingham, "Memorandum."

59. Doug Everingham, "Briefing Notes for the Prime Minister," March 1973, MS 7346, Everingham Papers, Box 21.

60. Australian Department of Health, "National Plan for Aboriginal Health," 43.

61. Everingham to Mayers, April 21, 1974, MS 7346, Everingham Papers, Box 21.

62. Mayers to Walton, April 15, 1974, MS 7346, Everingham Papers, Box 21.

63. See US Department of Health and Human Services, *Fact Sheet*.

64. Kaiser Family Foundation, *Health Coverage and Care*.

65. IHS enters into contracts and grants with forty-one nonprofit urban Indian organizations that provide health care services to urban Indians who lack access to IHS and tribally operated health care facilities. Urban Indian organizations often "provide the only affordable, culturally competent health care services available in urban areas." The budget for urban Indian health care, however, has failed to keep pace with inflation and the growing urban Indian population. For example, in 2019, according to the Tribal Budget Workgroup, the funding allocated for urban Indian health was "estimated at [only] 22 percent of the projected need for primary care services." The FY 2019 President's Budget requested $46.4 million for Urban Indian Health—down from the FY 2018 annualized amount of $47.3 million and the FY 2017 enacted level of $47.6 million. See National Tribal Budget Formulation Workgroup, *2019 Budget*.

66. Advocates of Native American health often point to the fact that the budget of the Veterans Administration is fourteen times that of the IHS while serving only four times the population. In a report published by the National Tribal Budget Formulation Group, which makes recommendations to the IHS, they noted that "our Indian communities are combatting ongoing historical trauma not unlike that of untreated PTSD due to war experiences. We have patients who have lost limbs due to untreated diabetes or unintentional injuries associated with the third world environments in which we live. Health care is rationed and expectations for quality care in outdated facilities and equipment are so low that patients have nearly lost all hope. . . . The message is clear: the Indian Health System has failed its mission." See National Tribal Budget Formulation Workgroup, *2020 Budget*.

67. Yashadhana et al., "Indigenous Australian," 2.

68. Yashadhana et al., "Indigenous Australians," 2.

69. O'Keefe and Walls, "Indigenous Communities Demonstrate Innovation," Brookings (website); Devon Haynie, "Native Americans in Minnesota Keep COVID-19 at Bay," *US News*, October 7, 2020; Yoav Litvin, "Indigenous Leadership Points the Way Out of the COVID Crisis," *Truthout*, May 5, 2020; Sukee Bennett, "American Indians Have the Highest Covid Vaccination Rate in the US," *PBS*, July 6, 2021; Rachel Hatzipanagos, "How Native Americans Launched Successful Coronavirus Vaccination Drives: 'A Story of Resilience,'" *Washington Post*, May 20, 2021; Fiona Stanley and Marcia Langton, "In the Early Days of Covid-19, Indigenous Leaders Used Their Voice and Averted a Catastrophe," *Guardian*, March 30, 2023; Teela

Reid, "Why Australia's Real Covid-19 Success Belongs to the First Nations," *Washington Post*, March 22, 2021.

70. Mayers, "Growing to Meet," 14.

71. Indian Health Service, "IHS Profile."

72. National Aboriginal Community Controlled Health Organizations, "Aboriginal Community Controlled."

73. See Panaretto et al., "Aboriginal Community-Controlled."

Epilogue

1. Echo-Hawk, Facebook post, December 14, 2020, www.facebook.com/perma-link.php?story_fbid=pfbidowPqbf1qHwFkPNDhtJvPiMfGopQqCFyZxZfswfWsiuirj pT9fyh8kQ2AS8uqcks2Pl&id=1260036730787825.

2. Echo-Hawk, Facebook post.

3. Echo-Hawk, Facebook post.

4. Echo-Hawk, Facebook post.

5. Cecilia Nowell, "They Asked for PPE and Got Body Bags Instead—She Turned Them into a Healing Dress," *Vogue Magazine*, February 4, 2021, www.vogue.com/article/body-bag-native-ribbon-dress.

6. Nowell, "They Asked for PPE."

7. Madigan, "How the Seattle Indian."

8. Madigan, "How the Seattle Indian."

9. Madigan, "How the Seattle Indian."

10. For example, in the United States, this was famously an early measure taken by the Navajo Nation to curb the rapid spread of the virus within their community. In Australia, Anangu Pitjantjatjara Yankunytjatjara (APY) Lands Traditional Owners restricted access to their region in early March 2020.

11. An example from this video series can be seen here: Northern Land Council, "WARLPIRI."

12. Urban Indian Health Commission and Robert Wood Johnson Foundation, *Invisible Tribes*; Eric Whitney, "Native Americans Feel Invisible in US Health Care System," *NPR*, December 12, 2017; Rebecca Nagle, "Native Americans Being Left out of US Coronavirus Data and Labelled as 'Other,'" *Guardian*, April 24, 2020; Kalen Goodluck, "The Erasure of Indigenous People in COVID-19 Data," *High Country News*, August 31, 2020; Kalen Goodluck, "Why the US Is Terrible at Collecting Indigenous Data," *High Country News*, December 14, 2020.

13. Rae Ellen Bichell, "Pandemic Complicates Tribes' Quest for Data Sovereignty," July 13, 2020, *KUNC*, www.kunc.org/health/2020-07-13/pandemic-complicates-tribes-quest-for-data-sovereignty.

14. Bichell, "Pandemic Complicates."

15. Bichell, "Pandemic Complicates."

16. Bichell, "Pandemic Complicates."

17. Bichell, "Pandemic Complicates."

18. Echo-Hawk, Facebook post.

Bibliography

Manuscript Collections

Australia

Canberra

Australian Institute for Aboriginal and Torres Strait Islander Studies
    Aboriginal Affairs Press Clipping Collection
    Aboriginal Health Problems
    [Papers of the] Workshop on Aboriginal Health Research, Canberra,
        November 9–10, 1973
    Proceedings of a National Seminar on Health Service for Aborigines, held at
        Monash University, May 14–17, 1972
National Library of Australia
    Hospital and Allied Services Advisory Council (Australia) Minutes,
        1970–79
    Papers of A. J. Metcalfe, 1961–71
    Papers of Dr. Barry Christophers, 1922–81
    Papers of Charles Duguid, 1884–1986
    Papers of Charles Perkins, 1936–2000
    Papers of Douglas Nixon Everingham, 1972–80
    Papers of Elizabeth Reid 1963–81
    Papers of Frank Gare, circa 1937–2004
    Papers of Jack and Jean Horner, 1956–2003
    Papers of Jessie Street, 1889–1970
    Papers of Sir Paul Hasluck, 1925–89
    Papers of Richard Emanuel Klugman, 1938–89
    Papers of Shirley Kral, 1971–92
    Papers of Shirley Andrews, 1917–2002
    Records of the Australian Council for Civil Liberties, 1963–71
    The Riley Collection 1888–1968, pamphlet material 1950–68
    Tomato Press Publications, 1971–76

Sydney

National Archives of Australia
    Aboriginal Health—radio and television programs referring to Aborigines
    Aboriginal Health—seminar on Aboriginal health problems, ANU, March/
        April 1974

Aboriginal Health—briefing notes for the prime minister and other ministers, 1974

Aboriginal Health—report of workshop on health and nutrition of Aboriginal children, 1974

Aboriginal Health Programs—liaison between state health authorities and aboriginal medical services, 1977

Personal papers of E. G. Whitlam [Health and Welfare: Aborigines—Australian Institute of Aboriginal Studies]

New South Wales State Records

Aborigines Welfare Board Records

Anti-Discrimination Board Records

Premier's Department Letters received, 1927–62

State Library of New South Wales (Mitchell Library)

Aboriginal-Australian Fellowship Records

Faith Bandler Papers

Federal Council for the Advancement of Aborigines and Torres Strait Islanders (FCAATSI) Records

Hannah Middleton Papers

Pamela Beasley Papers

Pearl Gibbs Papers

Reverend A. W. Grant Papers

Vivienne Abraham Papers

Sydney City Archives

Community Ephemera Collection

Records and research material of the Inner Sydney Regional Council for Social Development

South Sydney Municipal Council Development Application Files

South Sydney Municipal Council General Correspondence Files

South Sydney Municipal Council Building Application Files

The Sydney Reference Collection

Sydney University Archives

A. P. Elkin Papers

United States

Seattle, WA

King County Archives

Seattle-King County Department of Public Health Director's Files

Public Health History Files

National Archives and Records Administration (NARA)

Records of the Portland Area Office

Records of the Puget Sound Indian Agency

Records of the Tacoma Indian Hospital

Records of the Taholah Indian Agency

Records of the Tulalip Indian Agency

Records of the Western Washington Agency
Records of the Yakima Indian Agency
Seattle Municipal Archives
Department of Community Development
Model City Program Records
Office of the City Clerk
Seattle King County Health Department
Teresa Brownwolf-Powers, Private Collection
Papers of the American Indian Women's Service League
University of Washington Special Collections
Abraham Bergman Papers
Church Council of Greater Seattle Papers
Erna Gunther Papers
Frederick Haley Papers
Hank Adams Papers
Henry M. Jackson Papers
William Lewis Paul Papers

Washington, DC

US Department of the Interior
Branch of Health, Bureau of Indian Affairs Records
United States Division of Indian Health Records
United States Department of Health, Education, and Welfare Records

Washington, DC; College Park, MD

US National Archives and Records Administration, NARA I (DC) and NARA II (MD)
General Records of the Department of Health, Education, and Welfare
Records of the Indian Health Service
Records of the Public Health Service
Records of the Office of the Assistance Secretary for Health
Records of the Office of the Secretary of the Interior
Records of Temporary Committees, Commissions, and Boards
Records of the National Council on Indian Opportunity
Records of the American Indian Policy Review Commission
Records of the National Commission on America's Urban Families
Records of the National Commission on American Indian, Alaska Native,
and Native Hawaiian Housing
Records of the Bureau of Indian Affairs
Records of the Offices of the Chief Clerk and the Assistant Commissioner of
Indian Affairs
Records of Assistants to the Commissioner
Records of the Relocation Division
Records of the Health Division
Records of the Office of Indian Services

Oral History Collections

American Indian Women's Service League. "Strong Voices" oral history project. Seattle, WA
    Roque, Connie. Interview by Iris Friday, May 28, 2009
A History of Aboriginal Sydney
    www.historyofaboriginalsydney.edu.au/
National Library of Australia, Canberra
    Gordon Briscoe Collection
    Peter Read Collection
Redfern Oral History Project
    http://redfernoralhistory.org/OralHistory/tabid/70/Default.aspx
Seattle Civil Rights and Labor History Project
    http://depts.washington.edu/civilr/
Teresa Brownwolf-Powers. American Indian Women's Service League Interviews, private collection, Seattle, WA

Oral History Interviews

Bentz, Marilyn. Interview by Teresa Brownwolf-Powers, Seattle, WA, May 2001.
Butterfield, Mary Jo. Interview by Teresa Brownwolf-Powers, Seattle, WA, May 11, 2001.
Butterfield, Mary Jo. Interview by Iris Friday, December 7, 2008.
Chapelle, Lillilan. Interview by Teresa Brownwolf-Powers, Seattle, WA.
Chisholm, Pat. Interview by author, Canberra, August 16, 2014.*
Codd, Julie. Interview by author, Seattle, WA, August 15, 2013.
Corpuz, Becky. Interview by author, Seattle, WA, August 23, 2013.
Crowfeather, Ian (Standing Rock Sioux). Interview by author, Seattle, WA, August 27, 2013.
Elke, Letoi. Interview by Teresa Brownwolf-Powers, Seattle, WA, May 26, 2000.
Foley, Gary (Gumbainggir). Interview by author, Melbourne, August 27, 2014.
Forquera, Ralph (Juaneño Band of California Mission Indians). Interview by author, Seattle, WA, August 23, 2013.
Garcia, Adeline (Haida). Interview by Teresa Brownwolf-Powers, Seattle, WA, May 24, 2000.
Garcia, Jania (Haida). Interview by author, Seattle, WA, August 28, 2013.
Grey, Janine (Tlingit). Interview by author, Seattle, WA, August 5, 2013.
Hollow, Walt (Assiniboine/Sioux). Trainer, Steve. Interview by author, Seattle, WA, August 18, 2013.
Ingram, David (Bundjalung). Interview by author, Sydney, August 6, 2014.*
Johnny, Abe (Cowichan). Interview by author, Seattle, WA, August 16, 2013.
Jones, Jilpia Nappaljari (Wiradjari). Interview by author, Canberra, August 13, 2014.
Jones, Pearl (Wiradjuri). Interview by author, Sydney, August 10, 2014.

Kauffman, Claudia. Interview by Teresa Brownwolf-Powers, Seattle, WA.

Macleod, Ross. Interview by author, Sydney, August 9, 2014.

Norman, Bill (Yakama). Interview by author, Seattle, WA, August 11, 2013.*

Olsen, Polly (Yakama). Interview by author, Seattle, WA, August 13, 2013.

Red Elk, Arlene. Interview by Teresa Brownwolf-Powers, Seattle, WA.

Reyes, Luana (Colville). Interview by Teresa Brownwolf-Powers, Seattle, WA.

Sanidad, Michelle. Interview by Teresa Brownwolf-Powers, Seattle, WA.

Tongs, Julie (Wiradjuri). Interview by author, Canberra, August 12, 2014.

Trainer, Steve. Interview by author, Seattle, WA, August 10, 2013.

Trainer, Trish. Interview by author, Seattle, WA, August 10, 2013.

Troyer-Willson, Joyce (Tsimsian). Interview by author, Seattle, WA, August 10, 2013.

Tucker, Dorothy "Dot" (Wiradjuri). Interview by author, Canberra, August 12, 2014.

* Indicates the name has been changed at the request of the interviewee.

Newspapers, News Media, Newsletters, and Magazines

Aboriginal Medical Service Newsletter (Sydney)

Aboriginal Quarterly (Canberra)

Associated Press (New York)

Atlantic (Washington, DC)

Australian

Australian Woman's Weekly

Baffler (New York)

Black Belt Magazine (Los Angeles)

Black Liberation (Melbourne)

Black National Times (Sydney)

Black News Service (Brisbane)

Bulletin (Bend, OR)

Canberra Times (Canberra)

Dawn /New Dawn (Sydney)

Ellensburg (WA) Daily Record

Everett (WA) Herald

FCAATSI NEWS (Sydney)

Globe and Mail (Toronto)

Guardian

High Country News (Paonia, CO)

Indian Center News (Seattle, WA)

Koori-Bina: A Black Australian News Monthly (Sydney)

KUNC (Greeley, CO)

Lamp (Sydney)

Land Rights News (Alice Springs, NT)

Melbourne Sun (Melbourne)

Montreal Gazette (Montreal)

New Doctor (Sydney)

New Horizons (Seattle, WA)

New York Times

Northcote Leader (Melbourne)

Northwest Indian News (Seattle, WA)

NPR News

Race Relations News Letter (Sydney)

Reader's Digest

Redfern Voice (Sydney)

Scientific American

Seattle Post-Intelligencer

Seattle Times

Son of Lemark (Melbourne)

Sports Illustrated

Sunday Telegraph (Sydney)

Sydney Morning Herald

Truthout (Sacramento)

U.S. News & World Report

Vogue

Washington Post

Primary Sources

Aboriginal Medical Service. Seven-Year Progress Report, 1971–1978 (Sydney, 1979).

Aboriginal Medical Service Redfern. "About Us." Aboriginal Medical Service. Updated 2021. https://amsredfern.org.au/.

———. "History." Aboriginal Medical Service. Accessed July 1, 2015. www.amsredfern.org.au/?page_id=15 (site discontinued).

Australian Broadcasting Commission. Out of Sight, Out of Mind. August 30, 1969. www.abc.net.au/news/2011-08-08/out-of-sight-out-of-mind---1969/2833724.

Australian Bureau of Statistics. "Census of Population and Housing—Counts of Aboriginal and Torres Strait Islander Australians (Reference Period 2021)." Updated August 31, 2022. www.abs.gov.au/statistics/people/aboriginal-and-torres-strait-islander-peoples/census-population-and-housing-counts-aboriginal-and-torres-strait-islander-australians/2021.

Australian Department of Health. The National Plan for Aboriginal Health Submission to the House of Representatives Standing Committee on Aboriginal Affairs, Health Problems of Aboriginals, Hansard.

Australian Department of Territories. "Fringe Dwellers." Pamphlet, Canberra: Government Printers, 1959. Burke Library Special Collections, Columbia University, New York.

Baillie, Patricia. "Pictures from The Block, Redfern Sydney." Patricia Baillie. Accessed May 20, 2016. www.patriciab.com/blockpix.html (site discontinued).

Beasley, Pamela. "The Aboriginal Household in Sydney." In Attitudes and Social Conditions: Aborigines in Australian Society, by R. Taft, J. Dawson, and P. Beasley. Canberra: Australian National University Press, 1970.

Bennett, Mary M. The Australian Aboriginal as a Human Being. London: Alston Rivers, 1930.

Berndt, R. M., and C. H. Berndt. End of an Era: Aboriginal Labour in the Northern Territory. Canberra: AIAS, 1987.

Braasch, W. F., B. J. Branton, and A. J. Chesley. "Survey of Medical Care Among the Upper Midwest Indians." Journal of the American Medical Association 139, no. 4 (1949): 220–25.

Briscoe, Gordon. Racial Folly: A Twentieth-Century Aboriginal Family. Canberra: Australian National University Press, 2010.

Bryant, Hilda. The Red Man in America. Olympia, WA: Office of the State Superintendent of Public Instruction, 1970.

Cleland, J. B. "Disease amongst the Australian Aborigines." Journal of Tropical Medicine and Hygiene 2 (1928): 157–60.

Commissioner of Indian Affairs. Annual Report, Report of Field Matron, Pima Agency, Dated August 15, 1903. Washington, DC: Government Printing Office, 1903.

———. Commission on the Organization of the Executive Branch of Government: Functions and Activities of the National Government in the Field of Welfare. Washington, DC: Government Printing Office, 1949.

Community Access Video Centre. Aboriginal Activists and Organization and Events 1975. Australian Institute for Aboriginal and Torres Strait Islander Studies, Canberra.

Crotty, J. M. "Anaemia and Nutritional Disease in Northern Territory Native Children." *Medical Journal of Australia* 2 (1958): 322–25.

Duguid, Charles. *No Dying Race*. Adelaide: Rigby, 1963.

Earle, Augustus. *Natives of N. S. Wales as Seen in the Streets of Sydney*. Trove. Accessed April 12, 2024. https://nla.gov.au/nla.obj-135290431/view.

Foard, Fred. "The Health of the American Indians." *American Journal of Public Health* 39, no. 11 (November 1949): 1403–6.

Foley, Gary. "The Koori History Website Project." Accessed March 16, 2024. www.kooriweb.org.

Forte, Margaret. *Flight of An Eagle: The Dreaming of Ruby Hammond*. Adelaide: Wakefield Press, 1995.

Gale, Fay. *Urban Aborigines*. Canberra: Australian National University Press, 1972.

Gale, Fay, and Joy Wundersitz. *Adelaide Aborigines: A Case Study of Urban Life 1966–1981*. Canberra: Australian National University Press, 1982.

Garcia, Adeline. Quoted in KUOW interview transcript, January 13, 2014. Accessed July 14, 2015. www2.kuow.org/program.php?id=6995 (site discontinued).

Health Coverage and Care for American Indians and Alaska Natives. Menlo Park, CA: Kaiser Family Foundation, October 2013.

Health and Nutrition of Aboriginal Children: Report of a Workshop. Workshop held in Sydney, December 1–5, 1969.

Hollows, Fred. "On the Need to Implement Federal Policy in Aboriginal Health: An Address to the Department of Aboriginal Health." Unpublished paper, 1979.

Horner, Jack. *Seeking Racial Justice: An Insider's Memoir of the Movement for Aboriginal Advancement, 1938–1978*. Canberra: Aboriginal Studies Press, 2004.

Indian Health Service. "About Urban Indian Organizations." Indian Health Service. Accessed March 24, 2024. www.ihs.gov/Urban/aboutus/about-urban-indian-organizations/.

———. "IHS Profile (Based on 2015–2020 Census Data)." Indian Health Service. Updated August 2020. www.ihs.gov/newsroom/factsheets/ihsprofile/.

———. *Indian Health Service Office of Urban Indian Health Programs Strategic Plan 2017–2021*. Washington, DC: Indian Health Service, 2017.

———. "The Indians' Health and Public Health." *American Journal of Public Health* 44, no. 11 (1954): 1461–63.

Kalokerinos, Archie. "Aboriginal Infant Mortality and Ascorbic Acid Deficiency Patterns." *Medical Journal of Australia* 1 (January 1967).

———. "Some Aspects of Aboriginal Infant Mortality." *Medical Journal of Australia* 1 (January 1969).

Killington, Gary. *Similar Yet Distinctive: Aborigines in Urban Settings with Particular Reference to Adelaide*. BA Hons. thesis, University of Adelaide, 1973.

Langton, Marcia. "A Day Among Fringe Dwellers." *Social Alternatives* 1, no. 5 (September 1979): 72–74.

———. "Urbanizing Aborigines." *Social Alternatives* 2, no. 2 (August 1981): 16–22.

Lee, P. E. "Enteritis on Palm Island, North Queensland." *Queensland Institute of Medical Research, 8th Annual Report* (1953): 3.

Lickiss, J. Norelle. "The Aboriginal People of Sydney with Special Reference to Health of Their Children: A Study in Human Ecology." MD thesis, University of Sydney, 1971.

——. "Aboriginal Children in Sydney: The Socio-Economic Environment." *Oceania* 41, no. 3 (March 1971).

Lovejoy, Frances. "Costing the Aboriginal Housing Problem." *Australian Quarterly* 43, no. 1 (1971).

Madigan, Grace. "How the Seattle Indian Health Board Became a Model for Pandemic Response." Evergrey. April 13, 2021. https://theevergrey.com/how-the-seattle-indian-health-board-became-a-model-for-pandemic-response/.

Marsden, Gillian (Jill), Sharyne Shiu-Thornton, and Ralph Forquera. "The History of the Seattle Indian Health Board 1970–1975: The Early Years." Unpublished Paper, April 2007.

Mayers, Naomi. "Growing to Meet the Work's Demands." In *A Story to Tell: The Working Lives of Ten Aboriginal Australians*, by Nan Gallagher. Melbourne: Cambridge University Press, 1992.

Meriam, Lewis. *The Problem of Indian Administration: Report of a Survey Made at the Request of Honorable Hubert Work, Secretary of the Interior, and Submitted to Him, February 21, 1928.* Baltimore, MD: Johns Hopkins Press, 1928.

Missick Museum. "Power in Native Art: American Indian Artistic and Aesthetic Sovereignty." Accessed July 18, 2016. www.artsandsciences.sc.edu/mckissickmuseum/power-native-art-american-indian-artistic-and-aesthetic-sovereignty (site discontinued).

Mitchell, Ian S. "Aborigines in the Greater Sydney Area: Populations, Problems, and Possibilities." *Social Service* (November 1971–February 1972): 10–14.

Moodie, Peter M. *Aboriginal Health.* Aborigines in Australian Society 9. Canberra: Australian National University Press, 1973.

Mountford, C. P., ed. *Records of the American–Australian Scientific Expedition to Arnhem Land, Vol. 2, Anthropology and Nutrition.* Melbourne: Melbourne University Press, 1960.

National Aboriginal Community Controlled Health Organisations. "Aboriginal Community Controlled Health Organisations (ACCHOs)." National Aboriginal Community Controlled Health Organizations. Accessed March 16, 2024. www.naccho.org.au/acchos/.

——. "About Us." Updated 2022, www.naccho.org.au/about-us/.

National Council of Urban Indian Health (NCUIH). "Urban American Indian Undercount in the 2020 Census Went Underreported." NCUIH Research Blog. August 28, 2023. https://ncuih.org/2023/08/28/urban-american-indian-undercount-in-the-2020-census-went-underreported/.

National Museum of Australia. "Gordon Bryant," Collaborating for Indigenous Rights Website. Updated 2014. http://indigenousrights.net.au/people/pagination/gordon_bryant.

National Tribal Budget Formulation Workgroup. *The National Tribal Budget Formulation Workgroup's Recommendations on the IHS FY 2019 Budget.* March 2017.

———. *The National Tribal Budget Formulation Workgroup's Recommendations on the Indian Health Service Fiscal Year 2020 Budget*. April 2018.

Nixon, Richard. "Special Message to the Congress on Indian Affairs," July 8, 1970. *Public Papers of the Presidents of the United States: Richard Nixon, 1970*. Washington, DC: Government Printing Office.

Northern Land Council. *WARLPIRI—A Short Film Made by the NLC in the Warlpiri Language About COVID-19/Coronavirus*. April 5, 2020. www.youtube.com /watch?v=WO6AIjV5Qt8.

O'Keefe, Victoria M., and Melissa L. Walls. "Indigenous Communities Demonstrate Innovation and Strength Despite Unequal Losses During COVID-19." Brookings, April 2, 2021. www.brookings.edu/articles/indigenous -communities-demonstrate-innovation-and-strength-despite-unequal-losses -during-covid-19/.

Parron, Thomas. *Alaska's Health: A Survey*. Pittsburgh, PA: University of Pittsburgh, 1954.

Raup, Ruth M. *The Indian Health Program 1800–1955*. Washington, DC: Government Printing Office, United States Department of Health, Education, and Welfare, Public Health Service, 1959.

Richie, Chip, and Steven Heape. *Don't Get Sick After June: American Indian Healthcare*. Dallas, TX: Rich-Heape Films, 2010.

Rudge, P. F. (with the assistance of the Aboriginal and Torres Strait Island Unit). *Aboriginal Access to Welfare Services: A Response to the Report of the House of Representatives Standing Committee on Aboriginal Affairs Dealing with Aboriginal Legal Aid*. Australian Department of Social Security, Aboriginal Access to Welfare Services, 1982.

Seattle Indian Health Board "Position Paper on the BIA Relocation Program and Its Impact in the Greater Seattle Area." August 31, 1982.

———. "Thunderbird Treatment Center." Seattle Indian Health Board. Accessed March 13, 2024. www.sihb.org/ttc/.

———. "Vision, Missions, Values." Seattle Indian Health Board. Accessed March 16, 2024. www.sihb.org/mission-statement/.

Senate Committee on Indian Affairs. *Aspects of Indian Policy*. Senate Committee Print, Seventy-Ninth Congress, 1st Session. Washington, DC: Government Printing Office, 1945.

Shelton, Brett Lee. *Legal and Historical Roots of Health Care for American Indians and Alaska Natives in the United States*. Menlo Park, CA: Henry J. Kaiser Family Foundation, February 2004.

Smith, Shirley, and Bobbi Sykes. *Mum Shirl: An Autobiography with the Assistance of Bobbi Sykes*. Melbourne: Heinemann Educational Australia, 1981.

Sykes, Roberta (Bobbi). "Lecture to Monash University Black Australian Studies Course, 1974: Aboriginal Medical Service, Redfern." *Aboriginal Issues: Health* 1, no. 1 (June 1976).

Taylor, Theodore W. *The States and Their Indian Citizens*. Washington, DC: US Department of the Interior, 1972.

Thomson, Neil. "Aboriginal Health and Health-Care." *Social Science & Medicine* 18, no. 11 (1984): 939–48.

"Treaty of Medicine Creek, 1854." Governor's Office of Indian Affairs—Treaties. Accessed August 30, 2024. https://goia.wa.gov/tribal-government/treaty-medicine-creek-1854.

"Treaty of Neah Bay, January 31, 1855." Governor's Office of Indian Affairs—Treaties. Accessed August 30, 2024. https://goia.wa.gov/tribal-government/treaty-neah-bay-1855.

"Treaty with the Kiowa and Comanche, October 21, 1867." Tribal Treaties Database. Accessed August 30, 2024. https://treaties.okstate.edu/treaties/treaty-with-the-kiowa-and-comanche-1867-0977.

"Treaty with the Klamath, October 14, 1864." Tribal Treaties Database. Accessed August 30, 2024. https://treaties.okstate.edu/treaties/treaty-with-the-klamath-etc-1864-0865.

"Treaty with the Winnebago, 1832." Tribal Treaties Database. Accessed August 30, 2024. https://treaties.okstate.edu/treaties/treaty-with-the-winnebago-1832-0345.

"The Urban Aborigine." *Radio University*. University of Adelaide, 1969.

Urban Indian Health Commission and Robert Wood Johnson Foundation. *Invisible Tribes: Urban Indians and Their Health in a Changing World*. Seattle, WA: Urban Indian Health Commission, 2007.

Urban Indian Task Force. *The People Speak, Will You Listen? Report of the Governor's Indian Affairs Task Force: Urban and Landless Committees*. Olympia: State of Washington, 1973.

US Bureau of Indian Affairs. *Annual Report of the Commissioner of Indian Affairs 1941*. Washington, DC: Government Printing Office, 1941.

——. *Annual Report of the Commissioner of Indian Affairs 1954*. Washington, DC: Government Printing Office, 1954.

US Congress. *An Act to Transfer the Maintenance and Operation of Hospital and Health Facilities for Indians to the Public Health Service, and for Other Purposes, House Report no. 2430*. Eighty-Third Congress, 2nd session, July 21, 1954.

——. *Providing for Medical Services to Non-Indians in Indian Hospitals, House Report no. 797*. Eighty-First Congress, 1st Session, June 14, 1949.

——. *Providing for Medical Services to Non-Indians in Indian Hospitals, Senate Report no. 1095*. Eighty-First Congress, 1st Session, September 20, 1949.

US Congress, 67 stat. B132. "Concurrent Resolutions: Indians." Washington, DC: Government Printing Office, 1953.

US Congress, 52 stat. 311. *Providing for Medical Services to Non-Indians in Indian Hospitals, House Report no. 641*. Eighty-Second Congress, 1st Session, June 25, 1951.

US Department of Health, Education, and Welfare. *Annual Report of the Secretary of Health, Education and Welfare*. Washington, DC: Government Printing Office, 1955.

——. *Health Services for American Indians*. Washington, DC: Government Printing Office, 1957.

———. *Indian Health Highlights.* Washington, DC: Public Health Service Division of Indian Health, 1959.

US Department of Health and Human Services, Indian Health Service. *Fact Sheet: Basis for Health Services.* January 2015. www.ihs.gov/sites/newsroom /themes/responsive2017/display_objects/documents/factsheets/BasisforHealth Services.pdf.

———. *Indian Health Service Gold Book—The First 50 Years of the Indian Health Service: Caring and Curing.* Washington, DC: Indian Health Service, 2005.

US Department of the Interior. *Annual Report of the Secretary of the Interior.* Washington, DC: Government Printing Office, 1952.

———. *Annual Report of the Secretary of the Interior.* Washington, DC: Government Printing Office, 1955.

US Federal Government, PL 94-437 Indian Health Care Improvement Act, 90 Stat. 1400, Ninety-Fourth Congress. September 30, 1976. Washington, DC: Government Printing Office. Accessed March 16, 2024. www.govtrack.us /congress/bills/94/s522/text.

Victorian Curriculum and Assessment Authority. "1967 Referendum: Sample History Unit." State of Victoria. Updated 2018. www.vcaa.vic.edu.au /Documents/viccurric/history/1967_Referendum_History.pdf.

Wagner, H. "Aboriginal Infant Mortality." *Lamp* 38, no. 9 (1981): 5–16.

Wait, E. "The Migration of People of Aboriginal Ancestry to the Metropolitan Area and Their Assimilation." BA Hons. dissertation, University of Sydney, 1950.

White, Laurence W., et al. *Tuberculosis Among the North American Indians: Report of a Committee of the National Tuberculosis Association.* Washington, DC: Government Printing Office, 1923.

Whitebear, Bernie. "Taking Back Fort Lawton." *Race, Poverty and the Environment* (Spring-Summer 1994).

Whitlam, E. Gough. "Statement by Leader of the Opposition to the House of Representatives: 'Aboriginals. Discussion of Matter of Public Importance' 13 August 1968." Whitlam Institute E-collection. http://cem.uws.edu.au/R?RN =695437248.

———. "Aboriginals and Society: Statement to a Conference of Commonwealth and State Ministers Concerned with Aboriginal Affairs," Adelaide, April 6, 1973. Full Transcript available at: Australian Government Department of the Prime Minister and Cabinet website, "Press Statement No. 74, 6 April 1973: Aboriginals and Society." Accessed March 16, 2024. https://pmtranscripts .dpmc.gov.au/release/transcript-2886.

Secondary Sources

Ablon, Joan. "Relocated American Indians in the San Francisco Bay Area: Social Interaction and Indian Identity." *Human Organization* 23 (1964): 296–304.

———. "Retention of Cultural Values and Differential Urban Adaptation: Samoans and American Indians in a West Coast City." *Social Forces* 49 (1971): 385–93.

Adakai M., M. Sandoval-Rosario, F. Xu, Teresa Aseret-Manygoats, Michael Allison, Kurt J. Greenlund, and Kamil E. Barbour. "Health Disparities Among American Indians/Alaska Natives—Arizona, 2017." *Morbidity and Mortality Weekly Report* 67, no. 47 (November 30, 2018): 1314–18. http://dx.doi.org/10.15585/mmwr .mm6747a4.

Alexander, Fred. *Moving Frontiers: An American Theme and Its Application to Australian History*. Melbourne: Melbourne University Press, 1947.

Alfred, Taiaiake. *Peace, Power, Righteousness: An Indigenous Manifesto*. 2nd ed. New York: Oxford University Press, 2009.

Allen, H. C. *Bush and Backwoods: A Comparison of the Frontier in Australia and the United States*. Westport, CT: Greenwood Press, 1975.

Anderson, Benedict. *Imagined Communities: Reflections of the Origin and Spread of Nationalism*. London: Verso, 1983.

Anderson, Ian. *Koorie Health in Koorie Hands: An Orientation Manual in Aboriginal Health for Health-Care Providers*. Melbourne: Koorie Health Unit, Health Department, Victoria, 1988.

——. "Black Bit, White Bit." In *Blacklines: Contemporary Critical Writing by Indigenous Australians*, edited by I. Anderson, M. Grossman, M. Langton, and A. Moreton-Robinson, 43–57. Melbourne: Melbourne University Press, 2003.

Anderson, Kay, and Jane Jacobs. "Urban Aborigines to Aboriginality and the City: One Path Through the History of Australian Cultural Geography." *Australian Geographical Studies* 35, no. 1 (1997): 12–22.

Anderson, Warwick. *The Cultivation of Whiteness: Science, Health, and Racial Destiny in Australia*. Melbourne: Melbourne University Press, 2005.

——. *Colonial Pathologies: American Tropical Medicine, Race, and Hygiene in the Philippines*. Durham, NC: Duke University Press Books, 2006.

Andrews, Mildred Tanner. *Women's Place: A Guide to Seattle and King County*. Seattle, WA: Gemil Press, 1994.

Arndt, Grant. "Indigenous Agendas and Activist Genders: Chicago's American Indian Center, Social Welfare, and Native American Women's Urban Leadership." In *Keeping the Campfires Going: Native Women's Activism in Urban Communities*, edited by Susan Applegate Krouse and Heather A. Howard, 33–55. Lincoln: University of Nebraska Press, 2009.

Arnold, David. *Colonizing the Body: State Medicine and Epidemic Disease in Nineteenth Century India*. Berkeley: University of California Press, 1993.

——, ed. *Imperial Medicine and Indigenous Societies*. Manchester, UK: Manchester University Press, 1989.

Attwood, Bain. *The Making of the Aborigines*. Sydney: Allen & Unwin, 1989.

——. *Rights for Aborigines*. Sydney: Allen & Unwin, 2004.

Attwood, Bain, and Andrew Markus. *The 1967 Referendum: Race, Power and the Australian Constitution*. 2nd ed. Canberra: Aboriginal Studies Press, 2007.

——, eds. *The Struggle for Aboriginal Rights: A Documentary History*. Sydney: Allen & Unwin Academic, 1998.

Barker, Joanne, ed. *Sovereignty Matters: Locations of Contestation and Possibility in Indigenous Struggles for Self-Determination.* Lincoln: University of Nebraska Press, 2005.

———. *Native Acts: Law, Recognition, and Cultural Authenticity.* Durham, NC: Duke University Press, 2011.

Barr, Julianna. *Peace Came in the Form of a Woman: Indians and Spaniards in the Texas Borderlands.* Chapel Hill: University of North Carolina Press, 2007.

Basch, Linda, Nina Glick Schiller, and Cristina Szanton Blanc, eds. *Nations Unbound: Transnational Projects, Postcolonial Predicaments and Deterrritorialized Nation-States.* Langhorne, PA: Gordon and Breach, 1993.

Bashford, Alison. *Imperial Hygiene: A Critical History of Colonialism, Nationalism and Public Health.* New York: Palgrave Macmillan, 2004.

Beck, Eduard J. *The Enigma of Aboriginal Health: Interaction Between Biological, Social, and Economic Factors in Alice Springs Town-Camps.* Canberra: AIAS, 1985.

Belich, James. *Replenishing the Earth: The Settler Revolution and the Rise of the Anglo-World, 1783–1939.* New York: Oxford University Press, 2009.

Berezin, Mabel. "Politics and Culture: A Less Fissured Terrain." *Annual Review of Sociology* 23 (1997): 361–83.

Berger, Dan, ed. *The Hidden 1970s: Histories of Radicalism.* New Brunswick, NJ: Rutgers University Press, 2010.

Bergman, Abraham, David C. Grossman, Angela M. Erdrich, John G. Todd, and Ralph Forquera. "A Political History of the Indian Health Service." *Milbank Quarterly* 77, no. 4 (1999): 571–604.

Berndt, R. M., and C. H. Berndt. *End of an Era: Aboriginal Labour in the Northern Territory.* Canberra: AIAS, 1987.

Bernstein, Alison R. *American Indians and World War II: Toward a New Era in Indian Affairs.* Norman: University of Oklahoma Press, 1991.

Biskup, Peter. *Not Slaves, Not Citizens: The Aboriginal Problem in Western Australia, 1898–1954.* St. Lucia, Australia: University of Queensland Press, 1973.

Blackhawk, Ned. "I Can Carry On from Here: The Relocation of American Indians to Los Angeles." *Wicazo Sa Review* 11, no. 2 (Fall 1995): 16–30.

Briscoe, Gordon. *Counting, Health and Identity: A History of Aboriginal Health and Demography in Western Australia and Queensland, 1900–1940.* Canberra: Australian Institute of Aboriginal and Torres Strait Islander Studies, 2003.

Brubaker, Rogers. *Ethnicity without Groups.* Cambridge, MA: Harvard University Press, 2006.

Bruyneel, Kevin. *The Third Space of Sovereignty: The Postcolonial Politics of U.S.-Indigenous Relations.* Minneapolis: University of Minnesota Press, 2007.

Buff, Rachel. *Immigration and the Political Economy of Home: West Indian Brooklyn and American Indian Minneapolis, 1945–1992.* Berkeley: University of California Press, 2001.

Burgmann, Verity. *Power and Protest: Movements for Change in Australian Society.* Sydney: Allen & Unwin, 1993.

Burnley, Ian, and James Forrest, eds. *Living in Cities: Urbanism and Society in Metropolitan Australia*. Sydney: Allen & Unwin, 1985.

Cahill, Cathleen D. *Federal Fathers & Mothers: A Social History of the United States Indian Service, 1869–1933*. Chapel Hill: University of North Carolina Press, 2011.

Cahill, Cathleen, Kent Blansett, and Andrew Needham, eds. *Indian Cities: Histories of Indigenous Urbanization*. Norman: University of Oklahoma Press, 2022.

Cameron, Catherine, Paul Kelton, and Alan C. Swedlund, eds. *Beyond Germs: Native Depopulation in North America*. Tucson: University of Arizona Press, 2015.

Campbell, Judy. *Invisible Invaders: Smallpox and Other Diseases in Aboriginal Australia 1780–1880*. Melbourne: Melbourne University Publishing, 2002.

Carpio, Myla Vicenti. "The Lost Generation: American Indian Women and Sterilization Abuse." *Social Justice* 31, no. 4 (2004): 40–53.

——. *Indigenous Albuquerque*. Lubbock: Texas Tech University Press, 2011.

Case, John, and Rosemary C. R. Taylor. *Co-Ops, Communes & Collectives: Experiments in Social Change in the 1960s and 1970s*. New York: Pantheon Books, 1979.

Castile, George Pierre. *To Show Heart: Native American Self-Determination and Federal Indian Policy, 1960–1975*. Tucson: University of Arizona Press, 1998.

Castile, George Pierre, and Robert L. Bee, eds. *State and Reservation: New Perspectives on Federal Indian Policy*. Tucson: University of Arizona Press, 1992.

Cerwonka, Allaine. *Native to the Nation*. Minneapolis: University of Minnesota Press, 2004.

Child, Brenda. *Boarding School Seasons: American Indian Families*. Lincoln: University of Nebraska Press, 1998.

Chowkwanyun, Merlin. *All Health Politics Is Local: Community Battles for Medical Care and Environmental Health*. Chapel Hill: University of North Carolina Press, 2022.

Clark, Jennifer. *Aborigines & Activism: Race, Aborigines & the Coming of the Sixties to Australia*. Perth: University of Western Australia Press, 2008.

Cleaver, Kathleen, and George N. Katsiaficas, eds. *Liberation, Imagination, and the Black Panther Party: A New Look at the Panthers and Their Legacy*. New York: Routledge, 2001.

Clendinnen, Inga. *Dancing with Strangers: Europeans and Australians at First Contact*. New York: Cambridge University Press, 2005.

Cobb, Daniel M. *Native Activism in Cold War America*. Lawrence: University Press of Kansas, 2008.

Cobb, Daniel M., and Loretta Fowler, eds. *Beyond Red Power: American Indian Politics and Activism since 1900*. Santa Fe, NM: School for Advanced Research, 2007.

Confer, Clarissa, Andrae Marak, and Laura Tuennerman, eds. *Transnational Indians in the North American West*. College Station: Texas A&M University Press, 2015.

Conzen, Kathleen Neils, David A. Gerber, Ewa Morawska, George E. Pozzetta, and Rudolph J. Vecoli. "The Invention of Ethnicity: A Perspective from the U.S.A." *Journal of American Ethnic History* 12, no. 1 (Fall 1992): 4–41.

Cook, Kevin, and Heather Goodall, eds. *Making Change Happen: Black and White Activists Talk to Kevin Cook about Aboriginal, Union and Liberation Politics.* Canberra: ANU Press, 2013.

Cornell, Stephen. *The Return of the Native: American Indian Political Resurgence.* New York: Oxford University Press, 1988.

Coulthard, Glen. *Red Skin, White Masks: Rejecting the Colonial Politics of Recognition.* Minneapolis: University of Minnesota Press, 2014.

Cowlishaw, Gillian. *The City's Outback.* Sydney: University of New South Wales Press, 2009.

Crosby, Alfred. "Virgin Soil Epidemics as a Factor in the Aboriginal Depopulation in America." *William and Mary Quarterly* 33, no. 2 (1976): 289–99.

Danziger, Edmund J. *Survival and Regeneration: Detroit's American Indian Community.* Detroit, MI: Wayne State University Press, 1991.

Dashuk, James. *Clearing the Plains: Disease, Politics of Starvation, and the Loss of Aboriginal Life.* Regina, SK: University of Regina Press, 2013.

Davies, Wade. *Healing Ways: Navajo Health Care in the Twentieth Century.* Albuquerque: University of New Mexico Press, 2001.

Davis, Julie. *Survival Schools: The American Indian Movement and Community Education in the Twin Cities.* Minneapolis: University of Minnesota Press, 2013.

DeJong, David H. *If You Knew the Conditions: A Chronicle of the Indian Medical Service and American Indian Health Care, 1908–1955.* Lanham, MD: Lexington Books, 2008.

———. *Plagues, Politics, and Policy: A Chronicle of the Indian Health Service, 1955–2008.* Lanham, MD: Lexington Books, 2011.

DeLisle, Christine Taitano. *Placental Politics: CHamoru Women, White Womanhood, and Indigeneity under U.S. Colonialism in Guam.* Chapel Hill: University of North Carolina Press, 2022.

Deloria, Philip. *Playing Indian.* New Haven, CT: Yale University Press, 1998.

———. *Indians in Unexpected Places.* Lawrence: University Press of Kansas, 2004.

Dhillon, Jaskiran K. *Prairie Rising: Indigenous Youth, Decolonization, and the Politics of Intervention.* Toronto, ON: University of Toronto Press, 2017.

Diamond, Jared. *Guns, Germs, and Steel: The Fates of Human Societies.* New York: W. W. Norton, 1999.

Doenmez, Caroline Fidan Tyler. "Carrying Water: Indigenous Women Reclaiming Birthing Sovereignty along the Red River." Phd diss., University of Minnesota, 2023.

Doukakis, Anna. *Aboriginal People, Parliament and "Protection" in New South Wales, 1856–1916.* Sydney: The Federation Press, 2006.

Dudley-Shotwell, Hannah. *Revolutionizing Women's Healthcare: The Feminist Self-Help Movement in America.* New Brunswick, NJ: Rutgers University Press, 2020.

Dunbar-Ortiz, Roxanne, ed. *Economic Development in American Indian Reservations.* Albuquerque: University of New Mexico, 1979.

———. *An Indigenous Peoples' History of the United States.* Boston, MA: Beacon Press, 2014.

Edmonds, Penelope. *Urbanizing Frontiers: Indigenous Peoples and Settlers in 19th-Century Pacific Rim Cities.* Vancouver: University of British Columbia Press, 2010.

Ellinghaus, Katherine. *Taking Assimilation to Heart: Marriages of White Women and Indigenous Men in the United States and Australia, 1887–1937.* Lincoln: University of Nebraska Press, 2006.

Enke, Anne. *Finding the Movement: Sexuality, Contested Space, and Feminist Activism.* Durham, NC: Duke University Press, 2007.

Erdrich Heidi E., and Laura Tohe, eds. *Sister Nations: Native American Women Writers on Community.* Minneapolis-St. Paul: Minnesota Historical Society Press, 2002.

Estes, Nick. *Our History Is the Future: Standing Rock Versus the Dakota Access Pipeline, and the Long Tradition of Indigenous Resistance.* New York: Verso, 2019.

———. "The Empire of All Maladies: Colonial Contagions and Indigenous Resistance." *Baffler* 52 (July 2020).

Evans, Julie, ed. *Equal Subjects, Unequal Rights: Indigenous Peoples in British Settler Colonies, 1830–1910.* New York: Palgrave, 2003.

Evans, Raymond, Kay Saunders, and Kathryn Cronin. *Exclusion, Exploitation, and Extermination: Race Relations in Colonial Queensland.* Sydney: Australia & New Zealand Book Company, 1975.

Fels, Marie. *Good Men and True: The Aboriginal Police of the Port Phillip District, 1837–1853.* Melbourne: Melbourne University Press, 1988.

Ferreira, Mariana K. Leal, and Gretchen Chesley Lang, eds. *Indigenous Peoples and Diabetes: Community Empowerment and Wellness.* Durham, NC: Carolina Academic Press, 2006.

Fixico, Donald L. *American Indians in a Modern World.* Lanham, MD: AltaMira Press, 2008.

———. *Bureau of Indian Affairs.* Santa Barbara, CA: Greenwood, 2012.

Foley, Gary. *The First Twenty Years: Aboriginal Medical Service.* Sydney: Aboriginal Medical Service Cooperative, 1991.

———. *A Short History of the Australian Indigenous Resistance 1950–1990.* Subversion Press, January 2010, https://kooriweb.org/foley/resources/pdfs/229.pdf.

———. *Termination and Relocation: Federal Indian Policy, 1945–1960.* Albuquerque: University of New Mexico Press, 1990.

———. *The Urban Indian Experience in America.* Albuquerque: University of New Mexico Press, 2000.

Ford, Lisa. *Settler Sovereignty: Jurisdiction and Indigenous People in America and Australia, 1788–1836.* Cambridge, MA: Harvard University Press, 2010.

Forte, Margaret. *Flight of An Eagle: The Dreaming of Ruby Hammond.* Adelaide: Wakefield Press, 1995.

Forte, Maximilian C., ed. *Indigenous Cosmopolitans: Transnational and Transcultural Indigeneity in the Twenty-First Century.* New York: Peter Lang, 2010.

Fowler, Loretta. "Politics." In *A Companion to the Anthropology of American Indians,* edited by Thomas Biolsi, 69–94. Malden, MA: Blackwell Publishing, 2004.

Fox, Renée Claire. *Essays in Medical Sociology: Journeys Into the Field.* New Brunswick, NJ: Transaction Publishers, 1988.

Fox, Renée Claire, and Judith P. Swazey. *The Courage to Fail: A Social View of Organ Transplants and Dialysis.* Chicago: University of Chicago Press, 1978.

Franco, Jeré Bishop. *Crossing the Pond: The Native American Effort in World War II.* Denton: University of North Texas Press, 1999.

Franklin, Margaret-Ann, and Isobel White, "The History and Politics of Aboriginal Health." In *The Health of Aboriginal Australia,* edited by Janice Reid and Peggy Trompf, 1–37. Sydney: Harcourt Brace Jovanovich Publishers, 1991.

Fredrickson, George M. *Black Liberation: A Comparative History of Black Ideologies in the United States and South Africa.* New York: Oxford University Press, 1995.

Furlan, Laura. *Indigenous Cities: Urban Indian Fiction and the Histories of Relocation.* Lincoln: University of Nebraska Press, 2017.

Gale, Fay. *Urban Aborigines.* Canberra: ANU Press, 1972.

Gale, Fay, and Joy Wundersitz. *Adelaide Aborigines: A Case Study of Urban Life 1966–1981.* Canberra: ANU Press, 1982.

Gallagher, Nan. *A Story to Tell: The Working Lives of Ten Aboriginal Australians.* Melbourne: Cambridge University Press, 1992.

Geddes, Gary. *Medicine Unbundled: A Journey Through the Minefields of Indigenous Health Care.* Toronto, ON: Heritage House Publishing, 2017.

Gerring, John. "The Perils of Particularism: Political History after Hartz." *Journal of Policy History* 11, no. 3 (1999): 313–22.

Goodall, Heather. *Invasion to Embassy: Land in Aboriginal Politics in New South Wales, 1770–1972.* Sydney: Sydney University Press, 2008.

Goodman, David. *Gold Seeking: Victoria and California in the 1850s.* Sydney: Allen & Unwin, 1994.

Grande, Sandy. *Red Pedagogy: Native American Social and Political Thought.* Lanham, MD: Rowman & Littlefield, 2015.

Gray, Christine K. *The Tribal Moment in American Politics: The Struggle for Native American Sovereignty.* Lanham, MD: AltaMira Press, 2013.

Greenwood, Margo, Sarah de Leeuw, and Nicole Marie Lindsay, eds. *Determinants of Indigenous Peoples' Health: Beyond the Social.* 2nd ed. Toronto, ON: Canadian Scholar's Press, 2018.

Griffiths, Max. *Aboriginal Affairs: A Short History.* Sydney: Kangaroo Press, 1995.

Grosz, Elizabeth. *Space, Time, and Perversion: Essays on the Politics of Bodies.* New York: Routledge, 1995.

Guise, Holly Miowak. *Alaska Native Resilience: Voices from World War II.* Seattle: University of Washington Press, 2024.

Gurr, Barbara. *Reproductive Justice: The Politics of Health Care for Native American Women*. New Brunswick, NJ: Rutgers University Press, 2014.

Haebich, Anna. *For Their Own Good: Aborigines and Government in the South West of Western Australia, 1900–1940*. 2nd ed. Perth: University of Western Australia Press, 1992.

——. *Spinning the Dream: Assimilation in Australia 1950–1970*. Perth: Fremantle Press, 2008.

Hahn, Steven. *A Nation Under Our Feet: Black Political Struggles in the Rural South, from Slavery to the Great Migration*. Cambridge, MA: Belknap Press, 2003.

Harmon, Alexandra, ed. *The Power of Promises: Rethinking Indian Treaties in the Pacific Northwest*. Seattle: Center for the Study of the Pacific Northwest in association with University of Washington Press, 2008.

Hertzberg, Hazel W. *The Search for an American Indian Identity*. Syracuse, NY: Syracuse University Press, 1971.

Hirabayashi, James, William Willard, and Luis Kenmitzer. "Pan-Indianism in the Urban Setting." In *The Anthropology of Urban Environments*. Washington, DC: Society for Applied Anthropology, 1972.

Hobart, Hi'ilei, Julia Kawehipuaakahaopulani, and Tamara Kneese. "Radical Care: Survival Strategies for Uncertain Times." *Social Text* 38, no. 1 (2020).

Hoffman, Beatrix. *Health Care for Some: Rights and Rationing in the United States Since 1930*. Chicago: University of Chicago Press, 2012.

Holm, Tom. *The Great Confusion in Indian Affairs: Native Americans & Whites in the Progressive Era*. Austin: University of Texas Press, 2005.

Horner, Jack. *Seeking Racial Justice: An Insider's Memoir of the Movement for Aboriginal Advancement, 1938–1978*. Canberra: Aboriginal Studies Press, 2004.

Huhndorf, Shari. *Going Native: Indians in the American Cultural Imagination*. Ithaca, NY: Cornell University Press, 2001.

Hunter, Ernest. *Aboriginal Health and History: Power and Prejudice in Remote Australia*. Cambridge: Cambridge University Press, 1993.

Inglis, Kerri A. *Ma'i Lepera: A History of Leprosy in Nineteenth-Century Hawai'i*. Honolulu: University of Hawaii Press, 2013.

Iverson, Peter. "Building toward Self-Determination: Plains and Southwestern Indians in the 1940s and 1950s." *Western Historical Quarterly* 16, no. 2 (1985): 163–73.

Jackson, Peter. *Constructions of Race, Place, and Nation*. London: UCL Press, 1993.

Jacobs, Jane M. *Edge of Empire: Postcolonialism and the City*. London: Routledge, 1996.

Jacobs, Margaret D. *White Mother to a Dark Race: Settler Colonialism, Maternalism, and the Removal of Indigenous Children in the American West and Australia, 1880–1940*. Lincoln: University of Nebraska Press, 2009.

Joe, Jennie R., and Francine C. Gachupin, eds. *Health and Social Issues of Native American Women*. Santa Barbara, CA: Praeger, 2012.

John, Maria. "The Violence of Abandonment: Urban Indigenous Health and the Settler-Colonial Politics of Nonrecognition in the United States and Australia." *Native American and Indigenous Studies* 7, no. 1 (Spring 2020): 87–120.

Johnson, Miranda. *The Land Is Our History: Indigeneity, Law, and the Settler State.* New York: Oxford University Press, 2016.

Johnson, Troy R. *The Occupation of Alcatraz Island: Red Power and Self-Determination.* Lincoln: University of Nebraska Press, 2008.

Jones, D., and J. Hill-Burnett. "The Political Context of Ethnogenesis: An Australian Example." In *Aboriginal Power in Australian Society*, edited by M. Howard, 214–46. St. Lucia, Australia: University of Queensland Press, 1982.

Jones, David S. *Rationalizing Epidemics: Meanings and Uses of American Indian Mortality Since 1600.* Cambridge, MA: Harvard University Press, 2004.

Kane, Robert L., and Rosalie A. Kane. *Federal Health Care (With Reservations!).* New York: Springer Publishing Company, 1972.

Kaplan-Myrth, Nili. *Hard Yakka: Transforming Indigenous Health Policy and Politics.* Lanham, MD: Lexington Books, 2007.

Karskens, Grace. *The Colony: A History of Early Sydney.* Sydney: Allen & Unwin, 2010.

Kauanui, J. Kēhaulani. "Off-Island Hawaiians 'Making' Ourselves at 'Home': A (Gendered) Contradiction in Terms?" *Women's Studies International Forum* 21, no. 6 (1998): 681–93.

——. "'A Structure, Not an Event': Settler Colonialism and Enduring Indigeneity." *Lateral: Journal of the Cultural Studies Association* 5, no. 1 (Spring 2016).

——. *Paradoxes of Hawaiian Sovereignty: Land, Sex, and the Colonial Politics of State Nationalism.* Durham, NC: Duke University Press, 2018.

Keith, Michael C. *Signals in the Air: Native Broadcasting in America.* Westport, CT: Praeger, 1995.

Kelley, Robin D. "The Black Poor and the Politics of Opposition in a New South City, 1929–1970." In *"Underclass" Debate: Views from History*, edited by Michael B. Katz, 293–333. Princeton, NJ: Princeton University Press, 1993.

Kelly, Max, ed. *Sydney, City of Suburbs.* Sydney: New South Wales University Press in association with the Sydney History Group, 1987.

Kelm, Mary-Ellen. *Colonizing Bodies: Aboriginal Health and Healing in British Columbia, 1900–50.* Vancouver: UBC Press, 1998.

Kelton, Paul. *Epidemics and Enslavement: Biological Catastrophe in the Native Southeast, 1492–1715.* Lincoln: University of Nebraska Press, 2007.

——. *Cherokee Medicine, Colonial Germs: An Indigenous Nation's Fight Against Smallpox, 1518–1824.* Norman: University of Oklahoma Press, 2015.

Konzen, K. A. "The Invention of Ethnicity: A Perspective from the U.S.A." *Journal of American Ethnic History* 12, no. 1 (Fall 1992): 4–41.

Kowal, Emma. *Trapped in the Gap: Doing Good in Indigenous Australia.* New York: Berghahn, 2015.

Kristjansson, Margaux. "Refusing Child-Stealing States: Settler Capitalism and the Ends of Canada's Indigenous Child Removal System." *Theory & Event* 27, no. 3 (2024): 381–410.

Krouse, Susan Applegate. "Kinship and Identity: Mixed Bloods in Urban Indian Communities." *American Indian Culture & Research Journal* 23, no. 2 (June 1999): 73–89.

Krouse, Susan Applegate, and Heather A. Howard, eds. *Keeping the Campfires Going: Native Women's Activism in Urban Communities*. Lincoln: University of Nebraska Press, 2009.

Kunitz, Stephen. *Disease Change and the Role of Medicine: The Navajo Experience*. Berkeley: University of California Press, 1983.

———. "The History and Politics of U.S. Health Care Policy for Native Americans and Alaska Natives." *American Journal of Public Health* 86, no. 10 (1996): 1464–73.

———. "Historical Influences on Contemporary Tobacco Use by Northern Plains and Southwestern American Indians." *American Journal of Public Health* 106, no. 2 (February 2016): 246–55.

Kyrova, Lucie. "Native Americans, Socialist Propaganda, and the Politics of the Oppressed." Paper presented at the Annual Meeting of the Native American and Indigenous Studies Conference, Sacramento, CA, May 19–21, 2011.

LaGrand, James B. *Indian Metropolis: Native Americans in Chicago, 1945–75*. Urbana: University of Illinois Press, 2002.

Lake, Marilyn, and Henry Reynolds. *Drawing the Global Colour Line: White Men's Countries and the International Challenge of Racial Equality*. New York: Cambridge University Press, 2008.

Land, Claire. *Decolonizing Solidarity: Dilemmas and Directions for Supporters of Indigenous Struggles*. London: Zed Books, 2015.

Lande, Nancy. *Words, Wounds, Chasms: Native American Health Care Encounters*. 2nd ed. Bozeman, MT: WindyCreek Press, 2016.

LaPier, Rosalyn R., and David R. M. Beck. *City Indian: Native American Activism in Chicago, 1893–1934*. Lincoln: University of Nebraska Press, 2015.

La Potin, Armand Shelby, ed. *Native American Voluntary Organizations*. New York: Greenwood Press, 1987.

LaVeist, Thomas. *Minority Populations and Health: An Introduction to Health Disparities in the U.S.* San Francisco: Jossey-Bass, 2005.

Lawrence, Jane. "The Indian Health Service and the Sterilization of Native American Women." *American Indian Quarterly* 24, no. 3 (2000): 400–419.

Lea, Tess. *Bureaucrats and Bleeding Hearts: Indigenous Health in Northern Australia*. Sydney: University of New South Wales Press, 2008.

Leff, Mark J. "Revisioning U.S. Political History." *American Historical Review* 100, no. 3 (June 1995): 829–54.

Lefkowitz, Bonnie. *Community Health Centers: A Movement and the People Who Made It Happen*. New Brunswick, NJ: Rutgers University Press, 2007.

Lerner, Barron H. *Contagion and Confinement: Controlling Tuberculosis along the Skid Road*. Baltimore, MD: Johns Hopkins University Press, 1998.

Lewis, Milton James. *The People's Health: Public Health in Australia, 1950 to the Present*. Westport, CT: Praeger, 2003.

Lobo, Susan. "Is Urban a Person or Place? Characteristics of Urban Indian Country." *American Indian Research and Culture Journal* 22, no. 4 (1998): 89–103.

———, ed. *Urban Voices: The Bay Area American Indian Community*. Tucson: University of Arizona Press, 2002.

Lobo, Susan, and Kurt Peters, eds. *American Indians and the Urban Experience.* Walnut Creek, CA: AltaMira Press, 2001.

Loew, Patty, and Kelly Mella. "Black Ink and the New Red Power: Native American Newspapers and Tribal Sovereignty." *Journalism Communication Monographs* 7, no. 3 (August 2005).

Lomawaima, Tsianina. *They Called It Prairie Light: The Story of Chilocco Indian School.* Lincoln: University of Nebraska Press, 1994.

Lothian, Kathy. "Moving Blackwards: Black Power and the Aboriginal Embassy." In *Transgressions: Critical Australian Indigenous Histories*, edited by Ingereth Macfarlane and Mark Hannah, 19–34. Canberra: ANU E-Press, 2007.

Loyd, Jenna. *Health Rights Are Civil Rights: Peace and Justice Activism in Los Angeles, 1963–1978.* Minneapolis: University of Minnesota Press, 2014.

Lux, Maureen K. *Medicine That Walks: Disease, Medicine, and Canadian Plains Native People, 1880–1940.* Toronto, ON: University of Toronto Press, 2001.

———. "We Demand 'Unconditional Surrender': Making and Unmaking the Blackfoot Hospital." *Social History of Medicine* 25, no. 3 (2012): 665–84.

———. *Separate Beds: A History of Indian Hospitals in Canada, 1920s–1980s.* Toronto, ON: University of Toronto Press, 2016.

Lyons, Scott Richard. *X-Marks: Native Signatures of Assent.* Minneapolis: Minnesota University Press, 2010.

Macintyre, Stuart. *The Poor Relation.* Melbourne: Melbourne University Press, 2010.

Mackey, Mike. "Closing the Fort Washakie Hospital: A Case Study in Federal Termination Policy." *Wyoming History Journal* 67, no. 2 (1995): 36–42.

Markus, Andrew. *Fear and Hatred: Purifying Australia and California, 1850–1901.* Sydney: Hale & Iremonger, 1979.

———. *Australian Race Relations, 1788–1993.* Sydney: Allen & Unwin, 1994.

McBride, David. *From TB to AIDS: Epidemics Among Urban Blacks since 1900.* Albany: State University of New York Press, 1991.

McCallum, Mary Jane. "This Last Frontier: 'Isolation' and Aboriginal Health." *Canadian Bulletin of Medical History* 22, no. 1 (2005): 103–20.

McCallum, Mary Jane Logan, and Adele Perry. *Structures of Indifference: An Indigenous Life and Death in a Canadian City.* Winnipeg: University of Manitoba Press, 2018.

McGrath, Ann. *'Born in the Cattle': Aborigines in Cattle Country.* Sydney: Allen & Unwin, 1987.

McGregor, Russell. *Imagined Destinies: Aboriginal Australians and the Doomed Race Theory, 1880–1939.* Melbourne: Melbourne University Press, 1997.

———. *Indifferent Inclusion: Aboriginal People and the Australian Nation.* Canberra: Aboriginal Studies Press, 2011.

Mihesuah, Devon Abbott. *Indigenous American Women: Decolonization, Empowerment, Activism.* Lincoln: University of Nebraska Press, 2003.

Miller, Bruce Granville. *Invisible Indigenes: The Politics of Nonrecognition.* Lincoln: University of Nebraska Press, 2003.

Miller, Douglas K. *Indians on the Move: Native American Mobility and Urbanization in the Twentieth Century.* Chapel Hill: University of North Carolina Press, 2019.

Million, Dian. "Felt Theory: An Indigenous Feminist Approach to Affect and History." *Wicazo Sa Review* 24, no. 2 (2009): 53–76.

——. *Therapeutic Nations: Healing in an Age of Indigenous Human Rights.* Tucson: University of Arizona Press, 2013.

Molina, Natalia. *Fit to Be Citizens? Public Health and Race in Los Angeles, 1879–1939.* Berkeley: University of California Press, 2006.

Moodie, Peter M. *Aboriginal Health.* Canberra: ANU Press, 1973.

Moreton-Robinson, Aileen. *Sovereign Subjects: Indigenous Sovereignty Matters.* Sydney: Allen & Unwin, 2008.

——. *The White Possessive: Property, Power, and Indigenous Sovereignty.* Minneapolis: University of Minnesota Press, 2015.

Morgan, George. *Unsettled Places: Aboriginal People and Urbanisation in New South Wales.* Adelaide: Wakefield Press, 2006.

Morgan, Murray. *Skid Road: An Informal Portrait of Seattle.* New York: Viking Press, 1960.

Morgen, Sandra. *Into Our Own Hands: The Women's Health Movement in the United States, 1969–1990.* 1st ed. New Brunswick, NJ: Rutgers University Press, 2002.

Morgensen, Scott Lauria. *Spaces between Us: Queer Settler Colonialism and Indigenous Decolonization.* Minneapolis: University of Minnesota Press, 2011.

Morris, Barry. *Domesticating Resistance: The Dhan-Gadi Aborigines and the Australian State.* Oxford, UK: Berg, 1989.

Nagel, Joane. *American Indian Ethnic Renewal: Red Power and the Resurgence of Identity and Culture.* New York: Oxford University Press, 1996.

Nash, Gerald D., and Richard W. Etulain, eds. *The Twentieth-Century West: Historical Interpretations.* Albuquerque: University of New Mexico Press, 1989.

Neils, Elaine M. *Reservation to City: Indian Migration and Federal Relocation.* Chicago: University of Chicago Press, 1971.

Nelson, Alondra. *Body and Soul: The Black Panther Party and the Fight Against Medical Discrimination.* Minneapolis: University of Minnesota Press, 2011.

Neog, Prafulla, Richard G. Woods, and Arthur M. Harkins. *Chicago Indians: The Effect of Urban Migration.* Minneapolis: University of Minnesota Press, 1970.

Nickel, Sarah A. *Assembling Unity: Indigenous Politics, Gender, and the Union of BC Indian Chiefs.* Vancouver: UBC Press, 2019.

Norman, Heidi. *What Do We Want?: A Political History of Aboriginal Land Rights in New South Wales.* Canberra: Aboriginal Studies Press, 2015.

Nugent, Maria. *Botany Bay: Where Histories Meet.* Sydney: Allen & Unwin, 2005.

O'Brien, Jean M. *Firsting and Lasting: Writing Indians Out of Existence in New England.* Minneapolis: University of Minnesota Press, 2010.

Olson, James S., ed. *Encyclopedia of American Indian Civil Rights.* Westport, CT: Greenwood Press, 1997.

Ortner, Sherry B. "Resistance and the Problem of Ethnographic Refusal." *Comparative Studies in Society and History* 37, no. 1 (January 1995): 173–93.

O'Sullivan, Meg Devlin. "'We Worry about Survival': American Indian Women, Sovereignty, and the Right to Bear and Raise Children in the 1970s." PhD diss., University of North Carolina, 2007.

——. "Informing Red Power and Transforming the Second Wave: Native American Women and the Struggle against Coerced Sterilization in the 1970s." *Women's History Review* 25, no. 6 (2016): 965–82.

——. "More Destruction to These Family Ties: Native American Women, Child Welfare, and the Solution of Sovereignty." *Journal of Family History* 41, no. 1 (2016): 19–38.

Panaretto, Kathryn S., Mark Wenitong, Selwyn Button, and Ian T. Ring. "Aboriginal Community-Controlled Health Services: Leading the Way in Primary Care." *Medical Journal of Australia* 200, no. 11 (2014): 649–52.

Pelka, Fred. *What We Have Done: An Oral History of the Disability Rights Movement.* Amherst: University of Massachusetts Press, 2012.

Perdue, Theda. *Cherokee Women: Gender and Culture Change, 1700–1835.* Lincoln: University of Nebraska Press, 1998.

Perheentupa, Johanna. *Redfern: Aboriginal Activism in the 1970s.* Canberra: Aboriginal Studies Press, 2021.

Philp, Kenneth R. "Stride toward Freedom: The Relocation of Indians to Cities, 1952–1960." *Western Historical Quarterly* 16, no. 2 (1985): 175–90.

Pilkington, Lionel, and Fiona Bateman, eds. *Studies in Settler Colonialism: Politics, Identity and Culture.* New York: Palgrave Macmillan, 2011.

Povinelli, Elizabeth. *The Cunning of Recognition: Indigenous Alterities and the Making of Australian Multiculturalism.* Durham, NC: Duke University Press, 2002.

——. *Economies of Abandonment: Social Belonging and Endurance in Late Liberalism.* Durham, NC: Duke University Press, 2011.

Price, Charles Archibald. *The Great White Walls Are Built: Restrictive Immigration to North America and Australasia, 1836–1888.* Canberra: ANU Press, 1974.

Rademaker, Laura, and Tim Rowse, eds. *Indigenous Self-Determination in Australia: Histories and Historiographies.* Canberra: ANU Press, 2020.

Raftery, Judith. *Not Part of the Public: Non-Indigenous Policies and Practices and the Health of Indigenous South Australians, 1836–1973.* Adelaide: Wakefield Press, 2006.

Raheja, Michelle. *Reservation Reelism: Redfacing, Visual Sovereignty, and Representations of Native Americans in Film.* Lincoln: University of Nebraska Press, 2010.

Ramirez, Renya K. "Healing Through Grief: Urban Indians Reimagining Culture and Community." *American Indian Research and Culture Journal* 22, no. 4 (1998): 305–33.

——. *Native Hubs: Culture, Community, and Belonging in Silicon Valley and Beyond.* Durham, NC: Duke University Press, 2007.

Razack, Sherene H. *Dying from Improvement: Inquests and Inquiries into Indigenous Deaths in Custody.* Toronto, ON: University of Toronto Press, 2015.

———, ed. *Race, Space, and the Law: Unmapping a White Settler Society.* Toronto, ON: Between the Lines, 2002.

Reading, Charlotte. "Structural Determinants of Aboriginal Peoples' Health." In *Determinants of Indigenous Peoples' Health: Beyond the Social*, 2nd ed., edited by Margo Greenwood, Sarah de Leeuw, and Nicole Marie Lindsay, 3–15. Toronto, ON: Canadian Scholar's Press, 2018.

Redman, Eric. *The Dance of Legislation.* New York: Simon and Schuster, 1973.

Reece, R. H. W. "'Laws of the White People': The Frontier Authority in Perth in 1838." *Push from the Bush*, no. 17 (1984): 2–28.

———. "Inventing Aborigines." *Aboriginal History* 11, vol. 1/2 (1987): 15–18.

Reid, Janice, and Peggy Trompf, eds. *The Health of Aboriginal Australia.* Sydney: Harcourt Brace Jovanovich, 1991.

Reid, Joshua. *The Sea Is My Country: The Maritime World of the Makahs, an Indigenous Borderlands People.* New Haven, CT: Yale University Press, 2015.

Reséndez, Andrés. *The Other Slavery: The Uncovered Story of Indian Enslavement in America.* Boston, MA: Mariner Books, 2016.

Reyes, Lawney L. *Bernie Whitebear.* Tucson: University of Arizona Press, 2006.

Reynolds, Henry. *The Other Side of the Frontier: Aboriginal Resistance to the European Invasion of Australia.* Melbourne: Penguin Books, 1982.

Roberts, Samuel. *Infectious Fear: Politics, Disease, and the Health Effects of Segregation.* Chapel Hill: University of North Carolina Press, 2009.

Rose, Michael. *For the Record: 160 Years of Aboriginal Print Journalism.* Sydney: Allen & Unwin, 1996.

Rosenthal, Nicolas G. *Reimagining Indian Country: Native American Migration & Identity in Twentieth-Century Los Angeles.* Chapel Hill: University of North Carolina Press, 2012.

Rowley, Charles. *Outcasts in White Australia: Aboriginal Policy and Practice.* Canberra: ANU Press, 1971.

Rowse, Tim. *Obliged to be Difficult: Nugget Coombs' Legacy in Indigenous Affairs.* Melbourne: Cambridge University Press, 2000.

Ruby, Robert H., and John A. Brown. *A Guide to the Indian Tribes of the Pacific Northwest.* Norman: University of Oklahoma Press, 1986.

Russell, Lynette, ed. *Colonial Frontiers: Indigenous-European Encounters in Settler Societies.* New York: Palgrave, 2001.

Ruzek, Sheryl Burt. *The Women's Health Movement: Feminist Alternatives to Medical Control.* New York: Praeger, 1978.

Saggers, Sherry, and Dennis Gray. *Aboriginal Health and Society: The Traditional and Contemporary Aboriginal Struggle for Better Health.* Sydney: Allen & Unwin, 1991.

Sardell, Alice. *The U.S. Experiment in Social Medicine: The Community Health Center Program, 1965–1986.* Pittsburgh, PA: University of Pittsburgh Press, 1988.

Sawer, Marian. *Sisters in Suits: Women and Public Policy in Australia.* Sydney: Allen & Unwin, 1990.

Sawer, Marian, and Marian Simms. *A Woman's Place: Women and Politics in Australia*. Sydney: Allen & Unwin, 1993.

Schissel, Wendy. *Home/Bodies: Geographies of Self, Place, and Space*. Calgary, AB: University of Calgary Press, 2006.

Scott, James C. *Weapons of the Weak: Everyday Forms of Resistance*. New Haven, CT: Yale University Press, 1985.

Sewell, William H. "Marc Bloch and the Logic of Comparative History." *History and Theory* 6, no. 2 (January 1, 1967): 208–18.

Shah, Nayan. *Contagious Divides: Epidemics and Race in San Francisco's Chinatown*. Berkeley: University of California Press, 2001.

Shoemaker, Nancy. *Negotiators of Change: Historical Perspectives on Native American Women*. New York: Routledge, 1995.

——. *American Indian Population Recovery in the Twentieth Century*. Albuquerque: University of New Mexico Press, 1999.

——. "Urban Indians and Ethnic Choices: American Indian Organizations in Minneapolis, 1920–1950." *Western Historical Quarterly* 19, no. 4 (November 1, 1988): 431–47.

Shreve, Bradley Glenn. *Red Power Rising: The National Indian Youth Council and the Origins of Native Activism*. Norman: University of Oklahoma Press, 2011.

Silliman, Jael, Marlene Gerber Fried, Loretta Ross, and Elena R. Gutierrez. *Undivided Rights: Women of Color Organize for Reproductive Justice*. Boston, MA: South End Press, 2004.

Silva, Noenoe K. *Aloha Betrayed: Native Hawaiian Resistance to American Colonialism*. Durham, NC: Duke University Press, 2004.

Simpson, Audra. *Mohawk Interruptus: Political Life across the Borders of Settler States*. Durham, NC: Duke University Press, 2014.

Singler, Joan, Jean Durning, Bettylou Valentine, and Maid Adams. *Seattle in Black and White: The Congress of Racial Equality and the Fight for Equal Opportunity*. Seattle: University of Washington Press, 2011.

Skyring, Fiona. *Justice: A History of the Aboriginal Legal Service of Western Australia*. Perth: University of Western Australia Publishing, 2011.

Sleeper-Smith, Susan. *Indian Women and French Men: Rethinking Cultural Encounter in the Western Great Lakes*. Amherst: University of Massachusetts Press, 2001.

Smith, Linda Tuhiwai. *Decolonizing Methodologies: Research and Indigenous Peoples*. 2nd ed. London: Zed Books, 2012.

Smith, Marian W. *Indians of the Urban Northwest*. New York: Columbia University Press, 1949.

Smith, Paul Chaat, and Robert Allen Warrior. *Like a Hurricane: The Indian Movement from Alcatraz to Wounded Knee*. New York: New Press, 1997.

Smith, Sherry L. *Hippies, Indians, and the Fight for Red Power*. Oxford: Oxford University Press, 2012.

Smith, Susan. *Sick and Tired of Being Sick and Tired: Black Women's Health Activism in America, 1890–1950*. Philadelphia: University of Pennsylvania Press, 1995.

Sorkin, Alan L. *The Urban American Indian*. Lexington, MA: Lexington Books, 1978.

Spearritt, Peter. *Sydney since the Twenties*. Sydney: Hale and Iremonger, 1978.

——. *Sydney's Century*. Sydney: University of New South Wales Press, 1999.

Stanbury, W. T., assisted by Jay H. Siegel. *Success and Failure: Indians in Urban Society*. Vancouver: University of British Columbia Press, 1975.

Steeler, William. *Improving American Indian Health Care: The Western Cherokee Experience*. Norman: University of Oklahoma Press, 2001.

Stevens, F. *Aborigines in the Northern Territory Cattle Industry*. Canberra: ANU Press, 1974.

Stevenson, Lisa. *Life Beside Itself: Imagining Care in the Canadian Arctic*. Oakland: University of California Press, 2014.

Stoler, Ann Laura. *Carnal Knowledge and Imperial Power: Race and the Intimate in Colonial Rule*. Berkeley: University of California Press, 2002.

Strouthous, Andrew. *US Labor and Political Action, 1918–24: A Comparison of Independent Political Action in New York, Chicago, and Seattle*. New York: St. Martin's Press, 2000.

Suarez, Sasha Maria. "Indigenizing Minneapolis: Building American Indian Community Infrastructure in the Mid-Twentieth Century." In *Indian Cities: Histories of Indigenous Urbanization*, edited by Cathleen Cahill, Kent Blansett, and Andrew Needham, 198–218. Norman: University of Oklahoma Press, 2022.

Taffe, Sue. *Black and White Together: FCAATSI: The Federal Council for the Advancement of Aborigines and Torres Straight Islanders 1958–1972*. St. Lucia, AUS: University of Queensland Press, 2005.

Tanner, Mildred Tanner. *Women's Place: A Guide to Seattle and King County*. Seattle, WA: Gemil Press, 1994.

Tatz, Colin, and Keith McConnochie, eds. *Black Viewpoints: The Aboriginal Experience*. Sydney: Australia and New Zealand Book Company, 1975.

Taylor, Quintard. *The Forging of a Black Community: Seattle's Central District, from 1870 through the Civil Rights Era*. Seattle: University of Washington Press, 1994.

Theobald, Brianna. *Reproduction on the Reservation: Pregnancy, Childbirth, and Colonialism in the Long Twentieth Century*. Chapel Hill: University of North Carolina Press, 2019.

Thomas, David. *Reading Doctor's Writing: Race, Politics and Power in Indigenous Health Research 1870–1969*. Canberra: Aboriginal Studies Press, 2004.

Thornton, Russell. *The Urbanization of American Indians: A Critical Bibliography*. Bloomington: Indiana University Press, 1982.

Thrush, Coll. *Native Seattle: Histories from the Crossing-over Place*. Seattle: University of Washington Press, 2007.

Townsend, Kenneth William. *World War II and the American Indian*. Albuquerque: University of New Mexico Press, 2000.

Trafzer, Clifford E. *Death Stalks the Yakama: Epidemiological Transitions and Mortality on the Yakama Indian Reservation, 1888–1964*. East Lansing: Michigan State University Press, 1997.

Trafzer, Clifford E., and Diane Weiner, eds. *Medicine Ways: Disease, Health, and Survival among Native Americans*. Lanham, MD: AltaMira Press, 2001.

Trahant, Mark. *The Last Great Battle of the Indian Wars: Henry M. Jackson, Forrest J. Gerard, and the Campaign for the Self Determination of America's Indian Tribes*. Fort Hall, ID: Cedars Group, 2010.

Trennert, Robert A. *White Man's Medicine: Government Doctors and the Navajo, 1863–1955*. Albuquerque: University of New Mexico Press, 1998.

Trometter, Alyssa L. "Malcolm X and the Aboriginal Black Power Movement in Australia, 1967–1972." *Journal of African American History* 100, no. 2 (Spring 2015): 226–49.

Tyrrell, Ian R. *True Gardens of the Gods: Californian-Australian Environmental Reform, 1860–1930*. Berkeley: University of California Press, 1999.

Ulrich, Roberta. *American Indian Nations from Termination to Restoration, 1953–2006*. Lincoln: University of Nebraska Press, 2010.

Vaughan, Megan. *Curing Their Ills: Colonial Power and African Illness*. Redwood City, CA: Stanford University Press, 1991.

Veracini, Lorenzo. "'Settler Colonialism': Career of a Concept." *Journal of Imperial and Commonwealth History* 41, no. 2 (2013): 313–33.

Vernon, Irene. *Killing Us Quietly: Native Americans and HIV/AIDS*. Lincoln: University of Nebraska Press, 2001.

Vlahov, David, ed. *Urban Health: Global Perspectives*. San Francisco, CA: Jossey-Bass, 2010.

Voyles, Traci Brynne. *Wastelanding: Legacies of Uranium Mining in Navajo Country*. Minneapolis: University of Minnesota Press, 2015.

Waddell, Jack, and Michael Watson, eds. *The American Indian in Urban Society*. Boston, MA: Little, Brown and Company, 1971.

Watson, Irene. *Raw Law: Aboriginal Peoples, Colonialism and International Law*. New York: Routledge, 2015.

Weibel-Orlando, Joan. *Indian Country, L.A.: Maintaining Ethnic Community in Complex Society*. Rev. ed. Urbana: University of Illinois Press, 1999.

White, Richard, and John M. Findlay, eds. *Power and Place in the North American West*. Seattle: University of Washington Press, 1999.

Wilkins, David E. *American Indian Politics and the American Political System*. 2nd ed. Lanham, MD: Rowman & Littlefield Publishers, 2006.

Wilson, Deborah. *Different White People: Radical Activism for Aboriginal Rights, 1946–1972*. Perth: University of Western Australia Publishing, 2015.

Witko, Tawa. *Mental Health Care for Urban Indians*. Washington, DC: American Psychological Association, 2006.

Wolfe, Patrick. *Settler Colonialism and the Transformation of Anthropology: The Politics and Poetics of an Ethnographic Event*. New York: Cassell, 1999.

——. "Settler Colonialism and the Elimination of the Native." *Journal of Genocide Research* 8, no. 4 (Dec. 2006): 387–409.

——. "Against the Intentional Fallacy: Legocentrism and Continuity in the Rhetoric of Indian Dispossession." *American Indian Culture and Research Journal* 36, no. 1 (January 1, 2012): 1–46.

———. "Patrick Wolfe on Settler Colonialism." In *Speaking of Indigenous Politics: Conversations with Activists, Scholars, and Tribal Leaders*, edited by J. Kēhaulani Kauanui, 343–60. Minneapolis: University of Minnesota Press, 2018.

Wunder, John R., ed. *Native American Sovereignty*. New York: Garland Publishing, 1996.

———. *Native Americans and the Law: Contemporary and Historical Perspectives on American Indian Rights, Freedoms, and Sovereignty*. New York: Garland Publishing, 1996.

Yashadhana, Aryati, Nellie Pollard-Wharton, Anthony B. Zwi, and Brett Biles. "Indigenous Australians at Increased Risk of COVID-19 Due to Existing Health and Socioeconomic Inequities." *Lancet Regional Health—Western Pacific* 1 (2020).

Young, T. Kue. *The Health of Native Americans: Toward a Biocultural Epidemiology*. New York: Oxford University Press, 1994.

Zoller, Heather M. "Health Activism: Communication Theory and Action for Social Change." *Communication Theory* 15 (2005): 341–64.

Index

Italic page numbers refer to illustrations.

absconding, practice of, 169–70, 171, 260n103

activism: concept of, 20–21; funding cuts for health care, 216; health, 21, 231n58; political, 193, 196–97. *See also* Aboriginal activism; Native American activism

Akwesasne Notes (journal), 180

Alaska Natives: hospital eligibility rules, 83; medical migration, 51, 52; sanitary conditions, 50. *See also* Native Americans

Alcatraz Island occupation, 193, 196, 252n121

Alcatraz Proclamation, 134

alcoholism, 30–31, 178; treatment, 231–32n4

American Indian Center (Chicago), 109

American Indian movement, 103

American Indian Women's Service League (AIWSL), 105, 110–13, *112*, 116, 118, 120, 201; committees and subgroups, 120–21; community-building, 123–24; Hospital Committee, 120–21; Seattle Indian Center, 127–29

American Indians. *See* Native Americans

American Indians United, 129

Answering Your Questions About Aborigines (Aboriginal Affairs), 94

Aquino, Ella, 110, *112*

Armstrong, Dick, 157

assimilationist policies: Australian, 35, 85–87, 99, 160–61; and citizenship, 70–71; vs. Indigenous control, 98; health care, ability to pay for, 245n80; health outcomes, 4–5, 97; myths of, 124, 192, 197–98; *New Dawn* and *New Horizons*, 60–61, *61*, 64–65, 69–70; resistance to, 137, 201–2; urbanization and "authenticity," 16–17, 20, 71–72, 102, 230n39. *See also* relocation policies

Australia: Aborigines Welfare Board (AWB) activists' influence and impact,

212–15; census, 38; Commonwealth Constitution, 38; Constitution, referendum campaign, 152–53; Department of Aboriginal Affairs (DAA), 212–13; federal approaches to Aboriginal people, 235n34; health insurance systems, 84; Indigenous health policies (1950–70), 84–88; Nationality and Citizenship Act (1948), 39; Office of Aboriginal Affairs (OAA), 212; and relocation, 35; Ten-Year Plan for Aboriginal Health (1973), 208; universal health care, 239n144. *See also* Aboriginal activism; Aboriginal health care; Aboriginal populations

The Autobiography of Malcolm X, 180

Awashish, Georges-Hervé, 8, 228–29n28

Bainikolo, Gloria, 158, 160

Bandler, Faith, 155–56, 163, 176

barefoot doctors, 10

Barker, Joanne, 14

Beasley, Pamela, 39, 162

Because a White Man'll Never Do It (Gilbert), 180

Beck, Eduard J., 53–54

Bellear, Bob, 186

Bellear, Sol, 176, 205

Bennett, Robert L., 143

Bentz, Marilyn, 122–23

Berezin, Mabel, 19

Bergman, Abe, 210–11

Berndt, Catherine, 57–58

Berndt, Roland, 57–58

Blackhawk, Ned, 235n46

Black Liberation (news publication), 181

Black News Service (news publication), 180, 181, 182

Black Panther Party, 21, 143–44, 219; clinics, 10; People's Free Medical Clinics, 21, 219

Black Power movement, 174–75, *175*, 181, 183, 197

Blansett, Kent, 17, 235n46

blood banks and donors, 121

mortality rates. *See* infant mortality and morbidity; life expectancy

Mullewa Aboriginal Hospital, 55

Mumey, Meredith, 110

Myer, Dillon, 81

Nash, Philleo, 77–78, 79

National Aboriginal Community Controlled Health Organisation, 254–55n6

National Aborigines Day, 204

National Black Theatre Company, 202

National Council of American Indians, 106

National Council of Indian Opportunity, 75, 88–91

National Council on Indian Opportunity (NCIO), 105, 106, 247n1

National Health Service Corps (NHSC), 142

National Seminar on Health Services (Melbourne, 1972), 95–97

Native American activism: and civil rights movement, 143; clinics, 143–44; community-building, 123–24; federal funding, 208–9; Fort Lawton occupation, 133–36; health care, documentation of needs, 138–39; relationships, strategic, 140–41; rights-based frameworks, 138–39; synergy and cooperation among groups, 136–37, 144; visibility, politics of, 125; women's roles, 109–111

Native American Alcoholism and Drug Abuse Center, 178

Native American health care (general): Meriam Report (1928), 47–49; "ping-pong" phenomenon, 7–8, 9, 126, 192, 251n89; residency and responsibility for, 88–93, 100–101. *See also* Indigenous health care

Native American health care (Seattle): clinic, 125–37; growth and exposure, 108–125; overview, 105–8; rights to health care, 137–45

Native Americans: citizenship and rights of, 245n66; clinics, funding for, 138–40; cultural retention, urban areas, 124–25; cultural spaces, need for, 136–37; culture, 198; demographics and census data, 121–23; diabetes rates, 1; family size, 37; housing discrimination, 37; land rights and territorial claims, 134, 137; pan-Indian community, Seattle, 124, 144–45; sanitation, need for, 50–51; self-relocatees, 42–43; social space, need for, 126–27, 129; treaty-making, 44–45; urban Indians, federal funds for, 209–211; urbanization trends, 41–42, 235n46; urban/rural divide, 211, 216–17; World War II service, 81–82. *See also* Bureau of Indian Affairs (BIA); Indigenous peoples; reservations, US; Seattle, WA

Natives of New South Wales as Seen in the Streets of Sydney (Earle), 16

Navajo Nation, 50–51; relocation, 34

Needham, Andrew, 17, 235n46

Nelson, Alondra, 20, 21, 143

Neuman, Eddie, 167

New Dawn (propaganda magazine), 60–61, *61*

New Horizons (BIA newsletter), 61–62

New South Wales Aborigines Protection Board, 60

Nickel, Sarah, 109

Nixon, Richard, 105, 209, 247n2

Noonuccal, Oodgeroo, 162–63

Northern Territory Medical Service, 54

Northwest Indian News, 123–24

Nurcombe, B., 159

nutrition: communal feeding in Australia, 56–57; diet and nutrition, 50; malnutrition, 149, 156; for pastoral workers in Australia, 57–58; pregnant mothers, 58

O'Brien, Jean M., 17

Old, H. Norman, 50–51

Urban Indian Hearings (NCIO), 116
Urban Indian Relocation Program, 113
urbanization: cities built on Indigenous land, 17; urban migration, 71–74, 201; urban/rural divide, 197. *See also* medical migration

vaccination campaigns, 43–44, 224–25. *See also* COVID-19 pandemic
venereal diseases, 44
Viner, Ian, 213
violence: death by exhaustion and abandonment, 6; structural, in healthcare, 3, 192, 215–20, 226; structural, in settler-colonial framework, 179; "white violence," 182–83
virgin-soil epidemics, 1–2
vocational training, 36–37

Wait, E., 38
Walton, R. G., 213–14, 215
"wandering Indians," 16, 18
wardship status of Aboriginal peoples, 35, 39, 68, 71, 72, 240–41n10
War on Poverty programs, 130
Warren, Pearl, 22, 105–7, 110–13, *112*, 117, 122, 126–31, 133, 135, 139, 194–95, 199
Watson, Irene, 6
Watson, Lilla, 176
Wave Hill Station, 57–58
We Have Bugger All! (Buchanan), 180

Weibel-Orlando, Joan, 40
White, Laurence W., 45–46
Whitebear, Bernie, 7–8, 11, 121, 130, 133–36, 138–42, 203, 208, 210–11, 251n89
Whitlam, E. Gough, 146, 157, 175, 187, 212–14
Widders, Terry, 176
Wilbur, Tandy, 92
Willesee, Michael, 187
Williams, Don, 158–59, 160
Winder, Ken, 176
Wolfe, Patrick, 3, 179
women: in Aboriginal households, 234–35n33; homemaking, 67; as medical migrants, 232n14; Native women in Seattle, 109–111; self-care politics, 144; sterilization, unauthorized, 114; women in Native American activism, 109–111; women's health movement, 10, 219–20; women's roles in public health, 110–11
Wood, Edmund J., 123
Wounded Knee, 193
The Wretched of the Earth (Fanon), 180

Young, Nancy, 147–54, 257n39; case as catalyst for change, 160; legacy and impact, 182; press coverage of case, 155–56
Young Lords Party, 144

Zoller, Heather M., 20, 21

www.ingramcontent.com/pod-product-compliance
Lightning Source LLC
Chambersburg PA
CBHW020458270326
41926CB00008B/650